Health system efficiency

How to make measurement matter
for policy and management

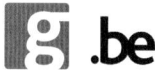

The European Observatory on Health Systems and Policies supports and promotes evidence-based health policy-making through comprehensive and rigorous analysis of health systems in Europe. It brings together a wide range of policy-makers, academics and practitioners to analyse trends in health reform, drawing on experience from across Europe to illuminate policy issues.

The Observatory is a partnership hosted by the WHO Regional Office for Europe; which includes the governments of Austria, Belgium, Finland, Ireland, Norway, Slovenia, Sweden, Switzerland, the United Kingdom, and the Veneto Region of Italy; the European Commission; the World Bank; UNCAM (French National Union of Health Insurance Funds); the London School of Economics and Political Science; and the London School of Hygiene & Tropical Medicine. The Observatory has a secretariat in Brussels and it has hubs in London (at LSE and LSHTM) and at the Technical University of Berlin.

Health system efficiency

How to make measurement matter
for policy and management

Edited by

Jonathan Cylus, Irene Papanicolas and Peter C. Smith

European
Observatory
on Health Systems and Policies
a partnership hosted by WHO

Keywords:

HEALTH CARE EVALUATION MECHANISMS
EFFICIENCY, ORGANIZATIONAL
DELIVERY OF HEALTH CARE
QUALITY OF HEALTH CARE
DECISION MAKING

ISBN 978 92 890 5041 8

Printed in the United Kingdom

Typeset by Tetragon, London

Cover design by M2M

Table of contents

Acknowledgements

We are indebted to the authors for their valuable contributions to the volume. We are very grateful to the Health Foundation for funding the author workshop. We would also like to thank Josep Figueras, Gaetan Lafortune, Ellen Nolte, Valerie Paris, Sarah Thomson, and Sebastian Salas-Vega for their support and feedback throughout, as well as Nataša Perić for reviewing the volume and providing helpful suggestions.

The production and copy-editing process for this book was coordinated by Jonathan North with the support of Caroline White. Additional support came from Sonia Cutler (copy-editing) and Tetragon Publishing Services (typesetting).

List of contributors

Reinhard Busse, Berlin University of Technology and European Observatory on Health Systems and Policies, Germany

Christopher S. Chapman, University of Bristol, United Kingdom

Kalipso Chalkidou, Imperial College London, United Kingdom

Anita Charlesworth, The Health Foundation, United Kingdom

Jonathan Cylus, European Observatory on Health Systems and Policies and London School of Economics & Political Science, United Kingdom

Alexander Geissler, Berlin University of Technology, Germany

Bruce Hollingsworth, Lancaster University, United Kingdom

Anja Kern, Baden-Württemberg Cooperative State University Mosbach, Germany

Aziza Laguecir, Kedge Business School, France

Alec Morton, University of Strathclyde, United Kingdom

Irene Papanicolas, London School of Economics & Political Science, United Kingdom

Mark Pearson, Organization for Economic Cooperation and Development, France

Wilm Quentin, Berlin University of Technology and European Observatory on Health Systems and Policies, Germany

Laura Schang, Ludwig-Maximilians-Universität München, Germany

Peter C. Smith, Imperial College Business School, United Kingdom

Emma Spencelayh, The Health Foundation, United Kingdom

Reijo Sund, University of Helsinki and University of Eastern Finland, Finland

Ranjeeta Thomas, Imperial College Business School, United Kingdom

Unto Häkkinen, Centre for Health and Social Economics (CHESS) and National Institute for Health and Welfare, Finland

Zeynep Or, Institut de Recherche et Documentation en Economie de la Santé (IRDES), France

List of tables, boxes and figures

Tables

Figures

Boxes

List of abbreviations

ACG	adjusted clinical group
AE	allocative efficiency
AMI	acute myocardial infarction
AN-SNAP	Australian subacute and non-acute care
APR-DRG	All-patient-refined diagnosis resource group
AR-DRG	Australian refined diagnosis resource group
ATV	added therapeutic value
BPH	benign prostatic hyperplasia
CAD	Canadian dollar
CAM	complementary and alternative medicine
CAPI	contracts for improved individual practice
CC	complications and/or comorbidities
CCG	clinical commissioning group
CEA	cost–effectiveness analysis
CHF	Swiss franc
CIHI	Canadian Institute for Health Information
CMG	case mix group
CMI	case mix index
CMS	Centers for Medicare & Medicaid Services
CPS	Care Pathway Simulator
CRS	constant returns to scale
DEA	data envelopment analysis
DHMA	Danish Health and Medicines Authority
DRG	diagnosis-related group
EQ-5D	EuroQol five dimensions questionnaire
EuroHOPE	European Health Care Outcomes, Performance and Efficiency
FFS	fee-for-service
FIM	functional independence measure
FTE	full-time equivalent
G-BA	*Gemeinsamer Bundesausschuss* (Federal Joint Committee) (Germany)
G-DRG	German diagnosis-related group
GHM	*groupe homogène de malades* (diagnosis-related group) (France)

GLM	generalized linear models
GP	general practitioner
HAS	*Haute Autorité de Santé* (National Health Authority) (France)
HCC	hierarchical condition category
HIF	health insurance fund
HRG	healthcare resource group
HSE	Health Service Executive (Ireland)
HTA	health technology assessment
ICD-9-CM	International Classification of Diseases, Ninth Revision, Clinical Modification
ICD-10	International Classification of Diseases, 10th revision
ICER	incremental cost effectiveness ratio
ICU	intensive care unit
IHPA	Independent Hospital Pricing Authority
IHPS	International Health Policy Survey
InEK	*Institut für das Entgeltsystem im Krankenhaus* (Institute for the Hospital Remuneration System) (Germany)
IPHA	Irish Pharmaceutical Healthcare Association
IQWiG	*Institut für Qualität und Wirtschaftlichkeit im Gesundheitswesen* (Institute for Quality and Efficiency in Health Care) (Germany)
IVF	in vitro fertilization
LOS	length of stay
MAQS	materiality and quality score
MDCs	Major Diagnostic Categories
MedPAC	Medicare Payment Advisory Commission
MHCC	mental health care cluster
MS-DRG	Medicare Severity Diagnosis Resource Group
NCPE	National Centre for Pharmacoeconomics (Ireland)
NICE	National Institute for Health and Care Excellence
NICU	neonatal intensive care unit
OECD	Organisation for Economic Co-operation and Development
OOP	out of pocket
PCI	percutaneous coronary intervention
P4P	pay-for-performance
PBM	performance-based management
PBMA	programme budgeting and marginal analysis
PCCL	patient clinical complexity level
PDA	patient decision aid
PHO	primary health organizations
PPP	purchasing power parity
PROM	patient-reported outcome measure

PSRA	priority-setting and resource allocation
QALY	quality-adjusted life year
QOF	Quality and Outcomes Framework
QOL	quality of life
REA	ratio-based efficiency analysis
ROM	risk of mortality
RPG	rehabilitation patient group
RUG-III	resource utilization group version III
SCIPP	System for Classification of In-Patient Psychiatry
SF-36	Short Form-36
SFA	stochastic frontier analysis
SHA	System of Health Accounts
SPOT	spend and outcome tool
STAR	socio-technical allocation of resources
TDABC	time-driven activity-based costing
TE	technical efficiency
USD	United States dollar
VBID	value-based insurance design
VLBW	very low birth weight
VLGA	very low gestational age
VRS	variable returns to scale
WHO	World Health Organization

Glossary

Allocative efficiency has two perspectives. On the output side, allocative efficiency examines whether limited resources are directed towards producing the correct mix of health care outputs, given the relative value attached to each. For example, these may reflect the preferences of funders (acting on behalf of society in general). On the input side, allocative efficiency examines whether an optimal mix of inputs is being used to produce its chosen outputs – for example, does the mix of labour skills minimize the costs of producing the outputs, given their relative wages.

Constant returns to scale occur when a given increase in inputs always gives rise to the same increase in outputs, regardless of the scale of operations.

Cost–effectiveness is a ratio of costs to the valued health care outputs (for example, outcomes) produced, often expressed as the cost per quality-adjusted life year.

Decreasing returns to scale occur when a proportionate increase in all inputs leads to a lower proportionate increase in outputs.

An **entity** is the accountable unit under scrutiny. At the finest micro level of analysis, an entity could be considered to be a single treatment, where the goal is to assess its cost relative to its expected benefit. At the meso level, an entity could be individuals or groups of practitioners, teams, hospitals or other organizations within the health system. The macro level entity could be considered as the entire health system.

External influences on the production of health care outputs or outcomes are beyond the control of entities; they could include case mix complexity, geography or the organization of the health system.

Health care efficiency measurement examines the extent to which the inputs to the health system, in the form of expenditure and other resources, are used to best effect to secure health system outputs and/or valued health system goals. It could embrace either allocative or technical efficiency, and is often conceptualized as waste.

Increasing returns to scale occur when a proportionate increase in all inputs leads to a greater proportionate increase in outputs.

Inputs are any resources that are used in the production of health care outputs and/or outcomes. They may include monetary or physical resources (for example, capital, labour, drugs) but also could include health care activities (for example, diagnostic tests or surgical procedures) if they are conceptualized as resources used to combine a more aggregate health care output.

Outputs are units of activity produced by combining health care inputs. They may include health care activities, such as surgical procedures (which are produced through combinations of labour, capital and other resources), or physical outputs, such as episodes of care (which are produced through combinations of health care activities).

Outcomes are valued health care outputs, such as quality-adjusted life years, patient-reported outcome measures or some other measure of health gain.

Production–possibility frontier indicates the maximum feasible level of outputs (or outcomes) that an entity could secure given the inputs at its disposal.

Quality-adjusted life years are a measure of life expectancy, expressed in terms of the number of years in full health (so the years in less than full health are given a lower weight than the years in full health). It is a generic measure, intended to be independent of the specific disease under scrutiny.

A **registry** is an information system that continuously records event-based data for a defined set of patients. A register contains a logically coherent collection of related data with some inherent meaning, typically reflecting events that have occurred, such as all treatment information for patients with a particular disease.

Scale efficiency is the extent to which an entity is operating at a scale that maximizes the ratio of outputs to inputs. If so, any higher level of scale would lead to decreasing returns to scale. Any lower level of scale would mean that the entity was operating under increasing returns to scale.

Technical efficiency indicates the extent to which the system is minimizing the use of inputs in producing its chosen outputs, regardless of the value placed on those outputs. An alternative formulation (which is equivalent when there are constant returns to scale) is to say that it is maximizing its outputs given its chosen level of inputs.

Preface

The pursuit of efficiency is one of the central preoccupations of health policymakers and managers, and it is justifiably a cause for such concern. Most immediately, inefficient care can lead to unnecessarily poor outcomes for the patients directly affected, measured either in terms of their health improvement, or in their broader satisfaction with the health system. More generally, inefficiency somewhere in the health system is likely to deny treatments and health improvement to patients who would otherwise have received treatment if resources had been better used, especially in systems operating with a fixed global budget. Taking an even broader perspective, inefficiency in the health system may divert resources from other productive sectors of the economy, including public services such as education, where the resources could be used productively.

Moreover, not only does increased efficiency allow money to be spent more effectively both inside and outside the health sector, but the ability to eliminate waste also demonstrates good stewardship of the health system. This may maintain and increase the willingness of governments and their citizens to pay for universal health coverage, through their taxes and social insurance premiums, and thereby secure the manifest social gains that such coverage brings. In contrast, a lack of evidence that a system or a provider is performing efficiently may damage confidence in these institutions, and compromise the social solidarity on which modern health systems depend.

There is ample evidence to suggest that inefficiency is a major problem in all health systems. The World Health Organization (WHO, 2000) pointed to very large apparent worldwide variations in efficiency at the system level, a finding replicated by subsequent work among high-income countries by the Organisation for Economic Co-operation and Development (OECD; Joumard et al., 2008). At a more forensic level, Berwick & Hackbarth (2012) identified six areas of waste in the US health system which, if addressed, could produce efficiency gains of at least 20% of total health care expenditures. The areas of waste they examined are particularly relevant for the US system, but can to some extent be found in all types of health systems, and include: failures of care delivery; failures of care coordination; overtreatment; administrative complexity; price failures; and fraud and abuse.

But what methods are most appropriate to measure health care efficiency, and how can efficiency metrics be used to make well-informed policy and managerial decisions? While the core idea of efficiency is easy to understand in principle – maximizing valued outputs relative to inputs – it often becomes more difficult to make operational when applied to a concrete situation, particularly at the system level. The difficulties of measuring and matching the inputs and outputs of health care organizations are well known. Furthermore, measuring the performance of the health sector is often greatly complicated by the influence of external factors, such as the social determinants of health. The health sector has little opportunity to influence many of these factors, so in principle any measure of efficiency must take account of their impact on measured levels of attainment.

Moreover, it is quite conceivable that there are efficiently functioning components operating within an inefficient broader health system. For example, the hospital sector – or parts of the hospital sector – may be operating extremely efficiently. However, those hospitals may be functioning within an extremely inefficient health system. In particular, it may be the case that inadequate attention is given to preventive and public health actions, or primary care may be poorly organized. The consequence may be unnecessarily high use of the hospital sector, with many patients using hospital care that a more cost-effective use of health system resources could have obviated. In short, it is often necessary to look at several levels and sectors of the health system to determine the magnitude and nature of inefficiency. This gives rise to a challenge in accommodating the needs of all the stakeholders interested in efficiency, which range from the general public to hospital managers to governmental policymakers. These stakeholders may require efficiency metrics for different purposes and decision-making objectives, and thus may be interested in different measures of output, outcome and input.

When considering efficiency, the general assumption in a great deal of the health economics literature is that the objective of the health system and its component parts is to improve the length and health-related quality of life (QOL) of the population. This is most famously embodied in the notion of a quality-adjusted life year. However, there may be other very important objectives attached to a health system, such as reducing disparities in health, protecting citizens from the financial consequences of illness and improving the responsiveness of health services to personal preferences. Furthermore, the valuations attached to these different health system outcomes may differ because of variations in individual preferences, the decision-making perspective being used or even because of the level of analysis being applied. As a result, a number of sometimes conflicting definitions for efficiency exist across stakeholders and even within the health economics literature itself.

Measuring the efficiency of health systems is therefore a challenging undertaking. This gives rise to two types of risk. On the one hand, decision-makers might conclude that identifying and addressing inefficiency is impossible, and therefore allow poor performance to persist, with the adverse consequences described earlier. Even worse, if expenditure reductions are required, decision-makers adopting this nihilistic perspective might adopt untargeted across-the-board cuts, with the danger of indiscriminately cutting highly cost-effective as well as inefficient activity. The second class of risk is that decision-makers rely on inadequate analysis or interpretation of efficiency metrics to implement reforms that target apparently inefficient practice. For example, an initiative to reduce the length of hospital inpatient stay may in some circumstances yield gains in terms of more efficient use of hospital resources. Yet, in other circumstances this may be at the expense of serious additional costs for ambulatory health services, or even future hospital readmissions. An important objective of this book is to try to help decision-makers to assess the balance of such risks when seeking to tackle inefficiency, and to make informed judgements about how they should reform their system to improve efficiency.

This volume sets out to review the state of the art of health system efficiency measurement, and to consider how existing metrics can influence policy formulation and managerial decision-making. The first section considers the different approaches for capturing data on health care inputs, outputs and outcomes, which are needed to formulate efficiency indicators. Next, the second section describes how these data can be combined to compare the efficiency of treatments, providers and systems. Finally, the third section of the volume explores how policymakers and managers might consider efficiency evidence when designing reforms and reconfiguring services.

Chapter 1 sets out a framework for thinking about efficiency that seeks to reconcile the different perspectives described earlier. The intention is to offer a unifying way of thinking about the construction and interpretation of efficiency metrics. The chapter recognizes that almost all efficiency metrics will be, to some extent, incomplete or contestable, so it argues that the important requirement is to be able to offer a balanced commentary on the strengths and weaknesses of any measure. The chapter's framework is intended to help in that endeavour.

In Chapter 2, Quentin et al. discuss the use of patient classification systems, including diagnosis-related groups, for efficiency measurement. Patient classification systems can be used to group types of patients (or health care products) in an effort to compare like-with-like, and to account for differences in patient complexity when measuring health care outputs.

Chapter 3 further explores the issue of comparing similar types of care, but does so by exploring the use of routine administrative registry data for measuring efficiency. Sund & Häkkinen describe a methodology for constructing patient episodes of care from registry data, which much like patient classification systems, allow for comparisons of similar patients. However, the benefit of using detailed linkable registry data is that comparisons can be made of full patient care pathways across multiple providers. The authors suggest that such data can allow for patient variations to be sufficiently accounted for so that observed variations in health care outputs can be more directly attributed to health care services.

In Chapter 4, Chapman et al. focus on the complexities associated with linking input costs to patient care, a fundamental concern for management accounting. While many types of costs are directly attributable to specific patient care episodes, other types of costs, such as overheads and other fixed costs, can be more problematic. These costs comprise a significant amount of health care resources and so clarity in terms of how they should be accounted for is essential. This chapter reviews different approaches to costing, highlighting a need for conceptual clarity over the costing methodologies appropriate to particular kinds of purposes and decision-making objectives.

Chapter 5 describes how outputs and inputs can be combined to form efficiency indicators. In this chapter, Hollingsworth concentrates on frontier-based methodologies, data envelopment analysis and stochastic frontier analysis, which seek to compare producers (for example, hospitals, countries) by constructing production possibilities frontiers that represent the highest levels of efficiency attainable, and assessing how far each producer is from the frontier. These methods appear frequently in the academic literature but have been used practically much more rarely. This chapter aims to make these methods more accessible so that they may perhaps play a greater role in policy and managerial circles, and includes guidelines for the application of these techniques that clearly set out how these methods can be of use to analysts, and to those who need to interpret and make use of the results generated.

In Chapter 6, Thomas & Chalkidou discuss the potential use of cost–effectiveness analysis – the holy grail of efficiency measurement – to achieve allocative efficiency at the health care organization (meso) level and the health system (macro) level. In particular, the authors discuss how cost–effectiveness analysis plays a central role prospectively in resource allocation decisions to ensure that the mix of health care services is chosen to maximize health, but less so in retrospective assessment of providers or treatments. They highlight potential areas for future research that will promote the application of cost–effectiveness analysis to meso-level and macro-level efficiency analysis, both in retrospective assessment of past performance, and as a tool for guiding future allocation decisions.

International comparison is becoming one of the most powerful tools for identifying performance weaknesses in health systems. However, there are numerous pitfalls in developing secure efficiency comparisons, caused, for example, by differences in definitions of inputs (such as human resources) and challenges in currency conversion. Chapter 7 provides a thorough review of available international efficiency comparisons. From regularly collected databases to one-off academic studies, Cylus & Pearson evaluate the extent to which the data provide sufficient evidence for comparing health care efficiency between countries.

Efficiency measurement is only useful if it plays a part in policy formulation and managerial decisions. Chapters 8 (Charlesworth, Or & Spencelayh) and 9 (Morton & Schang) review the role of efficiency information in these respective areas. The authors find, overwhelmingly, that while the desire for greater efficiency motivates decision-making, routine use of efficiency metrics to guide these decisions is severely lacking.

Chapter 10 summarizes and discusses the different threads of the book and highlights the promising opportunities for efficiency management. It also considers the potential for progress in using the information we have to guide the judgements we make about efficiency throughout the health system, thereby improving policy and managerial decisions.

The motivation for this book is that – in different ways – policymakers, managers, politicians and the general public have profound concerns about the efficiency of their health systems. In that context, there is a risk that decision-makers will make serious misjudgements about how to improve the system unless they have access to meaningful efficiency metrics that they can interpret in an informed manner. The book does not seek to put forward a set of prescriptive policy or managerial interventions that will improve efficiency. It is likely that such prescriptions will be highly specific to context, and in any case the evidence for many interventions is at best equivocal (OECD, 2010). Rather, the central purpose of this book is to promote a better understanding of the potential and limitations of efficiency metrics, examine the scope for developing better metrics and explore how they can be used to support good decision-making. We therefore hope that it provides a solid foundation for considering the efficiency of health systems and offers a good basis for those seeking to take concrete actions.

Jonathan Cylus, Irene Papanicolas, Peter C. Smith

References

Berwick DM, Hackbarth AD (2012). Eliminating waste in US health care. *JAMA*, 307(14):1513–1516.
Joumard I et al. (2008). *Health status determinants: lifestyle, environment, health care resources and efficiency.* OECD Economics Department Working Paper No. 627. Paris, OECD Publishing.
OECD (2010). *Value for money in health spending.* OECD Health Policy Studies. Paris, OECD Publishing.
WHO (2000). The World Health Report 2000. Health systems: improving performance. Geneva, WHO (http://www.who.int/whr/2000/en/whr00_en.pdf?ua=1, accessed 3 August 2016).

Chapter 1

A framework for thinking about health system efficiency

Jonathan Cylus, Irene Papanicolas, Peter C. Smith

This chapter takes up the challenge set out in the book's preface and offers a framework for thinking about the conceptualization and measurement of efficiency in health systems. The intention is to help those seeking to gain an understanding of the magnitude and nature of a system's inefficiencies. The chapter first reiterates why an understanding of health sector efficiency is important. We then explain what is meant by efficiency and explore in more depths the two fundamental concepts of allocative efficiency (AE) and technical efficiency (TE). We show that many metrics relating to efficiency are partial, and if viewed in isolation, can be misleading. We bring the discussion to a conclusion by presenting a framework for thinking about health efficiency metrics comprising five key issues: the entity to be scrutinized; the outputs; the inputs; the external influences on performance; and the impact of the entity on the broader health system.

1.1 Why is health sector efficiency important?

The notion of health sector efficiency – and related issues such as cost–effectiveness and value for money – are some of the most discussed dimensions of health care performance. These concepts seek to capture the extent to which the inputs to the health system, in the form of expenditure and other resources, are used to secure valued health system goals. In many other sectors of the economy, consumer preferences help to ensure that the most valued outputs are produced at market prices. However, there are numerous, well-rehearsed market failures in the health sector that mean that traditional market mechanisms cannot work, allowing poor quality or inappropriate care to persist at high prices if no policy action is taken. Most commentators would therefore agree that the pursuit of efficiency should be a central objective of policymakers and managers, and to that end better instruments for measuring and understanding efficiency are urgently needed.

Inefficient use of health system resources poses serious concerns, for a number of reasons:

- it may deny health gain to patients who have received treatment because they do not receive the best possible care available within the health system's resource limits;
- by consuming excess resources, inefficient treatment may deny treatment to other patients who could have benefited from treatment if the resources had been better used;
- inefficient use of resources in the health sector may sacrifice loss of consumption opportunities elsewhere in the economy, such as education or nutrition;
- wasting resources on inefficient care may reduce society's willingness to contribute to the funding of health services, thereby harming social solidarity, health system performance and social welfare.

Thus, as well as its instrumental value, tackling inefficiency has an important accountability value: to reassure payers that their money is being spent wisely, and to reassure patients, caregivers and the general population that their claims on the health system are being treated fairly and consistently. Also, health care funders including governments, insurance organizations and households are interested in knowing which systems, providers and treatments contribute the largest health gains in relation to the level of resources they consume. Efficiency becomes particularly important in the light of financial pressures and concerns over long-term financial sustainability experienced in many health systems, as decision-makers seek to demonstrate and ensure that health care resources are put to good use. When used appropriately, efficiency indicators can be important tools to help decision-makers determine whether resources are allocated optimally, and to pinpoint which parts of the health system are not performing as well as they should be.

1.2 What is inefficiency?

The concept of health system efficiency may seem beguilingly simple, represented at its simplest as a ratio of resources consumed (health system inputs) to some measure of the valued health system outputs that they create. In effect, this creates a metric of the generic type, the so-called resource use per unit of health system output. Yet, making this straightforward notion operational can give rise to considerable complexity. Within the health system as a whole, there exist a seemingly infinite set of interlinked processes that could be evaluated independently and found to be efficient or inefficient. This has given rise to a plethora of apparently disconnected indicators that give glimpses of certain aspects of inefficiency, but rarely offer a comprehensive overview.

Economists conceive the transformation of inputs into valued outputs as a 'production function', which indicates the maximum feasible level of output for a given set of inputs. Any failure to attain that maximum is an indication of inefficiency (Jacobs, Smith & Street, 2006). The concept of a production function can be applied to the functioning of very detailed micro units (such as a physician's office) through to huge macro units (such as the entire health system). Whatever level is chosen, the intention is to offer insights into the success with which health system resources are transformed into physical outputs (such as patient consultations), or (more ambitiously) into valued outcomes (such as improved health).

But why exactly might a health system not perform as well as it could? Processes in the health system may be inefficient for two distinct, but related reasons. The first reason is that health system inputs such as expenditure or other resources may be directed towards creating some outputs that are not priorities for society. For example, providing very high-cost end-of-life cancer treatments may create benefits for the individuals involved, but society may judge that the limited money available to the health system may be better spent on other interventions that create (in aggregate) larger health gains. The second reason for inefficiency is that there could be misuse of inputs in the process of producing valued health system outputs. Waste of inputs at any stage of the production process mean that there will be less output than what is possible for a given initial level of resources, leading to what can be loosely thought of as waste. For example, if a health system does not secure the minimum cost of medicines and other inputs, less output either in terms of quantity of patients treated or quality of care provided will be possible for a given level of expenditure. Likewise, if a patient's medical tests are unnecessarily ordered or duplicated, there is a waste of resources and other individuals may be forced to forego needed care.

Economists refer to these two concepts as as allocative efficiency (AE) and technical efficiency (TE). AE can be used to scrutinize either the choice of outputs or the choice of inputs. On the output side, it examines whether limited resources are directed towards producing the correct mix of health care outputs, given the preferences of funders (acting on behalf of society in general). AE can also examine whether the entity under scrutiny uses an optimal mix of inputs – for example, the mix of labour skills – to produce its chosen outputs, given the prices of those inputs.

In contrast, TE indicates the extent to which the system is minimizing the use of inputs in producing its chosen outputs, regardless of the value placed on those outputs. An alternative, but equivalent formulation is to say that it is maximizing its outputs given its chosen level of inputs. In either case, any variation in performance from the greatest feasible level of production is an indication of technical inefficiency, or waste. The prime interest in TE is therefore in the operational performance of the entity, rather than its strategic choices relating to what outputs it produces or what inputs it consumes.

The thesis underlying this book is that – whether inefficiency takes the form of inputs lost in the production of valued health outputs, or inputs misdirected towards relatively low-value health outputs – a first step towards remedial actions is to properly understand the magnitude and nature of any such inefficiency. To that end, it is important for decision-makers (whether clinicians, managers, regulators or policymakers) to understand the strengths and limitations of the many efficiency metrics that are becoming available.

We now therefore consider the concepts of allocative and TE in more detail.

1.3 Allocative inefficiency

AE is central to the work of health technology assessment (HTA) agencies, which often use expected gains in quality-adjusted life years (QALYs) as the central measure of the benefits of a treatment, and cost per QALY as a prime cost–effectiveness criterion for determining whether or not to mandate adoption of a treatment. The assumption underlying this approach is that payers wish to see their financial contributions used to maximize health gain. Under these circumstances, a provider would not be allocatively efficient if it produces treatments with low levels of cost–effectiveness, because the inputs used could be better deployed producing outputs with higher potential health gain (see Chapter 6).

Table 1.1 gives an example of a cost-per-QALY ranking, which indicates the relative value of a set of treatments being considered for introduction based on conventional estimates of incremental cost–effectiveness (compared to current practice). At the level of individual interventions, concentrating on introducing treatments with the lowest incremental cost per QALY maximizes the health benefits secured from limited funds. Of course, the volume of expenditure consumed by each intervention will depend on the incidence of the associated disease. In principle, the treatments under consideration should be prioritized in order of increasing cost per QALY, all of which should be included in the health benefits package until the available funds are exhausted. An equivalent perspective is to require that only treatments that lie below the system's cost-per-QALY threshold should be accepted, where the value of the threshold is determined by the size of the total budget available for the health system.

Table 1.1 *An example of an incremental cost-per-QALY league table*

Description	Cost
Pacemaker for atrioventricular heart block	£700
Hip replacement	£750
Valve replacement for aortic stenosis	£900
CABG (severe angina; left main disease)	£1040
CABG (severe angina; triple-vessel disease)	£1270
CABG (moderate angina; left main disease)	£1330
CABG (severe angina; left main disease)	£2280
CABG (moderate angina; triple-vessel disease)	£2400
CABG (mild angina; left main disease)	£2520
Kidney transplantation (cadaver)	£3000
CABG (moderate angina; double-vessel disease)	£4000
Heart transplantation	£5000
CABG (mild angina; triple-vessel disease)	£6300
Haemodialysis at home	£11 000
CABG (mild angina; double-vessel disease)	£12 600
Haemodialysis in hospital	£14 000

Sources: Briggs & Gray (2000), adapted from Williams (1985).
Note: CABG = coronary artery bypass graft.

AE can also be considered at a broad sectoral level to examine whether the correct mix of health services is funded, such that at a given aggregate level of expenditure, health outcomes are being maximized. For example, an allocatively efficient health system allocates funds between sectors like prevention, primary care, hospital care and long-term care so as to secure the maximum level of health-related outcomes in line with societal preferences. AE indicators at this level should indicate whether a health system is performing poorly because of a misallocation of resources between such health system sectors. Indicators such as the rate of avoidable hospital admissions might be considered an indicator of misallocation, perhaps suggesting that greater emphasis on primary care may yield efficiency improvements. Note that such principles can be equally applied to much smaller units of analysis, such as a primary care practice. Metrics such as excessive use of antibiotic prescribing, or excessive referrals to hospital specialists, might be indicators of allocative inefficiency.

Consideration of the different levels of AE highlights the fact that the health system may contain entities (such as clinical teams) that perform perfectly efficiently in producing what has been asked of them (for example, preventive treatments). However, consideration of a broader societal perspective may indicate that strategic decision-makers have misallocated resources between preventive and curative services, and that efficient teams are operating within an inefficient system.

Note that a great deal of emphasis on AE has hitherto been on *ex ante* guidelines on treatments and clinical pathways that should (or should not) be provided. Assuming those guidelines have been prepared in line with the principles of cost–effectiveness, they can also be used *ex post* to explore whether provider organizations and practitioners have deviated from policy intentions and delivered what can be thought of as inappropriate care. This may take the form of obviously suboptimal use of resources, such as hospital treatment of glue ear, a condition that does not typically require such a resource-intensive setting. However, it could also take the form of treatments that confer health benefits, but which policymakers have decided are not priorities, perhaps implicitly because their cost–effectiveness ratios are above the system's chosen cost–effectiveness threshold. End-of-life cancer drugs are emerging as a particularly challenging example of such treatments in some systems.

Of course, the inappropriate treatments might have been provided because the financial regime continues to reward such provision, or because clear guidelines have not been promulgated, in which case accountability for the efficiency failure may properly be assigned to policymakers rather than providers. The identification and measurement of inappropriate care is therefore a first step towards identifying inefficiency of this type and designing remedial policies. Note that some valuation of the health benefits of treatment is needed to determine whether or not an activity is cost-effective, and therefore appropriate.

On the input side, although given less attention, there may be potential for a wide range of indicators of allocative inefficiency, in the form of inappropriate use of health system resources. For example, metrics relating to the skill mix of labour inputs can be prepared at a whole system level or at a local level. It is also possible to envisage a wide range of metrics of treatment taking place in the wrong setting (for example, emergency department rather than primary care office), or using inappropriate inputs (such as emergency ambulance transport for non-urgent care).

1.4 Technical inefficiency

There is a sense in which the analysis and measurement of technical inefficiency is less demanding than that of allocative inefficiency. It does not require *ex ante* specification of norms, and instead is usually entirely an *ex post* examination of whether the outputs produced by the entity under scrutiny were maximized, given its inputs and external circumstances. Comparative performance therefore lies at the core of most analyses of technical inefficiency.

A major class of TE indicator examines the total costs of producing a specified unit of output, in the form, for example, of costs per patient within a specified disease category. The most celebrated form of such unit cost indicators forms the basis for the various systems of diagnosis-related groups (DRGs), initially developed by Fetter and colleagues at Yale University (Fetter, 1991) for use in the hospital sector (see Chapter 2). These methods cluster patients into a manageable number of groups that are homogeneous with regard to medical condition and expected costs. In the first instance, a hospital's average unit cost within a DRG category can be compared with a national reference cost for that DRG, often the mean of unit costs across all comparable institutions. This metric in itself may prove useful information on the functioning of specialities within the hospital.

Moreover, the number of cases in each DRG can then be multiplied by the relevant reference cost to derive the expected aggregate costs of treating all the hospital's patients (if reference costs applied). This can be compared with its actual costs to yield an index of the hospital's relative efficiency. This approach has usually been used in the hospital sector, but can be extended to many other units of analysis in the health system.

An important barrier to applying the DRG method effectively is the great complexity of hospital cost structures. This has led to major challenges in allocating many hospital costs to specific patients and activities, and the associated variations in accounting practice are one of the reasons for apparent variation in unit costs. To the extent that it is feasible, greater standardization of accounting practices would seem to be an important priority. Chapman et al. (Chapter 4) discuss these important management accounting issues further.

Unit cost metrics offer insights into the overall TE of the entity (relative to other such entities), but give little operational guidance as to the reasons why such inefficiency arises, nor any insights into the AE of the entity. Therefore, aggregate measures of technical inefficiency can usefully be augmented by more specific metrics of operational waste, either in some specified form, such as excessive prices paid for inputs, comparatively long lengths of stay, or unnecessary duplication. Here we seek to examine the various types of TE indicators in the context of a stylized example, based on hospital treatment.

For health production processes of any complexity, there are usually a number of stages in the transformation of resources to outcomes, and much of the confusion in discussing efficiency arises because commentators are discussing different parts of that process. To illustrate, Figure 1.1 represents a typical (but simplified) process associated with the treatment of hospital patients. The overarching concern is with cost–effectiveness, which summarizes the transformation of costs (on the left-hand side) into valued health outcomes (the right-hand side). However, the data demands of a full system cost–effectiveness analysis are often prohibitive, and the results of such endeavours may in any case not provide policymakers with relevant information on the causes of inefficiency, or where to make improvements. To take remedial action, decision-makers require more detailed diagnostic indicators of just part of the transformation process.

Figure 1.1 *The production process in hospital care*

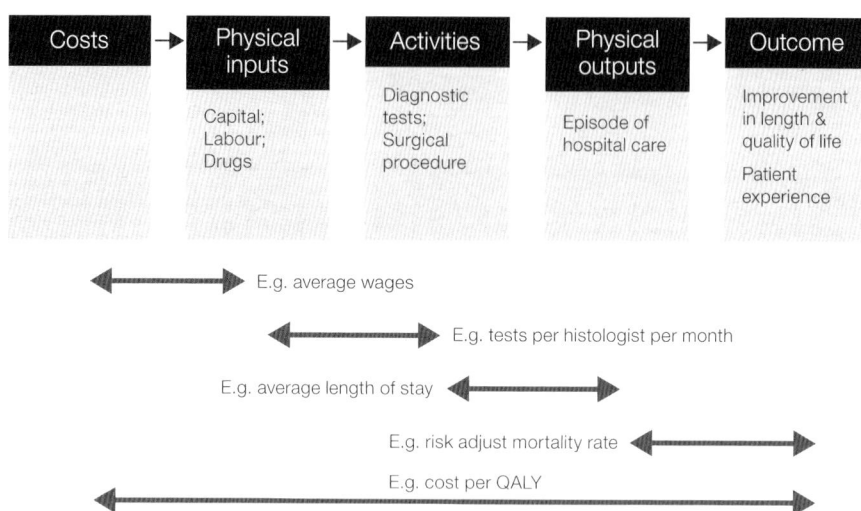

Note: QALY = quality-adjusted life year.

Inefficiency might occur at any stage of this transformation process. Take first the transformation of money into physical inputs. The principal question (given the mix of chosen inputs) is whether those inputs are purchased at minimum cost. For example, is the organization using branded rather than generic drugs, or paying wage rates in excess of local market rates? A metric such as the average hourly wage (adjusted for skill mix) might shed light on such issues. Note that if no adjustment is made for skill mix, the index may also capture information about the AE of input choices: is the right mix of doctors, other professionals and administrators being deployed? So, in many circumstances it may be helpful to prepare such indicators with and without adjustment.

The production process now moves to the creation of activities produced from those physical inputs, such as diagnostic tests or surgical procedures. Possible sources of waste here may include the use of highly skilled (and therefore costly) workers to produce activities that could be done by less specialized workers, or using excessive hours of labour or other physical inputs in the creation of a particular activity. We cite just one among countless numbers of such possible indicators – the number of tests undertaken by a histologist per month (see Figure 1.1). Note the manifest incompleteness of such an indicator (ignoring both the other outputs of the specialist and the other inputs to the testing function). However, the metric may in some circumstances prove useful when supporting broader efficiency metrics.

Next, physical outputs are created by aggregating activities for a particular service user. In a hospital setting, this usually refers to single episodes of patient care, an aggregation of many actions such as tests, procedures, nursing care and physician consultations. There is great scope for waste in this process, for example, in the form of duplicate or unnecessary diagnostic tests, use of branded rather than generic drugs, or unnecessarily long length of stay. Much depends on how the internal processes of the hospital are organized so as to maximize outputs using the given inputs. The well-known metric of length of stay, which indicates the number of bed days expended per case, falls into this category. (Of course, this will usually be adjusted for case mix complexity.)

The final stage of the health system production process is the quality of the outputs produced. Even when they employ the same physical inputs, activities or physical outputs, there is great scope for variation in effectiveness among providers. The notion of quality in health care has a number of connotations, including the clinical outcomes achieved (usually measured in terms of the gain in the length and quality of life) and the patient experience (a multidimensional concept). So, for example, even though two hospitals produce identical numbers of hip replacements, because of variations in clinical practice and competence, the value they confer on patients (in the form of length and quality of life, and patient experience) can vary considerably. Quality-adjusted output is usually referred to as the outcome of care in the literature. Quality of care has become a central concern of policymakers, and its measurement, while contentious, is usually essential if a comprehensive picture of efficiency is to be secured.

Note that the unit costs metric usually links costs to physical outputs. The numerous partial efficiency indicators that have been developed seek to shed some light on the reasons for variations in unit costs. Each metric gives an indication of the TE of part of the production process. Some, such as the labour productivity or length of stay examples, are based on only partial measures of inputs or outputs. Some are capable of adjustment for external influences on attainment (such as case mix complexity), others are not. None addresses the production process in its entirety, that is, the cost–effectiveness with which costly inputs are converted into valued outputs.

Furthermore, this stylized example looks only at the hospital sector, without reference to other aspects of the health system. It therefore focuses mainly on hospital TE, making no judgement on AE issues, such as whether patients might have been treated more cost-effectively in different settings (for example, primary care or nursing homes). And by focusing on the curative sector, it can shed no light on the success or otherwise of the health system's efforts to prevent or delay the onset of disease. A further aspect of whole system performance that is ignored is the impact of hospital performance on other sectors within the health system. For example, it may be the case that apparently high levels of efficiency in (say) average length of stay are being secured at the expense of heavy workloads for rehabilitative and primary care services, which may or may not be efficient from a whole system perspective.

1.5 An analytical framework for thinking about efficiency indicators

Figure 1.2 summarizes the principles underlying the simplistic viewpoint of efficiency referred, namely that it represents the ratio of the inputs an organization consumes in relation to the valued outputs it produces. The entity consumes a series of physical resources, referred to as inputs, often measured in terms of total costs. The organization then transforms those inputs into a series of valued outputs. Although measuring the aggregate value of inputs in terms of total costs is relatively uncontroversial, the valuation of aggregate outputs in the health sector depends on how much importance we place on different health system outputs, such as health improvement and quality of life, which are highly contested. Nevertheless, if we can agree on a measure of aggregate valued outputs, then we can calculate a summary measure of efficiency as the ratio of valued outputs to inputs, what is often referred to as cost–effectiveness, or how well the organization's costs are converted into valued benefits.

Figure 1.2 *The naive view of efficiency*

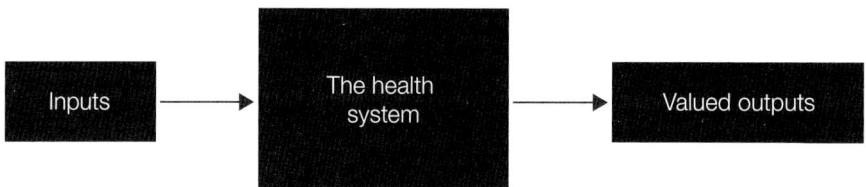

As discussed in the preceding section, any specific indicator of efficiency may seek to aggregate all inputs into a single measure of costs, or it may consider only a partial measure of inputs. For example, labour productivity measures such as patient consultations per full-time equivalent (FTE) physician per month ignore the many other inputs into the consultation, and the many outputs other than patient consultations produced by the physician. In effect, such partial measures create efficiency ratios using only a subset of the inputs and outputs represented by the arrows in Figure 1.2. Here the output measure is partial in several senses: a physician may undertake many other activities; there are many other inputs into the patient's care; and there is no information on the health gain achieved by the consultation. In short, the indicator shows only a fragment of the complete transformation of resources into the desired outcomes (improved health).

Numerous other issues arise when seeking to use the concept set out in Figure 1.2 to develop operational models of organizational efficiency in health care, reflecting the complexity of the health care production process. The production of the majority of health care outputs rarely conforms to a production-line type technology, in which a set of clearly identifiable inputs is used to produce a standard type of output. Instead, the majority of health care is tailor-made to the specific needs of an individual patient, with consequent variations in clinical needs, social circumstances and personal preferences. This means that there is often considerable variation among patients in how inputs are consumed and outputs or outcomes are produced. For example, contributions to the care process may be made by multiple organizations and caregivers, a package of care may be delivered over an extended period of time and in different settings, and the responsibilities for delivery may vary from place to place and over time.

In the light of these complexities, the objective of this section is to offer a framework for thinking more clearly about what a specific efficiency indicator tells us, and for identifying the respects in which the indicator may be informative, misleading or partial. Five aspects of any efficiency indicator are assessed in turn:

- the entity to be assessed;
- the outputs (or outcomes) under consideration;
- the inputs under consideration;
- the external influences on attainment;
- the links with the rest of the health system.

1.5.1 Identifying entities: what to evaluate?

Where then should an analyst begin? An assessment of efficiency first depends crucially on establishing the boundaries of the entity under scrutiny. At the finest micro level of analysis, an entity could be considered to be a single treatment, where the goal is to assess its cost relative to its expected benefit. At the other extreme, the macro level entity could be considered as the entire health system, defined by the WHO as "all the activities whose primary purpose is to promote, restore or maintain health" (WHO, 2000: p.5).

Most often, however, efficiency measurement takes place at some intermediate or meso level, where the actions of individuals or groups of practitioners, teams, hospitals or other organizations within the health system are assessed. Whatever the chosen level, as a general principle it is important that any analysis reflects an entity for which clear accountability can be determined, whether it is the whole health system, a health services organization or an individual physician. Only then can the relevant agent, whether it is the government, management board or physician, be held to account for the level of performance revealed by the analysis.

Almost all efficiency analysis relies on comparisons, so it is important to ensure that the entities being compared are genuinely similar. A great deal of efficiency analysis is concerned with securing such comparability. If organizational entities are operating in different circumstances, perhaps because the population cared for or the patients being treated differ markedly, some sort of adjustment will be needed to ensure like is being compared with like. We consider this in further detail when discussing external influences on attainment.

More generally, almost all organizations and practitioners operate within profound operational constraints, created by the legal, professional and financial environment within which they must operate. In assigning proper accountability for efficiency shortcomings, it is important to identify the real source of the weakness, which may lie beyond the control of the immediate entity under scrutiny. For example, a community nurse practising in a remote rural area may necessarily appear less efficient when assessed using a metric such as patient encounters per month. However, local geography may preclude any increase, and the nurse may be performing as well as can be expected within the constrained circumstances.

When choosing the entity to evaluate, there is often a difficult trade-off to be made between scrutiny of the detailed local performance of the system, and scrutiny of broader system-wide performance. In general terms, the performance of individual clinicians and clinical teams may be highly dependent on the inputs from other parts of the system (for example the performance of the emergency department in supporting the work of a maternity unit). Furthermore, determining the resources allocated to local teams can be challenging from an accountancy perspective. On the other hand, moving the analysis to a more aggregate level, while obviating the need to identify in detail who undertakes what activity, can make it difficult to identify what is causing apparently inefficient care.

1.5.2 *What are the outputs under consideration?*

In the context of efficiency analysis in the health sector, two fundamental issues need to be considered. How should the outputs of the health care sector be defined? And what value should be attached to these outputs? The consensus is that in principle health care outputs should properly be defined in terms of the health gains produced. However, organizations rarely collect relevant routine information about health gains and regardless, the construct of health gain has proved challenging to make operational. In most circumstances, it is rarely possible to observe a baseline, or counterfactual – the health status that would have been secured in the absence of an intervention. Furthermore, the heterogeneity of service users, the multidimensional nature of health, and the intrinsic measurement difficulties add to the complexity.

Recent progress in the use of patient-reported outcome measures (PROMs) offers some prospect of making more secure comparisons, at least of providers delivering a specific treatment (Smith & Street, 2013), and a number of well-established measurement instruments have been developed that could be used to collect before/after measures of treatment effects, such as the EuroQol five dimensions (EQ-5D) questionnaire and Short Form-36 (SF-36) (EuroQol Group, 1990; Ware & Sherbourne, 1992). Although many unresolved issues surrounding the precise specification and analysis of such instruments remain, their use should be considered whenever there are likely to be material differences in the clinical quality of different organizations.

In practice, however, analysts are often constrained to examining efficiency on the basis of measures of activities, for example, in the form of patients treated, operations undertaken or outpatients seen. Such measures are manifestly inadequate, as they fail to capture variations in the effectiveness (or quality) of the health care delivered. Yet there is often in practice no alternative to using such incomplete measures of activity in lieu of health care outcomes.

Measuring activities can also address a fundamental difficulty of outcome measurement – identifying how much of the variation in outcomes is directly attributable to the actions of the health care organization. For example, mortality after a surgical procedure is likely to be influenced by numerous factors beyond the control of the provider, or even the health system. In some circumstances such considerations can be accommodated by careful use of risk-adjustment methods. However, there is often no analytically satisfactory way of adjusting for environmental influences on outcomes, in which case analysing instead the activities of care may offer a more meaningful insight into organizational performance.

1.5.3 What are the inputs under consideration?

The input side of efficiency metrics is often considered less problematic than the output side. Physical inputs can often be measured more accurately than outputs, or can be summarized in the form of a measure of costs. However, even the specification of inputs can give rise to serious conceptual and practical difficulties.

A fundamental decision that must be taken is the level of disaggregation of inputs to be specified. At one extreme, a single measure of aggregate inputs (in the form of total costs) might be used. The input side of the efficiency ratio then effectively becomes costs. This approach assumes that the organizations under scrutiny are free to deploy inputs efficiently, taking account of relative prices. In practice, some aspects of the input mix are often beyond the control of the organization, at least in the short-term. For example, the stock of capital can usually be changed only in the longer-term. In these circumstances, it may be important to disaggregate to some extent the inputs to capture the different input mixes that organizations have inherited.

Labour inputs can usually be measured with some degree of accuracy, often disaggregated by skill level. An important issue is then how much aggregation of labour inputs to use before pursuing an efficiency analysis. Unless there is a specific interest in the deployment of different labour types, it may be appropriate to aggregate into a single measure of labour input, weighting the various labour inputs by their relative wages. There may be little merit in disaggregation unless there is a specific interest in the relationship between efficiency and the mix of labour inputs employed. Under such circumstances, metrics using measures of labour input disaggregated by skill type may be valuable. Such analysis may yield useful policy insights into the gains to be secured from (say) substituting some types of labour for others.

Although labour inputs can be measured readily at an organizational level, problems may arise if the interest is in examining the efficiency of subunits within organizations, such as (say) operating theatres within hospitals. It becomes increasingly difficult to attribute labour inputs as the unit of observation within the hospital becomes smaller (department, team, surgeon and patient). Staff often work across a number of subunits, but information systems cannot usually track their input across these units with any accuracy. Particular care should be exercised when developing metrics that rely heavily on input measures of self-reported allocations of professional time.

In general, capital is a key input whose misuse can be a major source of inefficiency. However, incorporating measures of capital into the efficiency analysis is challenging. This is partly because of the difficulty of measuring capital stock and partly because of problems in attributing its use to any particular activity or time period. Measures of capital are often very rudimentary and even misleading. For example, accounting measures of the depreciation of physical stock usually offer little meaningful indication of capital consumed. Indeed, in practice, analysts may have to resort to very crude measures, for example, the number of hospital beds or floor space as a proxy for physical capital. Furthermore, non-physical capital inputs, such as health promotion efforts, are important capital investments that can be difficult to attribute directly to health outcomes.

As with all modelling, efficiency metrics should be developed according to the intentions of the analysis. If the interest is in the narrow, short-term use of existing resources, then it may be relevant to disaggregate inputs to reflect the resources currently at the disposal of management. If a longer-term, less constrained analysis is required, then a single measure of total costs may be a perfectly adequate indicator of the entity's physical inputs.

1.5.4 *What are the external influences on performance?*

In many contexts, a separate class of factors affects organizational capacity, which we classify as the external or environmental determinants of performance. These are influences on the organization beyond its control that reflect the external environment within which it must operate. In particular, many of the outcomes secured by health care organizations are highly dependent on the characteristics of the population group they serve. For example:

- population mortality rates are heavily dependent on the demographic structure of the population under consideration and the broader social determinants of health;
- the intensity of resource use is usually highly contingent on the severity of disease of patient;
- hospital performance may be related to how primary care is organized in the local community;
- the costs to emergency ambulance services of satisfying service standards (such as speed of attendance) may depend on local geography and settlement patterns.

There is often considerable debate as to what environmental factors are considered controllable. This will be a key issue for any scrutiny of efficiency, and for holding relevant management to account. The choice of whether to adjust for such exogenous factors is likely to be heavily dependent on the degree of autonomy enjoyed by management, and whether the purpose of the analysis is short-term and tactical, or longer-term and strategic. In the short-term, almost all input factors and external constraints will be fixed. In the longer-term, depending on the level of autonomy, many may be changeable. In many circumstances it will be appropriate to consider efficiency metrics both with and without adjustment for external factors.

Broadly speaking, there are three ways in which environmental factors can be taken into account in efficiency analyses:

- restrict comparison only to entities operating within a similarly con-strained environment;
- model the constraints explicitly, using statistical methods such as regression analysis;
- undertake risk adjustment to adjust the outcomes achieved to reflect the external constraints.

The first approach to accommodating environmental influences is to select only entities in similar circumstances. Then, the intention is to compare only like-with-like. Of course this begs the question as to what criteria should be used to select the similar entities. They might simply be readily observable characteristics, such as urban/rural. Alternatively, statistical techniques such as cluster analysis might be used to identify similar organizations according to a larger number of observable characteristics (Everitt et al., 2001).

A shortcoming of comparing only similar entities is that it will reduce sample size, as it allows comparison of performance only with similar types. Therefore, a second approach is to incorporate environmental factors directly into a regression model of organizational efficiency. The regression analysis makes allowance for the uncontrollable factors at an organizational level, and the residual in the model (what cannot be explained) is the adjusted measure of efficiency. While leading to a more general specification of the efficiency model than the clustering approach, the use of such techniques gives rise to modelling challenges that are discussed in detail by Jacobs, Smith & Street (2006).

The final method to control for variation in environmental circumstances is the family of techniques known as risk adjustment. These methods adjust organizational outputs for differences in circumstances before they are used in any efficiency indicator, and are – where feasible – often the most sensible approach to deal with environmental factors. In particular, they permit the analyst to adjust each output for only those factors that apply specifically to that output, rather than use environmental factors as a general adjustment for all outputs.

Well-understood forms of risk adjustment include the various types of stand-ardized mortality rates routinely deployed in studies of population outcomes.

These adjust observed mortality rates for the demographic structure of the population, thereby seeking to account for the higher risk of mortality (ROM) among older people. Likewise, surgical lengths of stay might be adjusted for the severity of risk factors, such as the age, comorbidities and smoking status of the patients treated. The methods of risk adjustment, often based on multivariate regression methods, have been developed to a high level of refinement (Iezzoni, 2003). However, risk adjustment usually has demanding data requirements, generally in the form of information on the circumstances of individual patients.

1.5.5 Links with the rest of the health system

No outputs from a health service practitioner or organization can be considered in isolation from their impact on the rest of the health system in which they operate. For example:

- the effectiveness of preventive services will affect the nature of demand for curative services;
- the performance of hospital support services, such as diagnostic departments, will affect the efficiency of functional areas such as surgical services;
- the actions of hospitals, for example, in creating care plans for discharged patients, may have profound implications for primary care services;
- the performance of rehabilitative services may have important implications for future hospital readmissions.

Likewise, cost-effective treatment is often secured only if there is effective coordination between discrete organizations. The need for such coordination is becoming increasingly important as the number of people with complex comorbidities and care needs rises. The frequent calls for better integration of patient care reflect the concern that such coordination often fails to meet expectations. That failure may in itself be an important cause of inefficiency.

Scrutiny of a health system entity in isolation may ignore these important implications of the entity's impact on whole system efficiency. Thus, for example, if a primary care practice is held to account only by metrics of costs per patient, it might secure apparently good levels of efficiency by inappropriately shifting certain costs (such as emergency cover) onto other agencies, such as hospitals or ambulance services. The chosen metric creates perverse incentives for the practice, and may fail to capture its serious negative impact on other parts of the health system. That consequence should in principle be accounted for in any assessment of that practice's efficiency. In principle, it should be feasible to accommodate such negative effects – which economists conceive as externalities – within the analytic framework. However, in practice it is rarely done, with potentially important consequences for bias in efficiency assessment, perverse incentives and misdirected managerial responses.

Failures of integration of care for patients with complex, long-term needs pose an especially serious barrier to good efficiency assessment. Indeed, the very act of measuring the efficiency of separate entities may frustrate efforts to encourage cooperation between different parts of the health system unless successes of care integration are properly recognized in performance assessment. Organizations that are held to account with partial measures of efficiency that ignore coordination activities may be reluctant to divert efforts towards integration of future patient care. Linking patient data across multiple care settings (see Chapter 3) is an important prerequisite for beginning to address this issue.

1.6 Concluding comments

Two broad types of inefficiency have been discussed – allocative and technical inefficiency. Allocative inefficiency arises when the wrong mix of services is provided, given societal preferences, or when a suboptimal mix of inputs is used. Allocative inefficiency can occur at the level of the health system, the provider organization or the individual practitioner, and may arise from inadequate priority-setting, faulty payment mechanisms, lack of clinical guidelines, incomplete performance reporting or simply inadequate governance of the system. Technical inefficiency arises most notably at the provider and practitioner level, and may result from inappropriate incentives, weak or constrained management and inadequate information. Either type of inefficiency may have profoundly adverse consequences for payers, whose money is wasted, and for patients, who either receive poor care or are denied treatment because of the associated loss of resources.

This suggests that the simple notion of efficiency as the conversion of inputs into valued outputs disguises a series of thorny conceptual and methodological problems. Setting aside the obvious measurement difficulties, the structural problem can be illustrated as in Figure 1.3, which is a more realistic development of Figure 1.2. Naive efficiency analysis involves examining the ratio of health system outputs to health system inputs (the shaded boxes). Yet system inputs should also incorporate previous investments by the organization (which we call endowments) and external constraints (such as other organizations and population characteristics). System outputs should also include endowments for the future management of the organization, joint outputs and outputs not directly related to health, such as enhanced workforce productivity.

It will never be feasible to accommodate all the issues summarized in Figure 1.3 into a single efficiency metric. Rather, the analyst should be aware of which factors are likely to be material for the efficiency metric under consideration, and seek to offer guidance on the implications of serious omissions and weaknesses. The framework we have introduced seeks to deconstruct efficiency metrics into a manageable number of issues for analytical scrutiny. It is immediately relevant mainly for analysis of TE, although its discussion of external circumstances and broader impact on the health system raises issues relating to AE.

Figure 1.3 *A more complete model of efficiency*

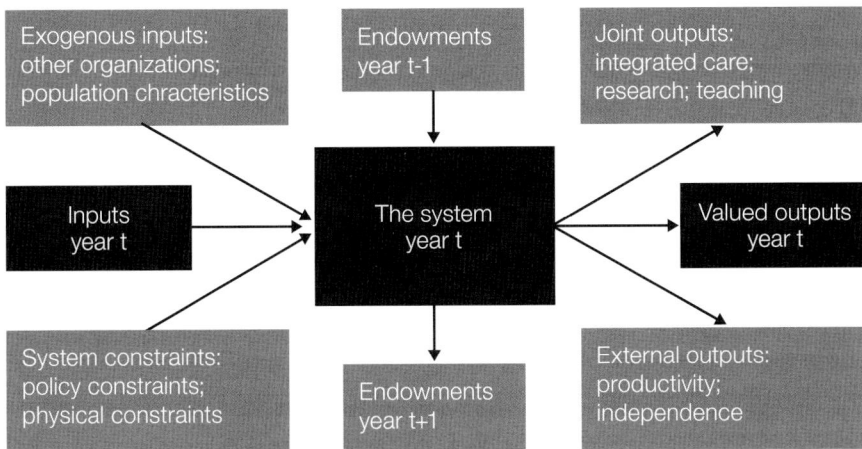

Source: Smith (2009).

The pursuit of health system efficiency is a central concern in all health systems, made strikingly more urgent in many countries by adverse economic circumstances and pressure on public finances. However, measurement methodology is, and will remain, highly contested and is at a developmental stage. Notwithstanding their complexity, the economic concepts of AE and TE offer the only currently available unifying framework for assessing all the diverse objectives of health systems within an efficiency framework. The numerous potential metrics of efficiency all have limitations. However, it is almost certainly preferable to steer the health system with the imperfect measures we have available, rather than to fly blind. In our view, efficiency analysis should be routinely embedded in all relevant functions of service delivery and policymaking. However, it is vital that decisions are taken in full recognition of the strengths and weakness of indicators, and that the search for improved metrics and better resources for comparison is pursued with vigour. The rest of this book offers insights into some of the most promising prospects for future improvement.

References

Briggs A, Gray A (2000). Using cost effectiveness information. *BMJ*, 320(7229):246.

EuroQol Group (1990). EuroQol: a new facility for the measurement of health-related quality of life. *Health Policy*, 16(3):199–208.

Everitt B et al. (2001). *Cluster analysis*. London, Arnold.

Fetter R (1991). Diagnosis related groups: understanding hospital performance. *Interfaces*, 21(1):6–26.

Iezzoni LI (2003). *Risk adjustment for measuring healthcare outcomes*. 3rd edn. Chicago, Health Administration Press.

Jacobs R, Smith P, Street A (2006). *Measuring efficiency in health care: analytic techniques and health policy*. Cambridge, CUP.

Smith PC (2009). Measuring for value for money in health care: concepts and tools. (http://www.health.org.uk/sites/health/files/MeasuringValueForMoneyInHealthcareConceptsAndTools.pdf, accessed 3 August 2016).

Smith PC, Street AD (2013). On the uses of routine patient-reported health outcome data. *Health Economics*, 22(2):119–131.

Ware JE Jr, Sherbourne CD (1992). The MOS 36-item short-form health survey (SF-36). I. Conceptual framework and item selection. *Medical Care*, 30(6):473–483.

WHO (2000). The World Health Report 2000. Health systems: improving performance. Geneva, WHO (http://www.who.int/whr/2000/en/whr00_en.pdf?ua=1, accessed 3 August 2016).

Williams A (1985). Economics of coronary artery bypass grafting. *British Medical Journal*, 291(6491):326–329.

Chapter 2

Measuring and comparing health system outputs: using patient classification systems for efficiency analyses

Wilm Quentin, Alexander Geissler, Reinhard Busse

2.1 Introduction: what are the benefits of classifying patients into groups?

As outlined in Chapter 1, health system efficiency measurement deals with measuring and analysing health system outputs in relation to inputs (or vice versa). While it is complex to quantify and to compare inputs into the health system (see Chapter 4), it is even more difficult to define and appropriately quantify and compare health system outputs. This is the focus of this chapter.

Researchers and practitioners have long struggled with defining an appropriate output measure for health systems, and for health care organizations (for example, hospitals) or other units of analyses (for example, individual physicians). The ultimate aim of health systems is improved population health (WHO, 2000). Consequently, the ideal output measure would be a measure of health improvement (Barer, 1982; Hollingsworth, 2008,). However, because this final output measure is almost never available in routine administrative data sets, efficiency analysis generally has to content itself with measuring other intermediate outputs (Linna, Häkkinen & Magnussen, 2006; Vitikainen, Street & Linna, 2009).

In the 1970s, a group of researchers led by Robert Fetter at Yale University were interested in understanding the outputs or products of hospitals (Fetter, 1991). At the time, hospital output or activity was usually reported on the basis of highly aggregated measures, such as the number of bed days provided and/or the number of discharged patients. However, these measures ignored the differences that existed in the types of patients – or the mix of cases – treated by different providers. Consequently, these measures could not be used for efficiency comparisons in a meaningful way.

At about the same time, hospitals started to routinely collect information on coded diagnoses and patient procedures. However, there were tens of thousands of different diagnoses and procedures. Fetter's basic idea was to condense the confusingly large number of different (individual) patients treated by hospitals into a manageable number of groups (Fetter et al., 1980). On the one hand, the aim was to create groups that should contain patients with similar clinical characteristics (similar diagnoses and procedures) to be medically meaningful. On the other hand, the aim was to group together patients with broadly similar resource consumption in terms of costs to be able to analyse the efficiency of production.

The efforts of Fetter and colleagues led to the development of the first system of diagnosis-related groups (DRGs), which has become the most widely used system for the classification of hospital inpatients (Busse et al., 2011; Fischer, 2000; Kimberly, Pouvourville & d'Aunno, 2008). Figure 2.1 illustrates the basic idea of classifying patients (or more precisely, cases) into DRGs by using a simple example: patients with appendicitis undergoing surgical removal of the appendix (appendectomy). The complexity (and costs) of treating patients undergoing an appendectomy differs depending on

Figure 2.1 *Classification of patients into DRGs: the example of appendectomy patients (based on Nordic DRGs, Estonian version)*

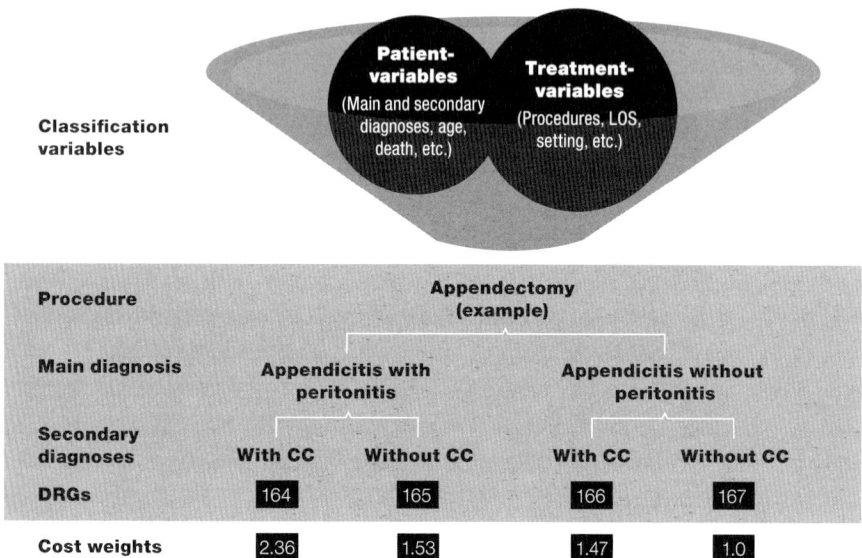

Source: Authors' own compilation based on Quentin et al. (2012).
Note: CC: complications and/or comorbidities; DRG: diagnosis-related group; LOS = length of stay.

whether patients have a generalized inflammation of the intestines (peritonitis) or not, and whether they have additional complications or comorbidities (CCs). Therefore, DRG systems often distinguish between these groups of patients by classifying patients into different DRGs (see Figure 2.1). As a result, each DRG contains patients with similar clinical characteristics and similar costs (Quentin et al., 2011). In addition, each DRG has a specific weight, which is a measure of the average cost of treating patients falling into that DRG.

There are several important benefits of classifying patients into DRGs or – more generally speaking – into groups. First, defining groups of patients reduces complexity and helps to establish a terminology (or common language) for clinicians and managers to think about what a hospital or department is actually doing. This definition of different types of patients or different hospital products is a prerequisite for clinicians and managers to collaborate in the optimization of treatment processes. Second, DRGs (or other groups of patients) can be used by providers and regulators to make comparisons of treatment costs for similar patients, that is, those falling into the same DRG. Third, because each DRG is characterized by a specific cost weight, it is possible to measure total hospital (or departmental) activity while adjusting for differences in resource consumption resulting from differences in the level of complexity of treated patients (cases).

This chapter reviews the use of patient classification systems for measuring and comparing health system outputs with a focus on DRGs. The next section provides further background information on DRG systems in Europe and defines certain terms, such as case mix and case mix adjustment. Subsequently, we present a few simple examples of how DRGs can be used to make comparisons of efficiency across providers. This is followed by a discussion of other patient classification systems that can be used to perform similar analyses for other health care sectors or entire populations. Finally, the conclusion draws together the main benefits of patient classification systems and highlights their limitations.

2.2 DRG systems in Europe: background and definitions

2.2.1 Origins and basic characteristics of different systems

Soon after the development of DRGs by Fetter and colleagues (Fetter, 1991), DRGs became widely used for reporting and payment purposes – first in the USA and later also in Europe. In the USA, Medicare soon realized the potential of DRGs (as definitions of hospital products) for payment purposes, and introduced the first DRG-based hospital payment system in 1983. Since then, DRGs have been adopted in most high-income countries (Paris, Devaux & Wei, 2010), and particularly in Europe (Busse et al., 2011), albeit with different purposes (Geissler et al., 2011).

Most countries use DRGs for hospital payment purposes although they differ both in the share of resources allocated via DRGs and payment method (case payment or budget allocation) (Cots et al., 2011). However, although most countries use a DRG system, these differ considerably across countries, thus complicating international comparisons of hospital outputs on the basis of DRGs. Table 2.1 summarizes some basic characteristics of a selection of DRG systems used in Europe and the USA.

In the USA, Medicare has continuously updated and refined its system, which is now known as the Medicare Severity (MS)-DRG system. France, Germany and the Nordic (Scandinavian) countries have developed national DRG systems based on DRG systems imported from abroad (Kobel et al., 2011). The groupes homogènes de malades (GHM) in France and the Nordic (Nord)-DRGs were

Table 2.1 *Basic characteristics of selected DRG systems used in Europe and the USA*

	AP-DRG (V.25)	APR-DRG (V26.1)	MS-DRG (2012)	AR-DRG (V.7)	G-DRG (2012)	GHM (2012)	HRG	Nord-DRG (2012)
Diagnosis coding	Before 1 October 2015: ICD-9-CM; after: ICD-10-CM			ICD-10-AM	ICD-10-GM	CIM-10	ICD-10	ICD-10
Procedure coding	Before 1 October 2015: ICD-9-CM; after: ICD-10-PCS			ACHI	OPS	CCAM	OPCS	NCSP
Groups	684	956	751	771	1193	2480	1389	798
Major diagnostic categories	27	27	27	25	27	28	23[a]	27
Partitions	2	2	2	3	3	4	2[a]	2
Severity/ complexity levels	3[b]	4/4[c]	3	4	Not limited	5[d]	3	2

Source: Authors' own compilation, partially based on Kobel et al. (2011).

Notes: [a]The HRG system does not define MDCs and partitions per se, but comparable categories exist. [b]Not explicitly mentioned (major CCs at the MDC level plus two levels of severity at the DRG level). [c]Base-DRGs can be split either based on severity of illness or on risk of mortality. [d]Four levels of severity plus one GHM for short stays or outpatient care. ACHI = Australian Classification of Health Interventions; AM = Australian Modification; AP = all-patient; APR = all-patient refined; AR = Australian refined; CCAM = Classification Commune des Actes Médicaux; CIM = Classification Internationale des Maladies, 10th edition; G-DRG = German DRG; GHM = groupe homogène de malades; GM = German modification; HRG = healthcare resource groups; ICD-9-CM = International Classification of Diseases, Ninth Revision, Clinical Modification; ICD-10-AM = International Classification of Diseases, 10th revision, Australian Modification; ICD-10-PCS = ICD-10 Procedure Coding System; MS-DRG = Medicare Severity DRG; NCSP = NOMESCO Classification of Surgical Procedures; NordDRG = Nordic DRG; OPCS = Operation and Procedure Coding System; OPS = Operationen- und Prozedurenschlüssel.

based on an earlier version of the Medicare DRG system. German (G)-DRGs were based on the Australian refined (AR)-DRGs. In addition, the AR-DRGs are used in Ireland and several Balkan countries without refinement. Other countries have developed their own DRG-like systems from scratch. In England, health-care resource groups (HRGs) were originally developed in the 1990s, because available DRG systems did not seem to adequately reflect English health care provision patterns.

Proprietary DRG systems have also been developed since the late 1980s, most notably by 3M Health Information Systems. Proprietary systems include the all-patient (AP)- and all-patient refined (APR)- DRG systems. These systems have been adopted by different institutions in the USA, both for payment purposes and for public quality reporting. In addition, several European countries, including Belgium, Portugal and Spain, have adopted these systems for payment and reporting purposes.

While the overall structure of most DRG systems is similar, there are large differences concerning the number of groups defined by these systems. Therefore, different systems vary in their ability to distinguish between different groups of patients or between different hospital products (Busse, 2012; Fischer, 2000).

In all countries, cases are assigned on the basis of coded information on diagnoses and procedures into a limited number of groups. In the USA, diagnoses and procedures were coded on the basis of the International Classification of Diseases and Related Health Problems, Ninth Revision, clinical modification (ICD-9-CM) until 2015. In Europe, most countries have used a national version of the 10th revision of the ICD (ICD-10) for diagnosis coding and a national system for procedure coding (see Table 2.1).

The number of DRGs ranges from 684 in the AP-DRG system to almost 2500 DRGs in the French GHM system (see Table 2.1). In all DRG systems, cases are first separated into a similar number of major diagnostic categories (MDCs), generally based on the main diagnosis of patients. In addition, all systems define at least two partitions, one for medical and one for surgical cases within each MDC. The AR-DRG and G-DRG systems introduced one additional partition into the classification algorithm to account for relevant procedures that do not need to be performed in an operating theatre.

One important difference across DRG systems is related to the ability of the systems to distinguish between different levels of severity. Many systems have evolved to separate cases into three levels of complications and comorbidities (minor, moderate, major) (see Table 2.1), usually assigning the severity level based on the most complicated secondary diagnosis. However, in the AR-DRG and G-DRG systems, all secondary diagnoses are simultaneously taken into account to compute a patient clinical complexity level (PCCL). The APR-DRG system is special in so far as it assigns each patient both a severity of illness level (reflecting resource intensity) and a risk of mortality level.

The differences in the exact classification process are evident when comparing the classification of patients with similar conditions across countries. For example, most appendectomy patients are classified into only 2 DRGs in the AR-DRG system, while 11 DRGs exist in the G-DRG system for the same patients (Quentin et al., 2011). Similarly, in the HRG system, all stroke patients are classified into only two DRGs, while they are classified into 10 different DRGs in the GHM and the G-DRG system (Peltola & Quentin, 2013).

It is important to be aware of the substantial differences that exist across national DRG systems. They illustrate that DRGs in one country are not the same as DRGs in another country, something that has to be taken into account when comparing outputs across countries (see Section 2.4). In addition, these differences highlight that hospital outputs defined by a national DRG system are only one (of many possible) options for defining hospital outputs. This means that efficiency analyses using one DRG system do not necessarily come to the same conclusion as efficiency analyses using a different DRG system.

2.2.2 Terminology: defining case mix, case mix index and case mix adjustment

Efficiency analyses have to control for relevant differences in the types of cases treated by a provider (for example, a hospital or a department) before making comparisons. The process of controlling for these differences is generally called case mix adjustment.

Case mix has been defined by Fetter (Fetter et al., 1980) as the relative proportions (the mix) of the different types of cases treated by a provider. DRGs make it easy to quantify the case mix of a provider as the DRG weight provides a measure for the complexity (or average cost) of patients in each DRG. In most countries, DRG weights are calculated so that a weight of 1 is equal to the average treatment costs of patients treated by all hospitals (or a subset of hospitals) in the country. Consequently, the average complexity of all cases treated by a specific provider can be measured with the DRG-based case mix index (CMI), which is calculated by summing up all DRG weights produced by a provider in a given period of time and dividing it by the number of treated cases. A hospital with a CMI <1 treats patients that are (on average) less complex than patients in other hospitals, while a hospital with a CMI >1 treats patients that are more complex than average.

The concept of case mix adjustment is closely related to the concept of risk adjustment; in fact, these terms are often used interchangeably (Iezzoni, 2009). Yet, there is a slight difference in their connotation: case mix adjustment implies a focus on the provider and on the relative proportions of different kinds of cases treated by that provider. By contrast, the term risk adjustment implies a shift in focus towards the distribution of risks in the underlying patient population.

Case mix adjustment can be used for different purposes (Hornbrook, 1982) and – depending on the specific purpose – it has to adjust for different factors. For example, when measuring and comparing efficiency or costs per case, case mix adjustment has to adjust for the differences in the risk of each provider's patient population requiring treatment that is less or more costly than average. This is what DRGs usually do because they are designed to group together patients (or cases) with similar costs. However, when measuring and comparing surgical mortality, case mix adjustment has to adjust for the differences in the risk of each provider's patient population having higher or lower mortality than average. While some DRG systems have been specifically developed to adjust for the risk of mortality (for example, the APR-DRG system), most systems are not made to do so.

2.3 Application of DRGs: indicators of efficiency

Several useful indicators of efficiency have been developed on the basis of DRGs. These allow assessments of hospital efficiency at different levels. First, DRGs can be used by regulators or purchasers at the macro level to compare total hospital costs per case, while adjusting for case mix. Second, DRGs can be used at the meso level to compare actual costs per DRG across different hospitals. Third, hospital managers can use DRGs at the micro level to compare their own cost structure against average costs of treatment in other hospitals or to identify those patients that have exceptionally high costs.

2.3.1 Macro level analyses: Measuring and comparing hospital costs per case

Table 2.2 shows how case mix-adjusted comparisons of average costs per case can be performed across a sample of hospitals. The table is based on an extract of Swiss hospital statistics for 20 hospitals located in the Canton of Zürich as reported by the Swiss Federal Office of Public Health (FOPH, 2014). The statistics include the total number of cases, total hospital costs and the CMI. When calculating costs per case without case mix adjustment (column 4), costs range from about CHF8000 in hospital 11, a relatively small municipal hospital, to about CHF20 700 in hospital 20, the University Hospital of Zürich.

Table 2.2 *Average costs per case (CHF) in 20 hospitals in the Canton of Zürich,* with *and without Swiss DRG-based case mix adjustment*

Hospital	Cases	Total costs	Costs per case	Rank	CMI	Case mix-adjusted costs per case	Case mix-adjusted rank
Hospital 1	9530	87 180 240	9148	18	0.83	11 040	15
Hospital 2	22 822	246 280 669	10 791	11	0.99	10 932	16
Hospital 3	7006	124 905 589	17 828	2	1.64	10 861	17
Hospital 4	15 151	255 497 225	16 863	3	1.21	13 947	3
Hospital 5	7294	113 805 086	15 603	4	1.20	13 002	7
Hospital 6	1541	15 216 743	9875	14	0.71	13 973	2
Hospital 7	1587	16 111 438	10 152	13	0.67	15 147	1
Hospital 8	3585	44 937 552	12 535	9	0.92	13 559	5
Hospital 9	7479	114 356 698	15 290	5	1.36	11 240	12
Hospital 10	10 091	98 605 272	9772	15	0.87	11 232	13
Hospital 11	3555	28 330 639	7969	20	0.76	10 508	18
Hospital 12	8879	84 771 197	9547	16	0.82	11 623	11
Hospital 13	9357	84 421 363	9022	19	0.86	10 506	19
Hospital 14	6863	72 103 253	10 506	12	0.83	12 586	8
Hospital 15	9550	88 431 583	9260	17	0.83	11 123	14
Hospital 16	7945	90 983 088	11 452	10	0.84	13 568	4
Hospital 17	19 732	268 798 867	13 622	7	1.11	12 260	9
Hospital 18	8767	111 660 180	12 736	8	1.06	11 962	10
Hospital 19	4711	65 063 193	13 811	6	1.37	10 064	20
Hospital 20	34 523	715 807 133	20 734	1	1.57	13 224	6

Source: Authors' own compilation based on FOPH (2014).
Note: CMI = case mix index; DRG = diagnosis-related group.

The CMI calculated on the basis of the Swiss DRGs in column 6 shows that hospitals treat very different types of patients. Not surprisingly, the Children's University Hospital (hospital 3), the University Hospital of Zürich (hospital 20) and the Orthopaedic University Hospital Balgrist (hospital 19) have the highest CMIs, indicating that these hospitals treat patients that are on average more complex than in other hospitals. By contrast, hospital 7, a small private hospital focused on complementary and alternative medicine (CAM) has the lowest CMI, while hospital 11 (the one with the lowest costs per case) has a relatively low CMI.

Dividing costs per case by the CMI provides the case mix-adjusted costs per case (second to last column). These are the costs that each hospital would have if it had a CMI of 1, that is, if it had an average patient case mix. (Another way of thinking about this is that these are the costs that the hospital needs for the production of 1 DRG weight.) After case mix adjustment, costs per case range from about CHF 10 000 to about CHF 15 000 and the ranking of hospitals in Table 2.2 changes considerably. For example, hospital 19 (the Orthopaedic University Hospital Balgrist) now has the lowest costs per case, while hospital 7 (the private CAM hospital) has the highest costs per case.

It is possible that certain patient characteristics are not appropriately accounted for by DRGs. For example, one hospital may have a larger proportion of more complex cases within each DRG. Therefore, even after case mix adjustment, comparisons of costs per case might not be entirely fair, and the exact position in the ranking could change because of random variation. Nevertheless, if hospitals have case mix-adjusted costs per case that are several thousand CHF higher than in other hospitals, there is likely to be room for improvement in efficiency.

2.3.2 Meso level analyses: measuring and comparing costs across hospitals for patients with certain diseases

As DRGs provide a definition for hospital products, the most straightforward DRG-based indicator of efficiency is that of average costs per DRG. Table 2.3 shows the average costs of patients in the most important acute myocardial infarction (AMI) DRGs of seven German hospitals (each treating more than 400 AMI patients per year). Average costs across all hospitals (last column) vary considerably depending on the DRG. Patients in F24B – AMI with percutaneous coronary intervention (PCI), treated with more than one stent and with a PCCL >3 – have the highest average costs (€6348), while patients in F60B – AMI treated without relevant procedures and with a PCCL <4 – have the lowest costs (€1993).

Each DRG contains a relatively narrowly defined group of patients. Yet, random variation may still lead to considerable variation of average costs per DRG if the number of patients per DRG is small. Therefore, cells containing <20 patients are left blank in the table and the number of patients treated in each DRG per hospital is indicated in brackets.

A comparison of the average costs per DRG across hospitals is useful because it can lead to questions about care processes in hospitals. For example, when looking at Table 2.3, it might be worth investigating why patients in G-DRG F24C in hospital 3 have on average costs that are more than €1300 above those of patients in hospital 8. If this kind of information is available, every hospital can identify those DRGs, where it has costs that are above the average of costs in other hospitals, and this can motivate efforts to optimize treatment processes.

Table 2.3 *Average costs (€) of patients with AMI classified into different G-DRGs in a sample of German hospitals, 2008*

G-DRG	Average costs in € (number of cases)							Average
	Hospital 1	Hospital 2	Hospital 3	Hospital 4	Hospital 5	Hospital 6	Hospital 7	
F24B	4835		9192	4166	6446			6348
	(33)		(38)	(26)	(31)			(143)
F24C	3346	4216	5253	3420	4713	5025	3897	4342
	(76)	(112)	(226)	(66)	(36)	(44)	(222)	(782)
F41A					4882			4350
					(27)			(72)
F41B	1811	3333	2155	1924	2892	2735	1602	2372
	(93)	(73)	(25)	(51)	(56)	(94)	(69)	(461)
F52A	4200	4942	5692	3622	5070			4789
	(49)	(42)	(38)	(75)	(92)			(326)
F52B	3127	3510	3368	2428	3753	4649	2952	3304
	(159)	(293)	(175)	(106)	(108)	(84)	(319)	(1244)
F60A	3060	3505		2173	4437	3744		3396
	(46)	(25)		(42)	(55)	(42)		(218)
F60B	1705	1792		1166	2117	2346	2178	1993
	(43)	(49)		(31)	(27)	(126)	(26)	(314)
Average	3159	3862	4884	3039	4328	3667	3313	3581
	(526)	(628)	(532)	(425)	(437)	(419)	(682)	(3560)

Source: Authors' own compilation based on EuroDRG research database.
Notes: Cells that would contain average costs of <20 cases have been left empty. AMI = acute myocardial infarction; G-DRG = German diagnosis-related group.

However, it is important to keep in mind that some differences in costs per DRG are justified, for example, if one hospital provides higher quality of care or has to ensure treatment availability in a relatively sparsely populated area. In addition, several studies have indicated that certain patient (for example, age, number of diagnoses), treatment (for example, number of procedures) and hospital characteristics (for example, available infrastructure or teaching status) beyond those considered by DRGs have an influence on hospital resource use (Busse, 2012; Mason, Street & Verzulli, 2010; Mason et al., 2012). Therefore, simple comparisons of costs per case have their limitations.

It is possible to conduct more complex regression-based analyses, taking into account additional patient and treatment level variables besides DRGs to control for these factors. Figure 2.2 shows an example of such an analysis, where unexplained variance in costs across English hospitals is shown after having controlled for HRGs and additional patient and treatment characteristics of patients undergoing hip replacement. As indicated by the relatively narrow confidence intervals (CIs), differences in costs across hospitals are significant also after controlling for these variables.

Figure 2.2 *Unexplained variance in cost of English hospitals treating hip replacement patients after controlling for HRGs and additional patient and treatment characteristics*

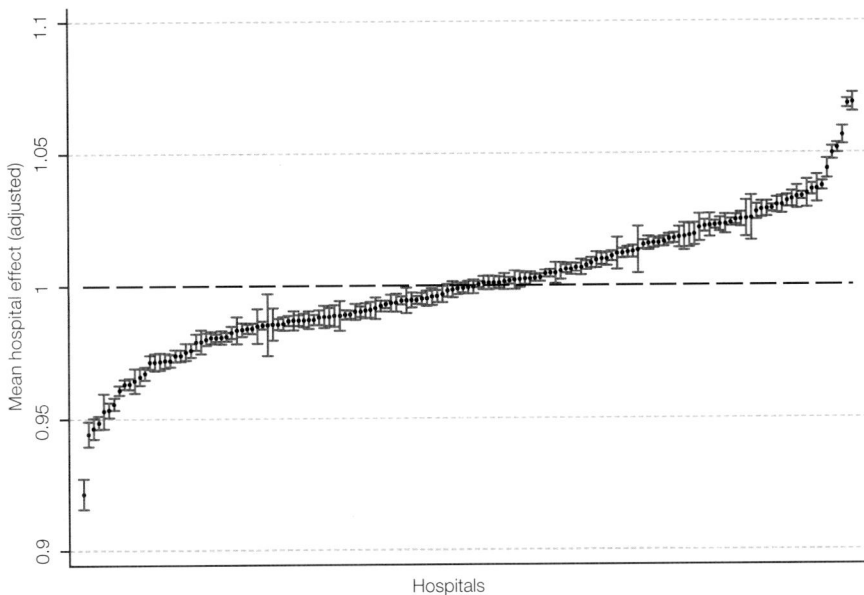

Source: Geissler, Scheller-Kreinsen & Quentin (2012).
Note: HRG = health care resource group.

2.3.3 *Micro level analyses: DRG-based comparisons of cost structures*

A more detailed DRG-based analysis of cost structures is necessary if the aim is to identify reasons for higher costs of treatment in individual hospitals. However, a prerequisite of such an analysis is that a high-quality cost accounting system is in place (see Chapter 4). In Germany, the annual update of DRG weights is based on cost data collected in a sample of about 250 hospitals that apply a standardized patient-level cost accounting system developed by the Institute for the Hospital Remuneration System (InEK) (InEK, 2014a).

Aggregated cost data broken down into individual DRGs is published by InEK and publicly available for download free of charge (see http://www.g-drg.de/cms/).

Table 2.4 shows an extract of this data for G-DRG I47B: revision or replacement of hip joint without complicating diagnosis, arthrodesis or very major CC (age >15 years). Cost data are broken down by cost elements (labour, materials, and infrastructure) and cost centres (normal ward, operating theatre and radiology). Each cell in the table shows the average treatment costs of patients falling into I47B for a specific cost element and cost centre. For example, the labour costs of physicians working on a normal ward for patients in I47B were €345.04.

Each hospital can compare its own cost structures with the national average if it follows the standard costing methodology published by InEK (InEK, 2007). Table 2.5 shows the difference in treatment cost of patients in G-DRG I47B in one German hospital compared with national average costs. Cost centres and cost elements, where the hospital has higher costs than the national average are highlighted in red. Total treatment costs per patient in G-DRG I47B are on average €553.72 above the German average. Most importantly, the hospital has on average €448.88 higher physician labour costs than the German average, because costs are higher in both normal ward and operating theatre.

Another useful DRG-based micro level analysis that can help to identify reasons for high costs is that of the distribution of costs of individual patients grouped into each DRG. As DRGs group together patients with similar costs, the costs of most patients should follow a normal distribution and only few cases should have costs that fall outside the normal ranges. These cases can then be analysed in more detail to identify (potentially modifiable) reasons for higher costs. Again, this type of analysis is possible only if the hospital's cost accounting system allows the calculation of costs at the level of individual patients.

Figure 2.3 shows the distribution of costs for 319 patients grouped into G-DRG F52B – AMI treated with PCI (0/1 stents) and PCCL <4 – treated in one German hospital. It shows that 96% of cases had costs below €5000. However, 4% of cases had higher costs and the most expensive patient had costs of €8248. Unfortunately, we do not have the full histories of these patients to identify the reasons why they had higher costs. However, some reasons can be ruled out because they would have led to the classification of patients into different DRGs. For example, if patients had required treatment on an intensive care unit (ICU) or multiple coronary interventions, these would have led to the classification into different DRGs.

Table 2.4 *Average hospital cost of DRG I47B in cost data sample of InEK*

German DRG catalogue — I47B — Revision or replacement of hip joint without complicating diagnosis, arthrodesis or major CC (age >15 years)

Cost-centre groups	Labour 1: Physicians	Labour 2: Nursing	Labour 3: Medical/technical staff	Material 4a: General drugs	Material 4b: Individual drugs	Material 5: Implants and grafts	Material 6a: Material (without drugs, implants and grafts)	Material 6b: Individual material (actual consumption, without drugs, implants/grafts)	Infrastructure 7: Medical infrastructure	Infrastructure 8: Non-medical infrastructure	Total
Units with beds											
1: Normal ward	345.04	863.19	46.95	75.72	4.87	–	72.41	7.16	171.25	806.71	2393.30
2: Intensive care unit	35.53	94.54	6.07	12.60	0.61	0.00	15.93	0.71	11.22	44.36	221.56
3: Dialysis unit	0.00	0.00	0.00	0.00	0.00	–	0.00	0.00	0.00	0.00	0.00
Diagnostics and treatments											
4: Operating theatre	351.15	–	224.70	15.86	6.36	1363.53	174.88	62.48	136.39	205.65	2541.01
5: Anaesthesia	204.47	–	130.68	18.55	0.63	–	47.91	1.80	24.18	67.11	495.32
6: Maternity room	0.00	–	0.00	0.00	0.00	–	0.00	0.00	0.00	0.00	0.00
7: Cardiac diagnostics/therapy	0.17	–	0.16	0.00	0.00	0.03	0.04	0.06	0.03	0.09	0.58
8: Endoscopic diagnostics/therapy	0.43	–	0.53	0.02	0.00	0.00	0.19	0.01	0.19	0.36	1.74
9: Radiology	17.41	–	35.12	0.45	0.02	0.01	8.49	13.89	10.07	24.99	110.45
10: Laboratories	5.81	–	44.89	3.18	40.38	0.00	33.63	20.79	4.65	21.14	174.47
11: Other diagnostics and therapies	16.42	2.06	150.58	1.85	0.01	0.01	10.82	7.40	7.15	68.31	264.60
Total	976.43	959.79	639.68	128.23	52.88	1363.58	364.30	114.30	365.13	1238.72	**6203.03**

Source: Authors' own compilation based on InEK (2010).
Note: CC = complications and/or comorbidities; DRG = diagnosis-related group.

Table 2.5 *Difference between an individual hospital's costs for G-DRG I47B and national average costs in €*

German DRG catalogue I47B		Revision or replacement of hip joint without complicating diagnosis, arthrodesis or major CC (age >15 years)	Labour			Material					Infrastructure		Total
Cost-centre groups			1 Physicians	2 Nursing	3 Medical/technical staff	4a General drugs	4b Individual drugs	5 Implants and grafts	6a Material (without drugs, implants and grafts)	6b Individual material (actual consumption, without drugs, implants/grafts)	7 Medical infrastructure	8 Non-medical infrastructure	
Units with beds	1: Normal ward		189.89	163.23	−1.04	−2.16	−4.87	–	−11.81	−1.99	−4.39	28.84	355.71
	2: Intensive care unit		5.42	16.73	−5.95	−7.45	−0.61	0.00	−9.47	−0.68	−6.88	−14.82	−23.71
	3: Dialysis unit		0.40	1.79	0.00	0.56	0.00	–	1.54	0.00	0.30	0.57	5.16
Diagnostics and treatments	4: Operating theatre		217.45	–	45.38	−2.26	−3.43	−3.73	−9.91	−39.58	−1.47	−10.52	191.92
	5: Anaesthesia		31.84	–	12.35	0.70	−0.48	–	7.88	−1.55	0.24	2.30	53.28
	6: Maternity room		0.00	–	0.00	0.00	0.00	–	0.00	0.00	0.00	0.00	0.00
	7: Cardiac diagnostics/therapy		0.60	–	−0.16	0.00	0.00	−0.03	−0.04	−0.06	−0.03	−0.09	0.19
	8: Endoscopic diagnostics/therapy		−0.34	–	−0.41	−0.01	0.00	0.00	−0.15	−0.01	−0.11	−0.30	−1.34
	9: Radiology		2.06	–	11.89	−0.35	0.05	0.00	−2.96	−0.01	−1.01	12.05	21.71
	10: Laboratories		0.75	–	−22.68	1.18	19.67	0.00	−14.48	42.05	−3.17	−11.09	12.23
	11: Other diagnostics and therapies		0.81	−2.05	3.36	−1.58	−0.01	−0.01	−7.37	1.29	3.73	−59.62	−61.44
Total			448.88	179.70	42.73	−11.36	10.31	−3.77	−46.78	−0.55	−12.78	−52.67	553.72

Source: Authors' own compilation based on the EuroDRG research database.

Note: CC = complications and/or comorbidities; DRG = diagnosis-related group.

Figure 2.3 *Distribution of costs for 319 Patients in G-DRG F52B in one German hospital*

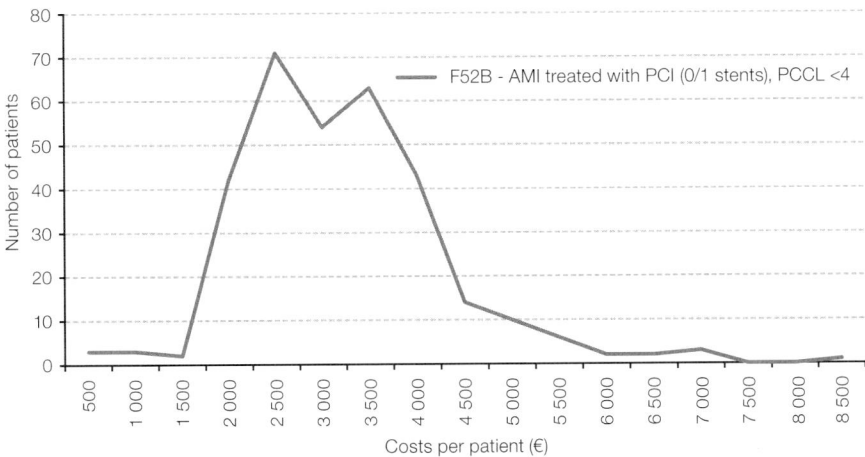

Source: Authors' own compilation based on the EuroDRG research database.
Note: G-DRG = German diagnosis-related group.

2.4 Patient classification systems for other areas of health care

In principle, any of the efficiency assessments shown for hospitals could be replicated (with the necessary adjustments) for other sectors using a classification system that has been developed for the sector, and the same is also possible for entire populations. Three countries that have systematically expanded the concept of patient classification (or case mix measurement) to almost all areas of health care are Australia, Canada and the USA. Table 2.6 provides an overview of the different patient classification systems used in these countries for different health care sectors.

All three countries have developed patient classification systems for most of the sectors shown in Table 2.6. Australia has developed one patient classification system for all subacute and non-acute care (AN-SNAP), applying to all patients receiving palliative care, rehabilitation and long-term or home care. Classification systems for psychiatric inpatient care are comparatively less developed. In Australia, a classification system is currently under development. In Canada, the System for Classification of In-Patient Psychiatry is currently used only for reporting purposes in the province of Ontario. In the USA, the MS-DRG system developed for acute inpatient care is used also for the classification of inpatient care days in psychiatric facilities.

Table 2.6 *Patient classification systems for different health care sectors in Australia, Canada and the USA*

	Australia	Canada	USA
Acute inpatient care	AR-DRG	CMG+[a]	MS-DRG
Acute outpatient care	Non-admitted care classification (under development)	CACS and DPG	APC
	URG		
Rehabilitation	AN-SNAP. Includes palliative care, rehabilitation, and long-term and psychogeriatric care	RPG	CMG
Long-term care (skilled nursing)		RUG-III	RUG-III
Psychiatric inpatient care	AMHCC (under development)	SCIPP, only in Ontario	MS-DRGs
Home care	AN-SNAP	RUG-III/HC	HHRG
Populations	–	–	CMS-HCC

Source: Authors' own compilation.
Notes: [a]CMG+ is a refined version of CMGs that accounts for additional factors affecting resource consumption. AMHCC = Australian mental health care classification; AN-SNAP = Australian subacute and non-acute care; APC = ambulatory payment classification; AR-DRG = Australian refined diagnosis-related group; CACS = comprehensive ambulatory classification system; CMG = case mix group; CMS = Centers for Medicare & Medicaid Services; DPG = day procedure group; HC = home care; HCC = hierarchical condition category; HHRG = home health resource group; MS-DRG = Medicare Severity DRG; RPG = rehabilitation patient group; RUG-III = resource utilization groups version III; SCIPP = System for Classification of Inpatient Psychiatry; URG = urgency-related group.

Some patient classification systems are developed by international networks. The most important such collaboration is the interRAI network, which has developed patient classification systems for long-term care facilities, home care and mental care. The Resource Utilization Group III (RUG-III) system developed by interRAI is used for long-term care facilities in Canada and the USA, and also in several European countries (OECD, 2013). Because the system is used in several countries, it can be used for cross-country analyses. The home care version of RUG-III (RUG-III/HC) is used only in Canada.

The concept of patient classification has also been expanded to entire populations. Instead of classifying patients, these systems classify the general population or a subset of the population into groups that are medically and economically homogeneous. In the USA, the Centres for Medicare and Medicaid Services (CMS) use the hierarchical condition category (HCC) system to adjust capitation payments to insurance plans providing coverage for older people opting for so-called Medicare advantage plans. Similarly, several European countries have developed population classification systems for risk-adjusted resource allocation purposes.

The following sections provide more details about different patient classification systems and highlight some of the differences across countries, which have to be taken into account in efficiency analyses.

2.4.1 Classification systems for patients treated by rehabilitation facilities

Several countries in Europe are working on developing patient classification systems for rehabilitation care (Kobel et al., 2011). Table 2.7 provides an overview to classification systems for rehabilitation care used in Australia, Canada, France and the USA. In Australia, Canada and the USA, classification systems were introduced slightly before or after the year 2000. In France, a classification system was introduced relatively recently in 2013.

Some systems are used only for the classification of inpatient stays, while others also include day cases and outpatients. Just as for acute care hospitals, the unit of analysis for all of these systems is a specified episode of care, for which similar resource use patterns can be identified.

The number of groups of different systems varies between 60 in Australia and 685 in France. In all countries, the principal diagnosis, that is, the diagnosis requiring rehabilitation, is used as a classification variable. As resource use in rehabilitation care depends strongly on the functional and cognitive status of patients, all systems also make use of these variables for the classification of patients into groups. Functional and cognitive status is assessed in Australia, Canada and the USA on the basis of the same instrument, that is, the functional independence measure (FIM). Only France uses a different instrument to determine the functional and cognitive status of patients. Unlike in acute care hospitals, where procedures always play an important role for the classification of patients, procedures are used only in France as classification variables for rehabilitation care.

In Australia, France and the USA, the systems have been primarily developed for payment purposes. However, they are also used with the purpose of improving transparency, for example, by comparing length of stay for similar groups of patients across providers (Meyer et al., 2012). In Canada, the main purpose of using rehabilitation patient groups (RPGs) is to facilitate the review of resource use by providers. The Canadian Institute for Health Information (CIHI) regularly produces resource use reports comparing resource use by RPGs at different providers (CIHI, 2011). In Australia, average length of stay by AN-SNAP category is published by the Independent Hospital Pricing Authority (IHPA), and rehabilitation facilities can benchmark themselves against the national averages (IHPA, 2014).

Efficiency measurement in rehabilitation care could potentially benefit considerably from the availability of FIM scores at admission and discharge in several routine databases, as these scores provide a meaningful measure for health improvement. Consequently, average health improvement can be compared for each case mix group across providers in relation to resource use (length of stay or costs) at different providers (Amatya & Khan, 2011).

Table 2.7 *Classification systems for rehabilitation facilities in selected countries*

System	Country	Year when introduced	Based on	Classification of	Number of groups	Classification variables	Principal purpose and use
AN-SNAP	Australia (also adopted by New Zealand)	1999	FIM	Inpatient stays, day cases, outpatients for other areas of care	60 classes for rehabilitation (45 inpatient, 3 day case, 12 outpatient), further classes	• Diagnosis requiring rehabilitation; • Cognitive status; • Functional status (based on FIM); • Age.	Payment (depends on region); transparency
RPG	Canada	2000	FIM	Inpatient stays	83 RPGs	• Diagnosis requiring rehabilitation; • Cognitive status (based on FIM); • Functional status (based on FIM); • Age.	Transparency (resource use review)
GME	France	2013	GHJ	Inpatient stays, day cases	685	• (Principal) diagnosis requiring rehabilitation; • Cognitive status; • Functional status; • Post-surgery indicator; • Medical and rehabilitation procedures; • Age; • Secondary diagnoses (comorbidities); • Day case status.	Payment (planned for 2016); transparency
CMG	USA (Medicare)	2002	FIM-FRG	Inpatient stays	92 CMGs	• Diagnosis requiring rehabilitation; • Cognitive status (based on FIM); • Functional status (based on FIM); • Age; • Comorbidities.	(IRF PPS)

Source: Authors' own compilation based on AHSRI (2012), CIHI (2011), MedPAC (2014a) and Ministère des Affaires sociales, de la Santé et des Droits des femmes (2015).

Note: AN-SNAP = Australian national subacute and non-acute patient classification; CMG = case mix group; FIM = functional independence measure; FIM-FRG = functional independence measure-functional related groups; GHJ = groupe homogène de journées; GME = groupe médico-économique; IRF PPS = inpatient rehabilitation facility prospective payment system; RPG = rehabilitation patient group.

2.4.2 Classification systems for psychiatric patients

Classification systems for psychiatric patients have been developed relatively recently and are still under development in several countries (Kobel et al., 2011). Table 2.8 shows an overview of patient classification systems used for psychiatric patients in a selection of countries. In Canada and the USA, classification systems were introduced in 2005. In Germany and England, they were introduced only in 2013. In Canada, a new classification system was developed for psychiatric patients on the basis of the interRAI Mental Health Assessment System, which is an instrument for evaluating the needs of adults with mental illnesses. In the USA, the MS-DRG system originally developed for acute care hospitals has simply been transferred to psychiatric hospitals, where it has been used since 2005 for adjusting per diem payments to providers.

In fact, compared with classification systems for acute or rehabilitation care, this is an important difference of classification systems for psychiatric patients. The unit of analysis of psychiatric patient classification systems is usually the (inpatient) care day, that is, the classification of patients does not lead to groups of patients with similar costs per stay but to groups of patients with similar costs per day. The reason for this is that the required length of stay of psychiatric patients is difficult to predict on the basis of diagnoses or other routinely available data (Cotterill & Thomas, 2004). Nevertheless, psychiatric patient classification systems allow comparisons of case mix across providers and enable case mix-adjusted assessments of costs per care day.

There are considerable differences in the classification systems of the four countries shown in Table 2.8. In the Canadian and English systems, it is possible to reclassify a patient into a different group after reassessment, if the clinical condition has changed over time. In England, a patient's mental health care cluster (MHCC) determines the time period after which a reassessment (and possible reclassification) becomes necessary, and the classification is independent of the setting where a patient is treated. In Germany and the USA, a patient is assigned to only one group for the duration of the entire stay in a psychiatric hospital. The number of groups varies between 21 in England and 77 in Germany. In addition, countries make numerous adjustments. In Canada, the 49 SCIPP groups are subdivided into admission, post-admission and long-term phases with different weights attached to each phase. In Germany, supplementary per diem payments exist for days or weeks with high-intensity care. In the USA, payments are adjusted for facility characteristics. Efficiency analyses should also take into account these adjustments because comparisons would otherwise be unfair. Classification variables vary considerably across countries. While Canada and England use variables that are related to patient functioning and patient needs, Germany and the USA place more emphasis on

Table 2.8 *Classification systems for patients treated by (inpatient) psychiatric care providers in selected countries*

System	Country	Year when introduced	Based on	Classification of	Number of groups	Classification variables	Principal purpose and use
SCIPP	Canada (Ontario)	2005	interRAI Mental Health Assessment System	Inpatient care days (acute, long-stay, forensic and geriatric); reclassification possible after reassessment	49 SCIPP groups (with episodes subdivided into admission, post-admission and long-term phase after 731 days)	• Primary and secondary diagnoses; • Mental and physical symptoms; • Social functioning; • Cognitive functioning; • Physical functioning; • Substance abuse; • Short-stay status; • Unemployed status; • Behaviours (harm to self and others).	Inpatient reporting; planned use for inpatient funding
MHCC	United Kingdom (England)	2013	HoNOS	Care days (which may include inpatient, outpatient and/or community-based care) + care periods (for fixed periods of time, varying by cluster); reclassification possible after reassessment	21 MHCC	• Severity; • Clinical need; • Non-clinical need; • All assessed via modified HoNOS instrument.	Purchasing; planned use for funding
PEPP	Germany	2013 (optional) 2017 (mandatory)	–	Inpatient (and semi-residential) care days, one PEPP per stay	77 PEPP (39 inpatient PEPP with weight, 18 inpatient PEPP without weight, 6 semi-residential PEPP with weight, 14 semi-residential PEPP without weight + supplementary payments for pharmaceuticals + supplementary payments per diem payments for high-intensity care)	• Type of stay (inpatient versus semi-residential); • Type of provider (child versus adult, psychiatric versus psychosomatic); • Diagnoses (primary and secondary); • Procedures (including codes for therapeutic interventions, intensity of care); • Age.	Provider payment (budget-neutral introduction for all hospitals in 2017)
MS-DRGs	USA (Medicare)	2005	CMS-DRGs	Inpatient care days, one MS-DRG per stay	17 DRGs + 17 comorbidity adjusters + electroconvulsive therapy adjuster + facility-based adjusters + degressive LOS adjusters	• Diagnoses • Procedures • Age	Provider payment (IPF PPS)

Source: Authors' own compilation based on DoH (2013), InEK (2014b), InEK (2014c), Mason & Goddard (2009), MedPAC (2014b), Monitor (2013), Ontario JPPC (2008), Perlman et al. (2013).
Note: CMS = case mix group; DRG = diagnosis-related group; HoNOS = Health of the Nation Outcome Scales; IPF PPS = inpatient psychiatric facility prospective payment system; LOS = length of stay; MHCC = mental health care clusters; MS-DRG = Medicare Severity diagnosis-related group; PEPP = Pauschalierendes Entgeltsystem Psychiatrie Psychosomatik; SCIPP = System for Classification of In-Patient Psychiatry.

diagnoses and procedures. In Germany, procedure codes capture the intensity of psychiatric care provided to patients, including the number of therapeutic sessions per week.

2.4.3 Classification systems for populations

Most countries with mandatory health insurance and competing health insurers have developed risk adjustment systems to allocate capitation payments to insurers. However, they can also be used for conducting case mix-adjusted efficiency analyses of all care provided to different populations. Table 2.9 provides an overview of the classification systems used for populations in Germany, the Netherlands and the USA, as well as the proprietary adjusted clinical group (ACG) system. A predecessor system of the ACGs had been developed in the 1980s as ambulatory care groups with the aim of facilitating utilization review and defining capitation-based reimbursement (Starfield et al., 1991). However, most of the population classification systems have been introduced only since the year 2000.

All systems shown in Table 2.9 classify the population into morbidity groups on the basis of diagnoses or pharmaceutical consumption in addition to considering certain demographic characteristics. In contrast to the patient classification systems for particular sectors, most population classification systems define groups that are cumulative. This means that multimorbidity is taken into account by classifying people into several groups (one for each type of morbidity) and the cost weights of each group are added up to calculate the total predicted costs of an individual. The ACG system is the only system that uses a different approach and classifies people into groups that are intended to account for the total morbidity of an individual patient.

Population classification systems can be used to calculate the CMI of entire populations by adding up the cost weights for covered individuals. This enables comparisons of the case mix-adjusted costs of coverage provided by different insurers or of the case mix-adjusted costs of treatment provided by networks of providers (for example, health maintenance organizations or accountable care organizations).

Figure 2.4 illustrates the importance of using an appropriate population classification system when making such comparisons to avoid organizations with a larger proportion of sick individuals being systematically disadvantaged in the comparison. The figure shows the predicted costs of German sickness funds in 2009 and 2013 in relation to actual expenditure in the same year. Predicted costs were calculated according to three different methods: 1) the old demographic risk adjustment model; 2) the HMG-RSA morbidity model of the year 2009;

Table 2.9 *Classification systems for populations in a selection of countries*

System	Country	Year when introduced	Based on	Classification of	Number of groups	Classification variables	Principal purpose and use
HMG of the RSA	Germany	2009	DCG/HCC	SHI-insured	V2015: 189 HMGs + Demographic adjustment + disability adjustment + residency abroad adjustment + sick pay adjustment. Grouping is cumulative (people can be grouped into several HMGs)	• Ambulatory and inpatient diagnoses; • Age; • Sex; • Disability (unable to work); • Residency abroad; • Sick pay status.	Capitation payments to sickness funds
PCG / DCG	Netherlands	2002 (PCGs), 2004 (DCGs)	CDS	People resident in the Netherlands	20 PCGs, + 13 DCGs, + demographic adjustment + nature of income + regional adjustment + socioeconomic status. Grouping is cumulative (people can be grouped into several DCGs/PCGs)	• Inpatient diagnoses; • Pharmaceutical consumption; • Age; • Sex; • Income type (social benefits); • Region; • Income; • Family size.	Capitation payments to insurance funds
CMS-HCC	USA (Medicare)	2004	DCG	Medicare Advantage enrollees	V2014: 79 HCCs + demographic adjustment + disability adjustment + Medicaid dual eligibility adjustment. Grouping is cumulative (people can be grouped into several HCCs)	• Ambulatory and inpatient diagnoses; • Age; • Sex; • Disability status; • Medicaid dual eligibility status.	Capitation payments to private insurance plans
ACG and various systems derived from it	Proprietary (Johns Hopkins), used in different countries/ settings at different times	Introduced in different countries/ settings at different times	Ambulatory care groups	Covered population	102 ACGs	• All diagnoses (ambulatory, inpatient, other) + additional variables depending on application, for example, for Dx-PM: ○ age; ○ sex; ○ complicated pregnancy; ○ pharmacy use; ○ hospital condition; ○ selected medical condition.	Population profiling; provider profiling; resource allocation

Source: Bundesversicherungsamt (BVA) (2014), MedPAC (2014c), Penno, Gauld & Audas (2013), Starfield & Kinder (2011), VWS (2011).

Note: ACG = adjusted clinical group; CDS = Chronic Disease Score; CMS = case mix group; DCG = diagnostic cost group; Dx-PM = diagnosis-based predictive model; HCC = Hierarchical Condition Category; HMG = Hierarchisierte Morbiditätsgruppen; PCG = pharmacy cost group; RSA = Risikostrukturausgleich; SHI = statutory health insurance.

and 3) the HMG-RSA morbidity model of the year 2013. The CMI of sickness funds (x-axis) is calculated based on the new model. Dots for individual sickness funds found at the same level of CMI provide coverage to populations with a similar average burden of morbidity. Differences in the expenditures of funds that have the same CMI levels cannot be explained by the diseases that are taken into account by the classification system, and must therefore be because of other reasons; these could include unaccounted differences in morbidity, or differences in efficiency. For example, one might consider that funds above the predicted lines in Figure 2.4 may be comparatively more efficient than the average fund, since they secure costs below the predicted values at given levels of case mix severity.

Figure 2.4 *Predicted costs of German sickness funds in relation to expenditure (predictive ratio) by CMI of funds, 2009 and 2013*

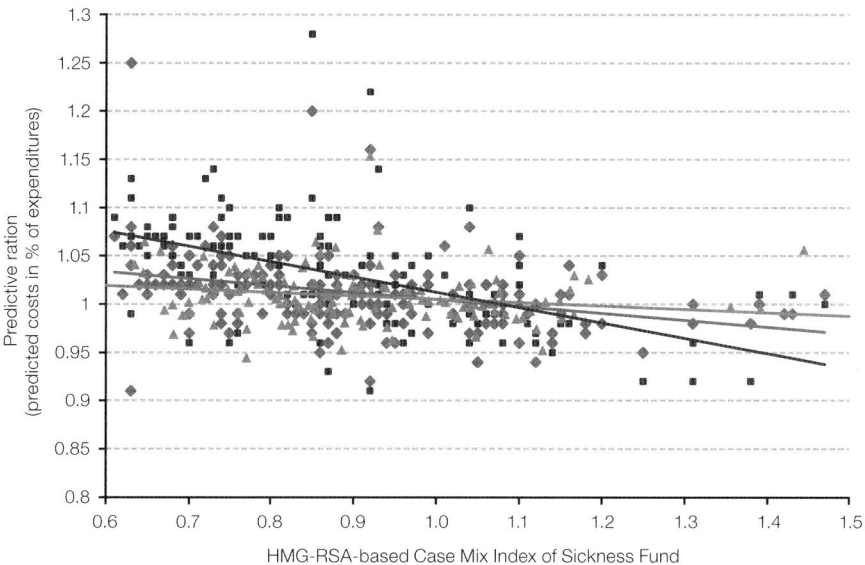

Key

- • Demographic adjustment (pre-2009)
- ◆ HMG-RSA morbidity adjustment (in 2009)
- ▲ HMG-RSA morbidity adjustment (in 2013)
- — Demographic adjustment (pre-2009)
- — HMG-RSA morbidity adjustment (in 2009)
- — HMG-RSA morbidity adjustment (in 2013)

Notes: Based on data provided by the Federal (Social) Insurance Office (BVA). CMI = case mix index; HMG = Hierarchisierte Morbiditätsgruppen; RSA = Risikostrukturausgleich.

As shown by the red (trend) line, the demographic risk adjustment model used before 2009 did not adequately adjust for the higher costs of treatment for funds insuring a larger proportion of sicker individuals, that is, funds with a high CMI tended to have a higher expenditure than predicted by the model. By contrast, funds with a low CMI (providing coverage for relatively healthy individuals) tended to have a lower expenditure than predicted. The introduction of the HMG-RSA-based morbidity adjustment in 2009 considerably improved the ability of the system to predict the expenditure of individuals insured by different sickness funds and reduced the systematic undercompensation of funds with a large proportion of sicker individuals. In subsequent years, the ability of the HMG-RSA to adjust for undercompensation of the system was improved even further (as indicated by the green trend line for the year 2013 in Figure 2.4).

2.5 Conclusion: advantages and limitations of patient classification systems

As stated at the beginning of this chapter, the ideal output measure for health systems and health care organizations is a measure of health improvement. However, most efficiency analysis has to content itself with measuring intermediate outputs, such as hospital inpatient stays or ambulatory care visits, which are meaningful only if they take into account the mix of different types of patients (or cases) treated by different providers.

Patient classification systems help to define different types of patients (or health care products) and to quantify differences in complexity on the basis of cost weights attached to each group of patients. As shown in Section 2.3, the classification of patients into DRGs enables several useful comparisons of hospital costs in relation to outputs to be made. Similar analyses are possible for other areas of health care by using classification systems that have been developed for different health care sectors and for entire populations (see Section 2.4). However, there are important limitations that have to be taken into account when using DRGs or other patient classification systems for case mix-adjusted efficiency analyses across providers or across populations.

2.5.1 Limitations of efficiency analyses based on DRGs or other patient classification systems

Case mix-adjusted comparisons of efficiency across providers should not be interpreted as perfectly accurate and fair. Just as with any other statistical analysis, random variation may contribute to considerable uncertainty concerning the estimated efficiency levels of providers. This is particularly problematic if providers treat only relatively small numbers of patients falling into a particular DRG (or any other group of patients). Consequently, efficiency comparisons should generally be published together with confidence intervals to indicate the level of uncertainty surrounding efficiency estimates. In addition, there are at least four other factors that may systematically bias estimates of efficiency analyses based on DRGs or other patient classification systems.

First, DRGs or other groups of patients defined by classification systems account for only a limited set of factors that influence the costs of care. If certain providers are more likely than others to attract more complex patients within each group of patients, they will inevitably have higher costs. Research has shown that certain patient-level factors beyond those captured by DRGs have a significant influence on costs of care (Busse, 2012; Laudicella, Olsen & Street, 2010) and hospitals can systematically differ concerning these characteristics (Mason et al., 2010). Recognizing that certain hospitals may attract a larger share of high-risk patients within each DRG, reimbursement systems usually adjust for outliers to protect providers from the risk of having cases with extremely high costs (Cots et al., 2011). Regression-based efficiency analyses can control for additional case mix factors (beyond those considered by DRGs) to enable fairer hospital comparisons (see Figure 2.2 and Street et al. (2012)) Nevertheless, even if such adjustments are made in efficiency comparisons, they will never be able to completely control for differences in case mix across providers.

Second, efficiency comparisons on the basis of DRGs do not take into account the quality of care provided by different hospitals. Certain hospitals may provide higher quality of care at higher costs, for example, by employing better skilled nurses or physicians, which would not be adequately reflected in efficiency comparisons. Parallel systems for comparisons of quality are needed to enable fair assessments of provider performance, taking into account both efficiency and quality, even if available studies have shown mixed results on the relationship between costs and quality (Gutacker et al., 2013; Häkkinen et al., 2014; Hussey, Wertheimer & Mehrotra, 2013). For example, as part of the EuroDRG project Häkkinen et al. (2014) compared both costs and quality (measured in terms of survival) in the treatment of patients with AMI and stroke in the hospitals of five European countries. They did not find a clear cost/quality trade-off except in Sweden, where hospitals with higher costs in the treatment of AMI patients also had higher-quality care.

Third, DRG systems and most other patient classification systems focus only on one particular care setting and ignore potential interactions between the costs in one setting and those in another (for example, higher rehabilitation costs related to lower costs because of earlier discharges in acute care hospitals). This is an important drawback, in particular when comparing efficiency of providers across countries. This drawback of classification systems focusing on particular settings could only be overcome by population-based analyses (see Chapter 3).

Fourth, data quality plays an important role. DRGs and other groups of patients are defined on the basis of administrative data generated by providers. On the one hand, inaccuracies in the registration of diagnoses and procedures by providers may lead to misclassification of patients into incorrect DRGs (Sutherland &

Botz, 2006), and consequently lead to biased comparisons. On the other hand, cost weights of individual DRGs can be incorrect if they are calculated on the basis of inaccurate hospital cost accounting systems (Tan et al., 2014). For example, if the allocation of overhead costs to patients is imprecise, the cost of high-complexity patients might be systematically underestimated (see Chapter 4), which would lead to inappropriately low weights for high-complexity DRGs. Therefore, data quality should be carefully monitored to ensure that comparisons are made on the basis of valid data.

Finally, while efficiency analyses can make transparent the differences in costs per DRG across providers, certain providers may have justifiably higher costs per DRG because of factors that are beyond their control. For example, certain providers may face higher input prices because they are located in areas where costs of land and salaries are higher. Other providers may have higher costs because of regulatory demands concerning the availability of equipment (for example, MRI scanners in rural areas), which may not be used at full capacity because of insufficient numbers of patients, thus leading to higher unit costs. DRG-based payment systems often adjust for these differences by adjusting payments for these factors, for example, a market forces factor in England or a wage index in the USA. Efficiency analyses across providers could use similar approaches if they aim to make fair comparisons across providers.

In summary, because of both random variation and potential systematic differences across providers, results of efficiency comparisons should not be taken as completely precise. Nevertheless, comparisons across providers are very useful because they may help to identify those providers with the greatest potential for improvements in efficiency, that is, those with substantially higher costs per unit of output.

2.5.2 Other benefits of patient classification systems and options for the future

A patient classification system defines clinically meaningful and economically (relatively) homogeneous groups of patients. These groups are useful for efficiency analyses as they allow adjusting for provider case mix. However, the most important benefit of having a patient classification system is that it provides a product definition for managers and clinicians who can consequently work together in optimizing treatment processes for a specified group of patients (Fetter, 1991). Some of the examples in Section 2.3 illustrate how DRGs can be used to improve hospital management, for example, by making higher costs of care for the treatment of similar patients transparent or by identifying high-cost outliers within DRGs. Regression-based case mix adjustment methods relying on multiple variables for individual risk factors are usually better at controlling for differences in case mix across providers than DRGs. However, because these methods do not provide a product definition, they do not provide a tool to analyse the patient case mix in a way that can improve treatment processes (Goldfield, 2010).

Patient classification systems always use routine administrative data sets to define groups of patients. As a result, data on all treated patients can be used for comparisons across providers. By contrast, case vignettes – explicitly defined patient care scenarios – always focus on only a very particular type of patient defined by specific criteria to identify identical cases across providers. On the one hand, the ability of vignettes to control for patient and treatment characteristics has important advantages when comparing costs across providers, in particular if located in different countries (Busse, Schreyögg & Smith, 2008). On the other hand, narrowly defined vignettes may be too restrictive for identifying differences in treatment processes across providers. Furthermore, a provider might have high costs for the treatment of one type of patient but might have low costs for the treatment of other types of patients. If efficiency is measured for only a few specific types of patients (vignettes), the results of efficiency comparisons might identify hospitals as providing inefficient care (for these patients), while they are, in fact, efficient when looking at all patients.

Comparing efficiency of providers across countries is particularly difficult (Busse, Schreyögg & Smith, 2008; Häkkinen & Joumard, 2007; Medin et al., 2013; Street et al., 2012). First, population differences beyond those measured by case mix adjustment, for example, concerning socioeconomic status or cultural expectations, may influence results. Second, treatment patterns differ across countries, for example, concerning whether rehabilitation takes place within the same hospital admission or at a different institution, implying that provider-based efficiency assessment can be misleading. Third, as shown in Section 2.2, many countries use their own national version of DRGs that cannot simply be used for international comparisons because of substantial differences concerning how groups of patients are defined in different systems. Fourth, coding systems and coding practices differ across countries (see Table 2.1), which means that diagnoses and procedures registered in different countries have to be mapped to a common coding system if the aim is to group patients into a common patient classification system. Fifth, cost accounting methods differ across countries, for example, concerning the inclusion of capital costs, physician costs or the apportionment of overheads, which means that costs are not comparable. Finally, adjusting for differences in input prices across countries is quite complex (Schreyögg et al., 2008).

Because of these problems, the EuroDRG project decided not to compare the efficiency of hospitals across countries but to limit comparisons to hospitals within the same country – although using a standardized methodology (Street et al., 2012). Countries that have a common patient classification system, such as the NordDRGs in Nordic countries, can use this system for cross-country comparisons (Medin et al., 2013). The OECD and Eurostat have recently developed a methodology for comparing the prices of hospital outputs across countries (Koechlin et al., 2014), using an approach similar to that used by the EuroDRG project for DRG price comparisons (Busse et al., 2013). The OECD/ Eurostat approach has defined 32 hospital products (or groups of patients) by using diagnosis and procedure codes that are translated into national coding systems. In a way, this approach creates 32 meta-DRGs that could be used as a starting-point for the development of methods for the comparison of hospital efficiency across Europe, for example, by developing a EuroDRG system.

The starting-point of this chapter was the observation that the ideal output measure for efficiency comparisons is a measure of health improvement. If it were possible to estimate average health improvement for different groups of patients, for example, the average number of QALYs gained per DRG, it would be possible to convert groups of patients defined by classification systems into measures of health improvement. However, current DRG systems are not designed to define groups of patients that benefit in a similar way from treatment. Nevertheless, adopting the basic idea of patient classification systems, future measures of health improvement are not inconceivable, at least for certain high-volume cases. For example, systems could be developed that would define groups of patients with similar characteristics (for example, based on diagnosis, severity and functional status) who would be likely to benefit in a similar way from particular types of treatment (medical or surgical procedures), while still having similar costs. Ultimately, such an approach could advance measurement of efficiency and move health systems towards more efficient delivery of care.

References

Australian Health Services Research Institute (AHSRI) (2012). AN-SNAP Version 3. (http://ahsri.uow.edu. au/content/idcplg?IdcService=GET_FILE&dDocName=UOW119626&RevisionSelectionMethod=lat estReleased, accessed 21 July 2016).

Amatya B, Khan F (2011). Rehabilitation for cerebral palsy: analysis of the Australian rehabilitation outcome dataset. *Journal of Neurosciences in Rural Practice*, 2(1):43–49.

Barer ML (1982). Case mix adjustment in hospital cost analysis: information theory revisited. *Journal of Health Economics*, 1(1):53–80.

Busse R (2012). Do diagnosis-related groups explain variations in hospital costs and length of stay? Analyses from the EuroDRG project for 10 episodes of care across 10 European countries. *Health Economics*, 21(Suppl. S2):S1–S5.

Busse R, Schreyögg J, Smith PC (2008). Variability in healthcare treatment costs amongst nine EU countries: results from the HealthBASKET project. *Health Economics*, 17(Suppl. S1):S1–S8.

Busse R et al., eds. (2011). *Diagnosis-related groups in Europe: moving towards transparency, efficiency, and quality in hospitals*. European Observatory on Health Systems and Policies Series. Maidenhead, Open University Press (http://www.euro.who.int/__data/assets/pdf_file/0004/162265/e96538.pdf (accessed 21 July 2016).

Busse R et al. (2013). Diagnosis related groups in Europe: moving towards transparency, efficiency, and quality in hospitals? *BMJ*, 346:f3197.

Bundesversicherungsamt (BVA) (2014). Festlegungen nach § 31 Absatz 4 RSAV für das Ausgleichsjahr 2015. Bonn, BVA (http://www.bundesversicherungsamt.de/fileadmin/redaktion/Risikostrukturausgleich/Festlegungen/AJ_2015/Festlegung_Klassifikationsmodell_2015.zip, accessed 21 July 2016).

Canadian Institute for Health Information (CIHI) (2011). RPG grouping methodology and rehabilitation cost weights. Ottawa, CIHI (http://www.cihi.ca/cihi-ext-portal/pdf/internet/info_rpg_method_costweight_en, accessed 21 July 2016).

Cots F et al. (2011). DRG-based hospital payment: intended and unintended consequences. In: Busse R et al., eds. *Diagnosis-related groups in Europe: moving towards transparency, efficiency and quality in hospitals.* European Observatory on Health Systems and Policies Series. Maidenhead, Open University Press (http://www.euro.who.int/__data/assets/pdf_file/0004/162265/e96538.pdf, accessed 24 July 2016).

Cotterill PG, Thomas FG (2004). Prospective payment for Medicare inpatient psychiatric care: assessing the alternatives. *Health Care Financing Review*, 26(1):85–101.

Department of Health (DoH) (2013). Mental health payment by results guidance for 2013–14. Leeds, DoH (https://www.gov.uk/government/uploads/system/uploads/attachment_data/file/232162/Mental_Health_PbR_Guidance_for_2013-14.pdf, accessed 21 July 2016).

Fetter RB (1991). Diagnosis related groups: understanding hospital performance. *Interfaces*, 21(1):6–26.

Fetter RB et al. (1980). Case mix definition by diagnosis-related groups. *Medical Care*, 18(Suppl. 2):iii, 1–53.

Fischer W, ed. (2000). Diagnosis Related Groups (DRGs) und verwandte Patientenklassifikationssysteme. Wolfertswil, Zentrum für Informatik und wirtschaftliche Medizin (http://fischer-zim.ch/studien/DRG-Systeme-0003-Info.htm, accessed 21 July 2016).

Federal Office of Public Health (FOPH) (2014). Kennzahlen der Schweizer Spitäler 2012 [Swiss hospitals key figures 2012]. Bern: FOPH (http://www.bag-anw.admin.ch/kuv/spitalstatistik/data/download/kzp12_publikation.pdf?version=1439213908&webgrab=ignore, accessed 21 July 2016).

Geissler A, Scheller-Kreinsen D, Quentin W (2012). Do diagnosis-related groups appropriately explain variations in costs and length of stay of hip replacement? A comparative assessment of DRG systems across 10 European countries. *Health Economics*, 21(Suppl. 2):103–115.

Geissler A et al. (2011). Germany: understanding G-DRGs. In: Busse R et al., eds. *Diagnosis-related groups in Europe: moving towards transparency, efficiency and quality in hospitals*. European Observatory on Health Systems and Policies Series. Maidenhead, Open University Press (http://www.euro.who.int/__data/assets/pdf_file/0004/162265/e96538.pdf, accessed 21 July 2016).

Goldfield N (2010). The evolution of diagnosis-related groups (DRGs): from its beginnings in case-mix and resource use theory, to its implementation for payment and now for its current utilization for quality within and outside the hospital. *Quality Management in Health Care*, 19(1):3–16.

Gutacker N et al. (2013). Truly inefficient or providing better quality of care? Analysing the relationship between risk-adjusted hospital costs and patients' health outcomes. *Health*

Häkkinen U, Joumard I (2007). Cross-country analysis of efficiency in OECD health care sectors. OECD Economics Department Working Papers No. 554. Paris, OECD Publishing (http://www.oecd-ilibrary.org/docserver/download/5l4nrhnfdlzq.pdf?expires=1469286000&id=id&accname=guest&checksum=24C8173BAC70D0B2BC9ECD5C6CE0BBC5, accessed 21 July 2016).

Häkkinen U et al. (2014). Quality, cost, and their trade-off in treating AMI and stroke patients in European hospitals. *Health Policy*, 117(1):15–27.

Hollingsworth B (2008). The measurement of efficiency and productivity of health care delivery. *Health Economics*, 17(10):1107–1128.

Hornbrook MC (1982). Hospital case mix: its definition, measurement and use. Part I. The conceptual framework. *Medical Care Review*, 39(1):1–43.

Hussey PS, Wertheimer S, Mehrotra A (2013). The association between health care quality and cost: a systematic review. *Annals of Internal Medicine*, 158(1):27–34.

Iezzoni LI (2009). Risk adjustment for performance measurement. In: Smith P et al., eds. *Performance measurement for health system improvement: experiences, challenges and prospects*. Cambridge, CUP.

Independent Hospital Pricing Authority (IHPA) (2014). Appendix G: subacute and non-acute admitted AN-SNAP V3.0. Darlinghurst, IHPA (http://www.health.gov.au/internet/ihpa/publishing.nsf/Content/nep-determination-2014-15-html~appendix~appendix-g, accessed 21 July 2016).

Institut für das Entgeltsystem im Krankenhaus (InEK) (2007). Kalkulationshandbuch. Sieburg, InEK (http://g-drg.de/cms/Kalkulation2/DRG-Fallpauschalen_17b_KHG/Kalkulationshandbuch, accessed 22 July 2016).

InEK (2010). G-DRG V2008/2010 HA-Report-Browser. Siegburg, InEK (http://www.g-drg.de/cms/content/view/full/2553, accessed 22 July 2016).

InEK (2014a). Abschlussbericht Weiterentwicklung des G-DRG-Systems für das Jahr 2015. Siegburg, InEK (http://g-drg.de/cms/content/download/5569/43022/version/1/file/Abschlussbericht_G-DRG-System2015.pdf, accessed 22 July 2016).

InEK (2014b). Abschlussbericht Weiterentwicklung des pauschalierenden Entgeltsystems für Psychiatrie und Psychosomatik (PEPP) für das Jahr 2015. Siegburg, InEK (http://www.gdrg.de/cms/content/download/5568/43014/version/2/file/Abschlussbericht_PEPP-System_2015.pdf, accessed 22 July 2016).

InEK (2014c). PEPP-Entgeltkatalog. Siegburg, InEK (http://g-drg.de/cms/content/download/5424/42049/version/1/file/PEPP-Entgeltkatalog_Version_2015_140923.xlsx, accessed 22 July 2016).

Kimberly JR, Pouvourville GD, d'Aunno TA, eds. (2008). *The globalization of managerial innovation in health care*. Cambridge, CUP.

Kobel C. et al. (2011). DRG systems and similar patient classification systems in Europe. In: Busse R, eds. *Diagnosis-related groups in Europe: moving towards transparency, efficiency and quality in hospitals*. European Observatory on Health Systems and Policies Series. Maidenhead, Open University Press (http://www.euro.who.int/__data/assets/pdf_file/0004/162265/e96538.pdf, accessed 24 July 2016).

Koechlin F et al. (2014). Comparing hospital and health prices and volumes internationally: results of a Eurostat/OECD project. Paris, OECD Publishing (http://ec.europa.eu/eurostat/documents/728703/728971/OECD-health-working-papers-75.pdf/a6e22472-95c4-4e77-bdb0-db3af4668e7f, accessed 22 July 2016).

Laudicella M, Olsen KR, Street A (2010). Examining cost variation across hospital departments: a two-stage multi-level approach using patient-level data. *Social Science & Medicine*, 71(10):1872–1881.

Linna M, Häkkinen U, Magnussen J (2006). Comparing hospital cost efficiency between Norway and Finland. *Health Policy*, 77(3):268–278.

Mason A, Goddard M (2009). Payment by results in mental health: a review of the international literature and economic assessment of the Integrated Packages Approach to Care (InPAC). York, Centre for Health Economics (http://www.cppconsortium.nhs.uk/admin/files/1426157927PbR%20MH%20report_June09%20pdfyorkuni.pdf, accessed 22 July 2016).

Mason A, Street A, Verzulli R (2010). Private sector treatment centres are treating less complex patients than the NHS. *Journal of the Royal Society of Medicine*, 103(8):322–331.

Mason A et al. (2012). How well do diagnosis-related groups for appendectomy explain variations in resource use? An analysis of patient-level data from 10 European countries. *Health Economics*, 21(Suppl. 2):30–40.

Medin E et al. (2013). International hospital productivity comparison: experiences from the Nordic countries. *Health Policy*, 112(1–2):80–87.

Medicare Payment Advisory Commission (MedPAC) (2014a). Inpatient rehabilitation facilities payment system. Washington, DC, MedPAC (http://www.medpac.gov/documents/payment-basics/inpatient-rehabilitation-facilities-payment-system-14.pdf?sfvrsn=0, accessed 22 July 2016).

MedPAC (2014b). Inpatient psychiatric facility services payment. Washington, DC, MedPAC (http://www.medpac.gov/documents/payment-basics/inpatient-psychiatric-facility-services-payment-system-14.pdf?sfvrsn=0, accessed 22 July 2016).

MedPAC (2014c). Medicare and the health care delivery system. Washington, DC, MedPAC (http://www.medpac.gov/documents/reports/jun14_entirereport.pdf?sfvrsn=0, accessed 22 July 2016).

Meyer M et al. (2012). Length of stay benchmarks for inpatient rehabilitation after stroke. *Disability and rehabilitation*, 34(13):1077–1081.

Ministère des Affaires sociales, de la Santé et des Droits des femmes (2015). Manuel des Groupes Médicoéconomiques en soins de suite et de réadaptation. Volume 1. Présentation et annexes générales. (http://www.sante.gouv.fr/fichiers/bos/2015/sts_20150001_0001_p000.pdf, accessed 21 July 2016).

Monitor (2013). Guidance on mental health currencies and payment. London, Monitor and NHS England (https://www.gov.uk/government/uploads/system/uploads/attachment_data/file/300864/Guidance_to_mental_health_currencies_and_payment.pdf, accessed 22 July 2016).

Organisation for Economic Co-operation and Development (OECD) (2013). A good life in old age: monitoring and improving quality in long-term care. OECD Health Policy Studies. Paris, OECD Publishing (http://ec.europa.eu/social/BlobServlet?docId=10292&langId=en, accessed 22 July 2016).

Ontario Joint Policy and Planning Committee (2008). Grouper and weighting methodology for adult inpatient mental health care in Ontario. Toronto, Ontario JPPC (http://booksnow1.scholarsportal.info/ebooks/ebooks2/ogdc/2014-02-25/3/286769/286769.pdf, accessed 22 July 2016).

Paris V, Devaux M, Wei L (2010). Health systems institutional characteristics: a survey of 29 OECD countries. OECD Health Working Papers, No. 50. Paris, OECD Publishing (http://www.oecd-ilibrary.org/docserver/download/5kmfxfq9qbnr.pdf?expires=1469322352&id=id&accname=guest&checksum=5A7778874202616C68F19D5E221917B0, accessed 22 July 2016).

Peltola M, Quentin W (2013). Diagnosis-related groups for stroke in Europe: patient classification and hospital reimbursement in 11 countries. *Cerebrovascular Diseases*, 35(2): 113–123.

Penno E, Gauld R, Audas R (2013). How are population-based funding formulae for healthcare composed? A comparative analysis of seven models. *BMC Health Services Research*, 13:470.

Perlman CM et al. (2013). Development of mental health quality indicators (MHQIs) for inpatient psychiatry based on the interRAI mental health assessment. *BMC Health Services Research*, 13:15.

Quentin W et al. (2011). Understanding DRGs and DRG-based hospital payment in Europe. In: Busse R, eds. *Diagnosis-related groups in Europe: moving towards transparency, efficiency and quality in hospitals*. European Observatory on Health Systems and Policies Series. Maidenhead, Open University Press (http://www. euro.who.int/__data/assets/pdf_file/0004/162265/e96538.pdf, accessed 24 July 2016).

Quentin W et al. (2012). Appendectomy and diagnosis-related groups (DRGs): patient classification and hospital reimbursement in 11 European countries. *Langenbeck's archives of surgery/Deutsche Gesellschaft für Chirurgie*, 397(2):317–326.

Schreyögg J et al. (2008). Cross-country comparisons of costs: the use of episode-specific transitive purchasing power parities with standardised cost categories. *Health Economics*, 17(Suppl. S1):S95–S103.

Starfield B, Kinder K (2011). Multimorbidity and its measurement. *Health Policy*, 103(1):3–8.

Starfield B et al. (1991). Ambulatory care groups: a categorization of diagnoses for research and management. *Health Services Research*, 26(1):53–74.

Street A et al. (2012). How well do diagnosis-related groups explain variations in costs or length of stay among patients and across hospitals? Methods for analysing routine patient data. *Health Economics*, 21(Suppl. S2):6–18.

Sutherland JM, Botz CK (2006). The effect of misclassification errors on case mix measurement. *Health Policy*, 79(2–3):195–202.

Tan SS et al. (2014). DRG systems in Europe: variations in cost accounting systems among 12 countries. *European Journal of Public Health*, 24(6):1023–1028.

Vitikainen K, Street A, Linna M (2009). Estimation of hospital efficiency: do different definitions and casemix measures for hospital output affect the results? *Health Policy*, 89(2):149–159.

Ministerie van Volksgezondheid, Welzijn en Sport (VWS) (2011). Health insurance in the Netherlands. The Hague, VWS (http://www.government.nl/files/documents-and-publications/leaflets/2012/09/26/ health-insurance-in-the-netherlands/health-insurance-in-the-netherlands.pdf, accessed 22 July 2016).

WHO (2000). The World Health Report 2000. Health systems: improving performance. Geneva, WHO (http://www.who.int/whr/2000/en/whr00_en.pdf?ua=1, accessed 3 August 2016).

Chapter 3

Using registry data to compare health care efficiency

Reijo Sund and Unto Häkkinen

3.1 Introduction

One of the main hurdles in efficiency measurement is figuring out how to evaluate the specific role of health services as a determinant of health outcome or disease progression. Variations in health occur not only because of differences in treatment and provider-level factors, but also because of person-level variations; a key challenge is to distinguish between the two, with treatment- and provider-level variations being of primary importance for analysts interested in assessing health care efficiency.

In this chapter, we describe a methodological approach with this objective in mind that makes use of routine registry data. The general idea is that by using detailed registry data, patient variations can be better accounted for so that variations in health care output are measured more accurately. This is accomplished by accounting for detailed patient information and following the treatment pathways of patients both over time and across multiple providers. Information on patient episodes of care can be used to derive adjusted measures that are then comparable between appropriate subpopulations, regions or providers.

Previously, this type of data on the relative performance of service providers was used to identify best practices or what worked (Häkkinen & Joumard, 2007). More recently, this kind of information has been used as a basis for paying for performance (Cashin et al., 2014). In addition, reliable information on provider effectiveness is essential in systems in which patients can choose their provider. In this chapter we focus on meso level analysis (that is, to the case mix- or risk-adjusted comparisons of service providers) and use a disease-based approach, because the health gains of activities can be measured most accurately at disease level (Häkkinen, 2011; Häkkinen et al., 2013).

One of the main obstacles to institutionalizing this type of measurement has been the lack of appropriate data in most countries. While advances in information technology have made it easier to produce and store all kinds of data, the emphasis has commonly been on the technical aspects of data collection and not on the information itself (Shani, 2000). As the data were originally produced for other purposes than for performance assessment, the transformation of secondary data into useful information is challenging (Sund et al., 2014).

Essentially registry data is a type of big data. A register is an information system that continuously records event-based data for a particular, complete set of patients. A register contains a logically coherent collection of related data with some inherent meaning, typically reflecting events that have occurred, such as all treatment information for patients with a particular disease. Register data are micro level data and each event can be linked to some individual and all events that have occurred for some individual can be linked together. Most of the registers are either administrative or quality registers. To be useful for research purposes, the structure and completeness of the data sources must be well documented and stable (Sund et al., 2014).

Recent OECD reports indicate that the infrastructure of national data is improving across countries and the technical capacity to analyse and report from personal health information data assets is greater today than it was even just five years ago (OECD, 2013, 2015). As this data infrastructure grows and more suitable data become available, the real bottleneck emerging is the ability to transform these data into useful information (Sund, 2003). In this chapter we present an approach to use routinely collected register-based data to its greatest potential. First, we give a general description of our methodological approach to develop selected indicators from registry data, and describe how to use these to profile the efficiency of providers. We then consider how this approach can be extended to international comparisons; finally, we discuss possible implications for the future.

3.2 Using registry data to define episodes of care

Registers, and particularly administrative registers, generally contain data on observable events that reflect whether an individual used certain health services at a particular moment in time. These event data provide a good sense of a patient's pathway through the health system. By linking patient-specific event data for a series of events that are linked to a particular health problem or disease, we can construct what we call a single patient's episode of care. Grouping patient events into disease-specific episodes of care can be useful for evaluating simple health care processes. It also moves the focus of quality of care away from a discrete service to an examination of the trajectory of patient care across providers, thus highlighting the challenges of care coordination.

All of the conditions detailed in this chapter are typically treated in hospitals, which in many countries have detailed data available for analysis. There are also possibilities to evaluate chronic diseases, such as diabetes, which are mainly treated in primary care using this type of approach. However, in such cases determining interesting events is quite different from the basic application of the methodological approach described herein.

A central consideration in defining an episode of care is to identify the starting and end-point of the episode. For particular conditions or patients, this may be easier than others. For example, acute disorders such as hip fractures, stroke and AMIs, have well-defined starting points and are resolved in a rather short time. Other conditions that also have well-defined follow-up times include care related to childbirth and care of pre-term infants. However, other disorders may have fuzzier starting points or require a longer follow-up, making the episode of care more complicated to construct. Such conditions include breast cancer, knee and hip arthroplasty, back surgery and schizophrenia.

A further challenge in defining the episode of care relates to dealing with the heterogeneity of patient needs, which may lead to different patterns of care emerging for patients with the same condition. For example, some patients may suffer from more than one condition, and thus also require acute or elective care that is unrelated to the episode, which can complicate the interpretation of the data.

In practice, the aim of constructing an episode of care is to use the data available in the registers to make the process of care visible across the entire treatment pathway. The main observable events in the register data are (re)admissions, operations, discharges, deaths, outpatient visits and medication purchases. To model the episode of care appropriately, the nature of the disease and the characteristics of the patient must be taken into account, since these are key factors affecting treatment decisions. An example of a possible episode of care is presented in Figure 3.1. This figure illustrates how different observable events in the data can be joined to form a total episode of care, which outlines the entire treatment pathway comprising distinct episodes of care across separate care settings (such as inpatient and outpatient care).

The next step is to categorize the service usage data available, and identify the level of care and the need for care. The idea is to identify a patient's possible state at each point in time based on transitions across a set of loci of care. Heterogeneity among patients may account for variations in the levels of care, in terms of the intensity of care and type of service (for example, if one patient has a more severe case) and thus are important to consider, while information on patient characteristics will allow differentiation in determining the need for care.

Figure 3.1 *Example of a care episode*

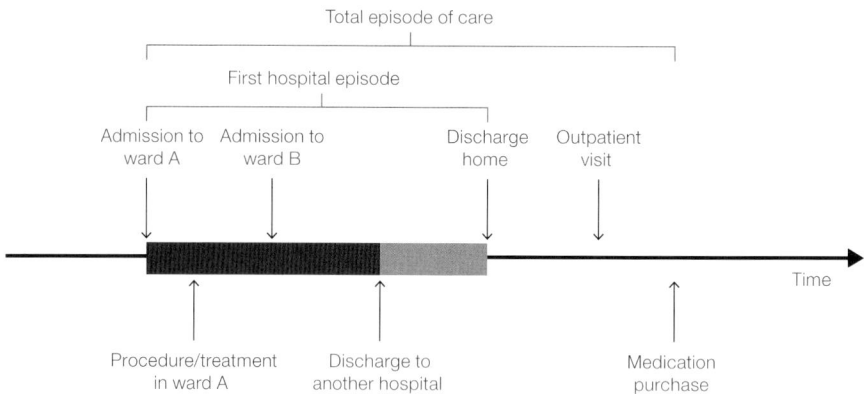

Hypothetical state spaces are well suited to describing general care episodes, but in practice, separating the care processes from the outcomes using this approach turns out to be more challenging. One way to conceptualize health outcomes using this approach is to consider possible changes in health status according to the available process data, since direct measures of health status are usually not available in registry data. In general, by assuming that patients are not treated randomly, one can assume that the decision to treat a patient in a given care setting reflects the appraised need for care. In other words, admissions and discharges from different types of institutions or the type of home care provided (home services/caregiver) can be considered to reflect some kind of qualitative changes in health status. For example, discharge to home usually means that a patient's health status is considered good enough that they probably can manage at home, while prolonged care or acute admission after discharge home typically reflects some kind of problem. Death is also a clear indication of health status. Box 3.1 provides a detailed illustration of an episode of care for a hip fracture.

3.3 Constructing indicators based on episodes of care

Once the care episode has been defined, it is possible to construct indicators that describe and evaluate interesting aspects of the treatment pathway, particularly regarding processes, costs and outcomes. The details of the indicators will likely vary depending on the health condition being investigated, but in general the main types of process and outcome measures extractable from register-based data remain similar. Example indicators for the hip fracture case are briefly described in Box 3.2 (Sund et al., 2011).

Box 3.1 *Illustration of the construction of an episode of care for a hip fracture*

To illustrate the construction of an episode of care, consider the example of a hip fracture case. The first task in the construction of a hip fracture episode is to identify the beginning of the episode. A natural choice for an index event to signal the beginning of the episode could be the hospitalization of the patient after their first hip fracture, as shown by the data.

The next step is to categorize the service usage data available from the point of view of the hip fracture, and identify the level of care and the need for care. The patient's possible state at each point in time is based on transitions across a set of loci of care. In this example, classifying patients according their residence (home or institution) before the fracture is one way to ensure the study population is sufficiently homogeneous, and account for differences in care.

In the case of a hip fracture, the following four different loci of care can be identified from the data. These can be considered to correspond to different levels of care, and are listed in increasing order of intensity:

1. home (including different types of home care, ordinary assisted living facilities and outpatient care);
2. nursing home (service houses with 24-hour assistance and residential homes);
3. health centre (inpatient ward of local primary care unit);
4. hospital.

In addition, a death state can be considered as the fifth possible state. More detailed classification (separating, for example, the types of home care and assisted living) may be possible if such data are available. Using these loci, we can construct different potential care pathways. The state space describing possible movements for a model of hip fracture care pathway is presented graphically in Figure 3.2.

Figure 3.2 *State space for the hip fracture care episode*

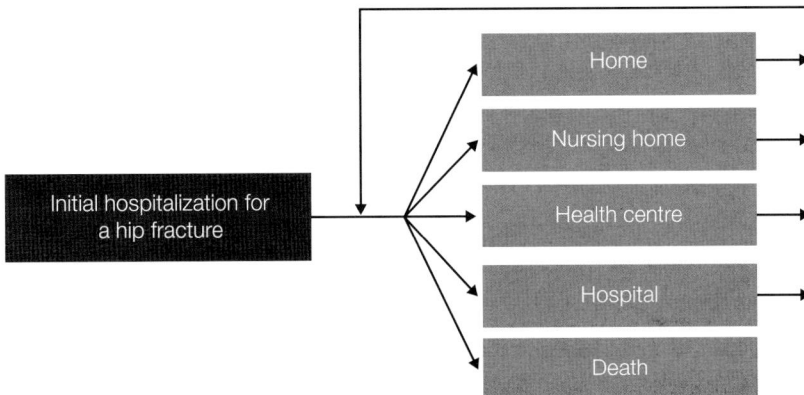

These steps allow us to put together the key events in the hip fracture treatment episode, as illustrated in Figure 3.3. In Figure 3.3, the hip fracture care episode is defined as starting on the index day, that is, the date of first admission to a surgical ward after the hip fracture. The next interesting event is surgery; the time between admission to a surgical ward and surgery is called the operative delay. The following event in Figure 3.3 is a kind of double event showing that the patient was discharged from the surgical ward to the rehabilitation ward. The time between the index day and first discharge (or death) is known as the index period and it usually corresponds to the length of stay in the surgical ward. The first hospital episode is defined as beginning on the index day and terminating at the first discharge to home, death or after four months of continuous inpatient care. The first hospital episode describes the acute phase of hip fracture treatment. If treatment continues for more than four months without discharge home, the patient is defined as a long-term care patient, because most discharges home are known to happen before four months. The follow-up period ends one year after the index day or at death, whichever happens first. In the example in Figure 3.3, the patient stays at home for some time after the first hospital episode, but is then admitted to hospital where they finally die and the follow-up terminates.

Figure 3.3 *Example of key events in the hip fracture treatment episode*

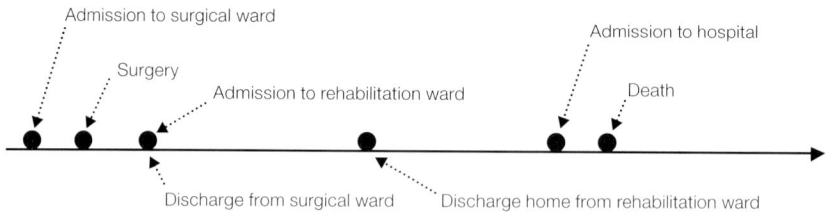

Box 3.2 *Examples of register-based indicators for the hip fracture case*

Background

- Number of patients
- Mean age
- Male share
- Distribution of fracture types:
  - femoral neck fracture;
  - pertrochanteric fracture;
  - subtrochanteric fracture.

- Proportion of patients in long-term care
- Proportion of patients admitted from home
- Number of days in home during 90 days before the fracture
- Proportion of patients with certain comorbidities

Process and cost

- Proportion of patients with operative delay longer than 2 days
- Type of operation:
  - non-cemented semi-prosthesis;
  - cemented semi-prosthesis;
  - total prosthesis;
  - osteosynthesis;
  - no operation.
- The length of index admission, days (first surgical hospitalization without hospital transfers)
- Length of first hospital episode, days
- Use of services during the first year following fracture:
  - specialized hospital inpatient care, days;
  - health centre inpatient care, days;
  - nursing home type of care, days;
  - number of outpatient visits in specialized hospital.
- Costs of index admission (€ per patient)
- Costs of first hospitalization (€ per patient)
- One-year hospital costs (€ per patient) including outpatient visits
- Proportion becoming long-term care patients (proportion of patients with at least 120 days of ontinuous inpatient care after the hip fracture)

Outcome

- 30-day mortality (%)
- 120-day mortality (%)
- One-year mortality (%)
- Proportion of patients at home (day 30)
- Proportion of patients at home (day 120)
- Proportion of patients at home after 365 days following the fracture
- Occurrence of a complication
- Readmission/reoperation

Special indicators

- State diagram

Indicators related to process and cost describe the treatments provided during the care episode. Register-based data are a fruitful resource for these kinds of indicators. Some of these indicators are descriptive, such as the type of surgery or prescriptions for certain types of medication. Others are pseudo-outcome indicators that can be derived from the observed admission states of the patients, such as the proportion of patients at home since a given time from the index event. Another type of indicator reflects the time between interesting events, such as the time from initial admission to surgery or length of stay in hospital or rehabilitation ward; comparing variations in the time between such events among similar groups of patients may provide an indication of efficiency. Finally, cumulative measures, such as the number of hospital days, outpatient visits and home visits during the year can also be of interest.

One challenge in using registry data is that there are limited outcome indicators available in register-based data. Thus, the actual effectiveness of treatment (change in health status) must usually be inferred indirectly from the process measures, as mentioned earlier. The few outcome indicators that are available are mortality and occurrence of adverse events, such as complication or reoperation. In certain cases, the ability to return to the same or lower level of care than before the beginning of the care episode may be considered to reflect a successful outcome, but usually this still describes the process rather than the outcome. A possible outcome indicator in the case of hip fractures is days at home with and without receiving additional care.

One special type of indicator that can be constructed using this approach is a state diagram. The idea is to use the defined state space of patients during the care episode and then simply calculate the proportions of patients in each state at each given point in time. An example of a state diagram for a hip fracture is illustrated in Figure 3.4. State diagrams capture a lot of easily interpreted information in a compact visual form. Similar approaches can be extended to reporting of even more detailed data in simple but informative visualizations. It is also possible to calculate some kind of crude approximation for health status by using suitably weighted daily states, that is, the observed levels of care can be associated with the average health status of patients.

The costs of treatment are very important, particularly for the construction of efficiency metrics using this approach. Unfortunately, in most cases the exact costs incurred at the patient level are not available. Instead, costs must be estimated by weighting the available data on resource use appropriately, that is, by giving each identifiable cost item (surgery, hospital days, medication purchases) a certain price (based on DRGs or mean per diem costs in a DRG group) and then simply summing these up to estimate the costs of treatment (Geue et al.,

Figure 3.4 *State diagram for hip fracture patients in Finland*

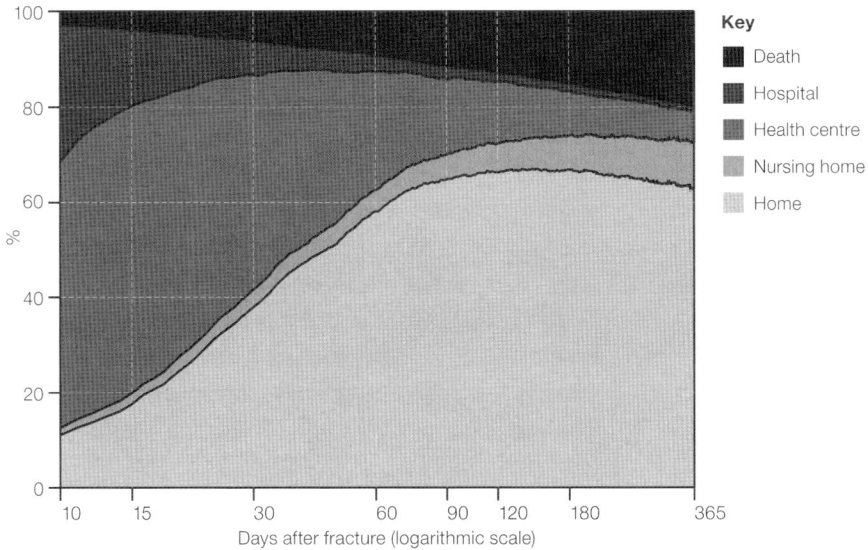

2012; Iversen et al., 2015; Peltola et al., 2011). This inevitably means that such treatment costs are only crude approximations that are certainly wrong for each individual, but still useful for group-level comparisons between care providers. An extra challenge when deriving costs is that after the death of a patient, costs drop to zero, which will severely bias comparisons (that is, bad effectiveness may result in low costs because so many patients died in the early phase). This must be taken into account (Häkkinen et al., 2014).

To evaluate performance of the entire treatment pathway, it is also important to have information on costs after the initial hospital episode. Such costs can account for about 50% of total hip fracture costs in the year after index admission (Figure 3.5). Moreover, differences in costs over one year across the four cities in Figure 3.5 seem to be explained by institutional care costs that occurred after the first hospital episode.

3.4 Comparing provider performance: the need for risk adjustment

In addition to using register-based data to describe the processes, outcomes and costs related to certain diseases and conditions, data can be used to assess and compare the effectiveness or efficiency of providers. To assess providers, some benchmark of good performance is required. Since absolute benchmarks may be difficult to define, it is much more common to compare service providers to each other.

Figure 3.5 *Hip fracture costs per patient in four Finnish cities 2009–2010*

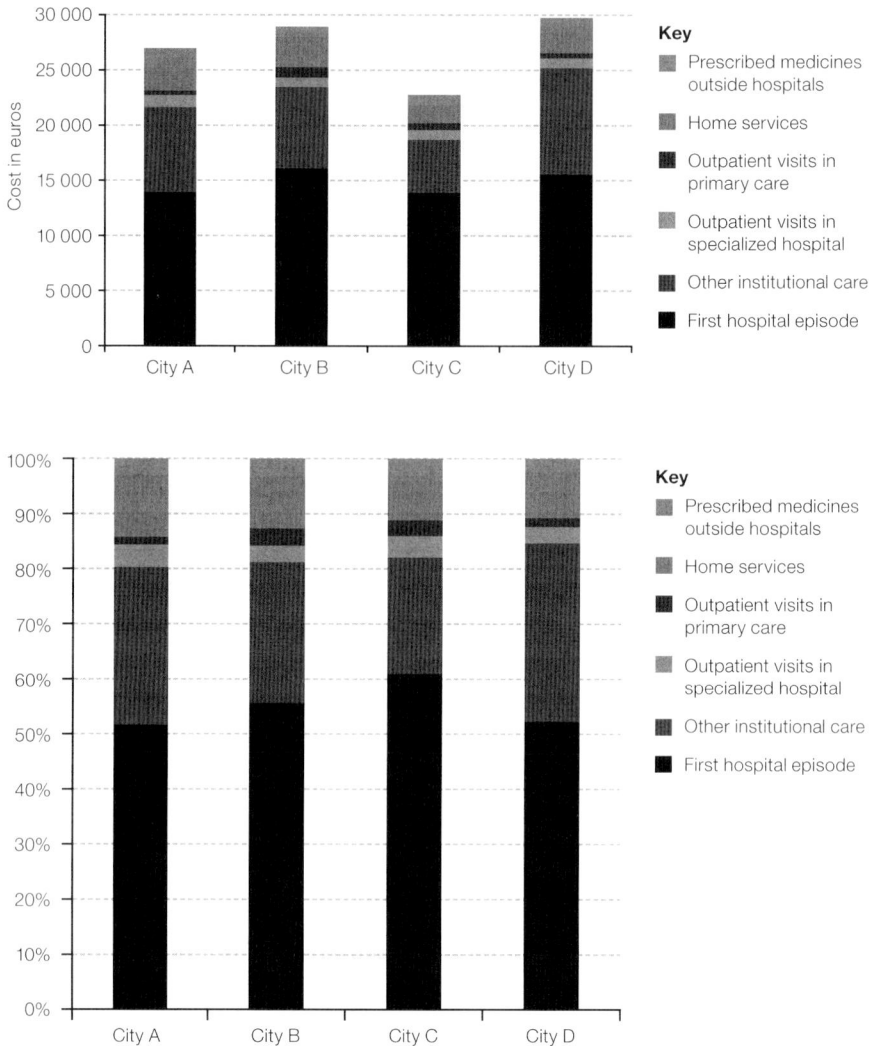

Key
- Prescribed medicines outside hospitals
- Home services
- Outpatient visits in primary care
- Outpatient visits in specialized hospital
- Other institutional care
- First hospital episode

The challenge is that variations across providers may occur for a number of reasons, and not be explained only by differences in provider performance. Differences may result from random variation related to the size of the provider, or data errors or differential coding practices. Differences may also result from variations in patient case mix from provider to provider. Variations could also be attributable to external environmental factors (for example, geography). Since, the main interest to policymakers is usually to identify performance variations, it is important to control for sources of variation as much as possible. This can be done by using risk adjustment.

Without risk adjustment, any observational study will be biased if the populations to be compared have differences in observed or unobserved background factors in ways that confound the outcomes of interest. In practice, risk adjustment involves controlling for differences in external factors that may hide the interesting variation. The challenge (and solution) is to find data on background variables, such as comorbidities, that can explain these variations. While background variables may be interesting to report in their own right, they are particularly useful for risk adjustment.

Register-based data cannot identify all potentially interesting variables to adjust for, but as long as linking the registry across to other registries is possible, so that the historical events of an individual can be extracted from the registers, then there is a potential breadth of suitable individual-level data available. In general, it is useful to develop a conceptual model that identifies the relevant factors that are known to have a potential confounding effect on the outcome of interest, and then evaluate the possibility to find relevant data from the registries.

In the case of a hip fracture, these confounders could theoretically include background variables such as biological measures, demographics, socioeconomic status, health-related behaviour, subjective quality of life, objective need for care, use of care, accident/fall history and hip fracture event. Of these, some biological factors do not change over time and therefore only one measurement can apply for all time periods. Biological events, accident/fall history and hip fracture events represent dimensions for which values are recorded in the proximity of some actual event. All other dimensions relate to phenomena that potentially change over time and should be continuously monitored. In practice, these are likely to be collected separately from the registry and only recorded at fixed intervals (rather than corresponding to particular events of interest).

Comorbidities are always important background variables to control for. The traditional approach is to use data on certain diagnoses to identify comorbidities. The most common comorbidity conditions are the ones defined for the purposes of the Charlson and Elixhauser indices. Because the data in many databases (for example, hospital discharge registries) are recorded at the time of discharge (that is, after surgery), they may include information that is related to the actual care delivered and thus reflect the quality of care provided; this would not be suitable for risk adjustment. Rather, only comorbidity data gathered from close to the time of index admission should be used. Another source to identify comorbidity conditions are the prescriptions registers, because for many drugs, there is only one primary condition for which that drug is prescribed. There may also be comorbidity clues in reimbursement system data; for example, in Finland, people receive compensation for the purchase of drugs if they have certain chronic diseases.

3.5 Adjustment techniques

Risk adjustment is not without challenges. It can only be done for covariates that are observed and for which data is available. Moreover, it is not always straightforward to select the suitable adjustment method, because many exist. If the outcomes of interest are not fixed beforehand or are multivariate responses, the easiest and most convenient approach is to perform matching based solely on the descriptive background variables. This results in (hopefully) comparable subpopulation groups. Propensity score methods may prove useful if several variables are to be matched. Unfortunately, matching with more than two groups (that is, with several providers) is often difficult.

A common approach is to adjust using regression techniques. The drawback to these techniques is that they require the outcome variable to be fixed beforehand, as the adjustment requires modelling for each outcome separately. The problem with regression-based adjustment is that it distorts the reality reflected in the observed data by converting the numbers to predictions given by a model that is designed to eliminate uninteresting variation from the outcome. Crudely, the intuitive idea in such adjustment is to do the comparison by treating similar patients in each provider using the model.

The standard approach in such modelling is to calculate the predicted values given by the model for the providers and compare observed versus predicted ratio. Logistic regression can be used for the binary outcomes and other generalized linear models (GLMs) for other types of outcomes. For example, costs are commonly modelled using GLMs with gamma distribution and logarithmic link function. Time-to-event analyses are more difficult to perform with an observed versus predicted technique.

When the different providers are concerned, it is easy to claim that there is a hierarchical structure that should be taken into account in comparisons, that is, that patients treated by the same provider might be somehow correlated. As a possible solution, hierarchical multilevel models have been suggested (Ash, Schwartz & Peköz, 2003), but in practice the use of complicated models may be out of the question because they are demanding and require an analyst to be responsive in the case of (common) convergence problems while estimating hundreds or thousands of models.

3.6 Examples of efficiency considerations

In efficiency analyses, the main interest is typically the connection between inputs and outputs, and often the connection between costs and outcomes. With register-based data, some outcome indicators are available, but as described earlier, costs are not usually directly observed, but rather, are only approximations calculated on the basis of the observed resource use. For example, if we consider the care episode for hip fracture patients, we know that that there are two main components contributing to costs: the surgery-related costs and the costs of follow-up care. However, often only the normative or expected costs are available.

From the Finnish data, we can observe the DRG group of the performed procedure as well as the actual procedure code. Based on the detailed costing data from one hospital district, we estimated the expected costs for each combination. These surgery costs are not the real costs of any single surgery, but estimated average costs of the same types of surgery. Although the DRG-based prices contain all of the acute surgery-related costs, they do not reflect differences in follow-up care including rehabilitation. Therefore, we also calculated the costs of all observed inpatient treatment and outpatient visits to hospitals. We know the level of care and the actual institution and can attach average prices for that type of care for each day to calculate the per diem costs. In the Finnish data, the costs of medication purchases are also available and we can include those that are relevant for the current disease group. Summing up the procedure, per diem costs and other observed costs result in estimated total costs. It is obvious that these costs are only approximations as they are nothing but weighted sums of observed resource use. As we are using averages, all individual-level costs are actually incorrect, but at the group level costs are fair approximations of costs. In actuality, this reflects the fact that costs are often less objective or observable measures than commonly thought (see Chapter 4).

Among hip fracture patients in Finland, there is only a small correlation between costs and outcomes. This may well be the case, but we must remember that in the conceptual sense the use of all observed care to calculate costs in a way is mixed up with the observed outcome, which is also an observable event of care history. So, in reality, such analyses may not get at the input–output relationship we are interested in when looking at efficiency analyses.

It may also be interesting to model the contribution of certain provider-specific factors to outcomes as a way to better understand provider efficiency. One potentially interesting factor could be the connection between the volume and outcomes of the provider. In the case of a hip fracture, the most obvious choice is to consider how the volume of hip fracture surgeries is related to outcomes. This could potentially provide an indication of allocative efficiency (AE) if policymakers are trying to decide whether it is better to allocate resources for hip fracture surgery to certain providers (that is, those with greater experience), or whether experience is not a major factor determining health outcomes.

Somewhat surprisingly, the hip fracture surgery volume was not associated with better or worse outcomes in Finland (Sund, 2010). However, when the volume of hip fracture patients at rehabilitation units was considered, statistically significant volume relation was found: in units where >25 hip fracture patients per year were rehabilitated, their outcomes were better (Figure 3.6). The actual reasons can only be speculated on, but are likely related to greater experience in hip fracture treatment among these providers.

Figure 3.6 *Association between the volume of the rehabilitation unit and mortality among Finnish hip fracture patients aged ≥65 years living at home before the fracture in 1998–2001*

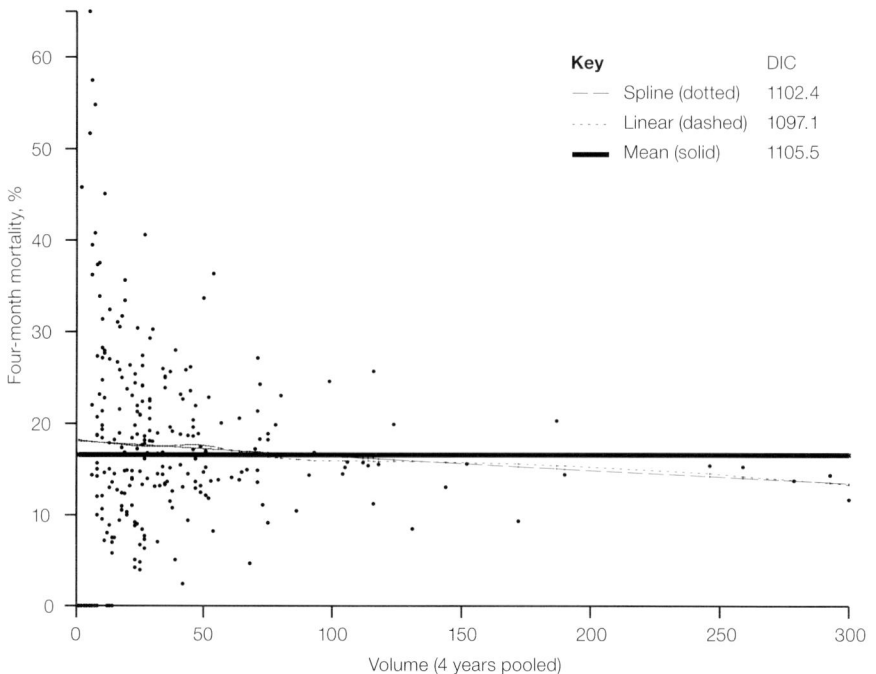

Notes: The x-axis represents the volume of the pooled number of treated hip fracture patients in a rehabilitation unit during 1998–2001 in Finland, and the y-axis represents the four-month risk-adjusted mortality. The dots represent the rehabilitation units (*n*=272). The solid line is the trend from the mean model, the dashed line is the trend from the linear model and the dotted line is the trend from the spline model. DIC = deviance information criterion.

3.7 International comparisons

The approach outlined in this chapter to construct episodes of care has worked very well in Finland. As applied through the PERFormance, Effectiveness, and Costs of Treatment episodes (PERFECT) project, this method produced hospital and district indicators annually for several conditions (Häkkinen, 2011). Implementation of such register-based performance evaluation systems requires – in addition to the availability of comprehensive data and methodological understanding – a multidisciplinary approach. Specific health system knowledge is essential for deciding the scope and specific questions to be addressed, and must be supplemented with clear understanding of the possibilities and limitations of register information. Clinical knowledge is needed when appraising details of the indication and management of a disease, and economic, epidemiological, statistical and data processing expertise are required to ensure that the methodology is appropriate. All of the expertise must be integrated during the entire process.

The whole analysis procedure has been extended to international performance monitoring in the European Union (EU)-funded European Health Care Outcomes, Performance and Efficiency (EuroHOPE) project (Häkkinen et al., 2013, 2015a). EuroHOPE is the first project to concretely map the possibilities to perform register-based performance monitoring in several European countries in a comparable way, that is, by allowing international comparisons in addition to national comparisons. Another pioneering project that has examined the possibilities to extend a similar approach to longer follow-up of diabetes patients in an international context is the EuroREACH diabetes case study.

3.8 The EuroHOPE project

In the EuroHOPE project (Häkkinen et al., 2013, 2015a), an international comparative database was constructed that allows performance indicators to be calculated at national, regional and hospital levels for several different disease groups (Figure 3.7). In the EuroHOPE project, the performance indicators were developed in collaboration with clinical experts in the different disease groups, and with experts in health economics, epidemiology and statistics.

The disease-based approach requires patient-level data covering the whole population and the possibility to deterministically link records from different national registers. In the seven countries (Finland, Hungary, Italy, the Netherlands, Norway, Scotland and Sweden) included in the EuroHOPE project, it was possible to link national hospital discharge registers with mortality registers and with registers of medicines prescribed. In Italy, similar data were available for two geographical areas. All databases present population data that reflect patterns of care and outcomes for the entire population residing in the defined territories.

Figure 3.7 *The EuroHOPE international comparative database*

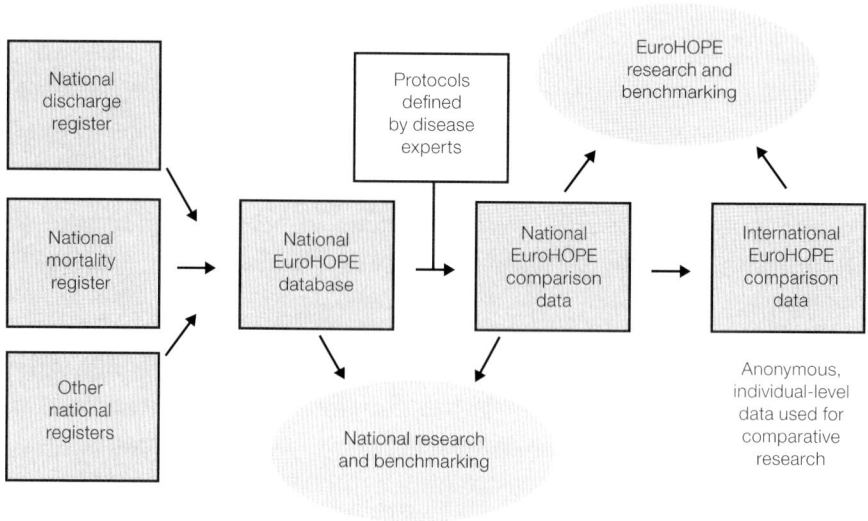

Source: Häkkinen et al. (2013)

The EuroHOPE project followed the ideas of the PERFECT project so that database creation was based on several general stages: 1) define the patient population; 2) collect the register material for the relevant patient population; 3) define the start and end of the episode (by defining and using the index admission and deciding how referrals should be treated) for the patients from the available variables concerning the care given; 4) check the history and follow-up on the use of health care services to define state and time variables for each patient; 5) construct the comorbidity variables; 6) calculate the direct health care costs; and finally, 7) combine the information from the previous stages to generate the comparison database.

This can be very challenging in an international context because of variations across data sources and differences in health system structures and practices. It may be extremely difficult to find compromises that work in each country and allow for cross-country comparability.

Also, in the estimation of the risk adjustment models, even after the standardized definition and data collection, a complication arises from the involvement of many different countries. Ideally, the individual-level data from all participating countries should be pooled before estimating the risk adjustment models, but that is not feasible because not all countries allow individual-level data to be shared because of privacy regulations. To avoid such problems, parameter estimates for the confounding factors are first estimated for every process or outcome measure using the broadest possible pooled data for each disease. Then, the coefficients of each model are made available to all partners who then calculate individual-level-predicted values for the indicators. The predicted values are then summed up at the country and regional level. The ratio of observed and the predicted value of the dependent variable in the comparable unit can be multiplied by the average value of the indicator in the pooled data to calculate the risk-adjusted indicator (Moger & Peltola, 2014).

In practice, after definitions have been agreed for the required standard form of comparison data, each national partner was individually responsible for producing its own national EuroHOPE comparison data, with the principles stated in the disease-specific study protocols. After this, the partners used a common statistical code which automatically processed the data, extracted the coefficients for the models from the EuroHOPE server and calculated the predicted and risk-adjusted values at all levels. Finally, the descriptive statistics along with the country-, regional- and hospital-level indicators and their confidence intervals were automatically transferred to a reporting template.

Figure 3.8 illustrates the regional-level variation in one-year mortality in the seven countries (EuroHOPE study group, 2014). For five countries, it was possible to pool individual-level data and, using a more sophisticated methodology (multilevel modelling), analyse the hospital-level variation in 30-day survival and the cost of the first hospital episodes, as well as the relationship between the measures, that is, the existence of cost–quality trade-off (Häkkinen et al., 2015b). Generally, the study did not find a positive correlation in the pooled analysis and in the separate country-level analysis. The only exception was Sweden where an increase of cost from €5000 to €20 000 was associated with an increase in 30-day survival from 90% to almost 100% (Figure 3.9). Further research could assess whether such spending increases provide good value for money.

Figure 3.8 *Age- and sex-adjusted one-year mortality by region, hip fracture*

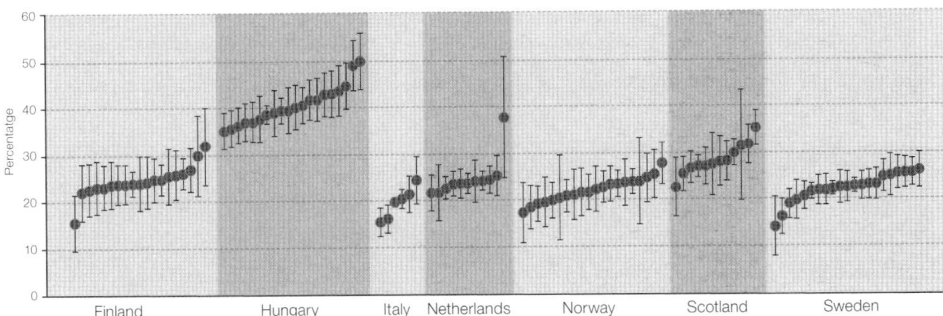

Source: EuroHOPE study group (2014).

Figure 3.9 *Relationship between cost and 30-day survival among hip fracture patients in Sweden in 2007–2008*

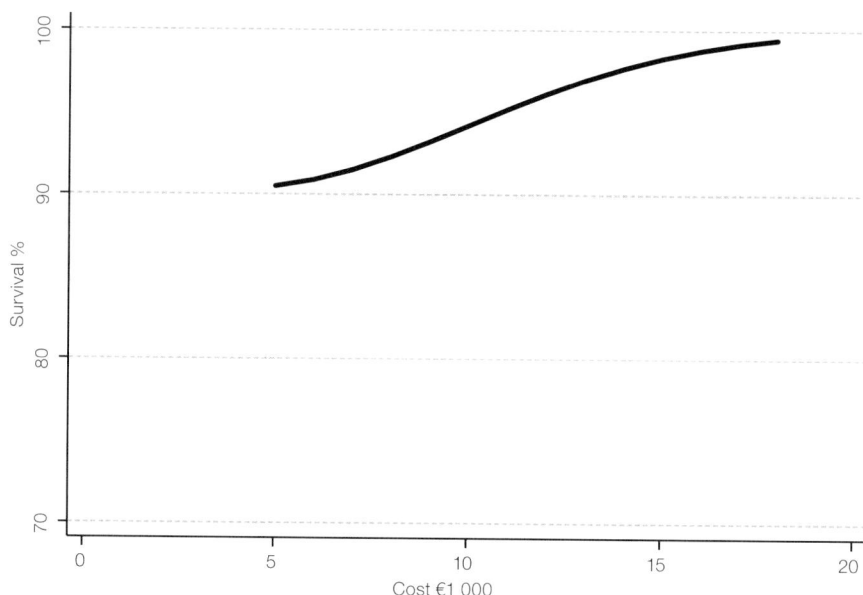

Source: Häkkinen et al. (2015b)

3.9 The EuroREACH diabetes case study

The EuroHOPE project showed that disease-based, risk-adjusted performance monitoring using register data is feasible in the international context, and several countries already have the necessary data. The focus was on the definition of the care episode and related processes and outcomes. As discussed, such an approach works well for disorders that have a clear beginning and relatively short acute phase so that it becomes feasible to see the main outcomes with relatively short follow-up times; hip fracture is again an example of such a condition.

There are, however, other diseases with a chronic course, and it would be interesting to see what can be done in the international context with the approach used in the EuroHOPE project. In the EuroREACH project, a case study for diabetes was conducted. One possible approach would have been to collect data on all persons with diabetes in a certain year, but that would have been problematic since comparisons would have been between very heterogeneous populations in varying disease states. Therefore, it was decided that a more appropriate and novel approach would be to follow a newly diagnosed diabetic cohort for a longer time period. This would show how recently diagnosed persons with diabetes are treated in the long term. Here the episode of care is much longer and less detailed than in acute diseases, but it may tell even more about the structural differences in treatment practices between different countries.

Three countries participated in the case study: Estonia, Finland and Israel (Kiivet et al., 2013). A structured study protocol and detailed data specifications were developed to generate standardized data sets in each country, for the long-term follow-up of an incident cohort of diabetic persons. It was not easy to agree on the definitions to be used, because the limitations and common properties of the data had to be carefully evaluated as the raw data were so different in each country: reimbursement data were used in Estonia; administrative register data in Finland; and very comprehensive electronic patient record data in Israel. Some compromises had to be made, but it was still possible to set certain standards.

In practice, a standardized common data format was defined. Common data definitions required expertise and (tacit) knowledge about the details and possibilities of the data (that is, persons who have used the data) for defining the care episodes.

The only feasible way to identify an incident diabetic cohort in a standardized way from these data sources was to determine the persons who had initiated their antidiabetic medication at the index year. This does not completely correspond to the clinical definition of the incident diabetes population, but it is the best approximation available and suitable for health system-specific comparisons. Analyses were conducted using the shared statistical programs on standardized data sets, so the results reflect the actual differences rather than unknown methodological details as in meta-analyses.

The case study showed that several clinically important aspects of quality of care as well as cost–effectiveness and health system efficiency can be assessed with the national administrative health data systems. By working with actual patient-level data it was possible to refine the existing indicators of performance and quality of care of diabetes and even propose some new ones, such as regular use of medication and event-free time from the start of diabetes treatment (Table 3.1). This stepwise, decentralized approach and use of anonymous person-level data allowed us to mitigate any legal, ownership, confidentiality and privacy concerns and create internationally comparative data with the extent of detail that has seldom been seen before (Kiivet et al., 2013).

Table 3.1 *Selected outcomes and service measures as provided to diabetes patients during eight years of follow-up*

	Year 1	Year 2	Year 3	Year 4	Year5	Year 6	Year 7	Year 8
Study population alive at the end of year (%)								
Estonia	96%	93%	89%	86%	82%	79%	75%	72%
Finland	98%	95%	92%	89%	86%	83%	80%	78%
Israel	98%	96%	94%	92%	90%	88%	86%	83%
Hospitalized for myocardial infarction, males 45-64, rate per 1000 per year								
Estonia	16	13	12	23	9	15	19	12
Finland	5	8	6	8	6	6	6	5
Israel	6	6	8	7	4	8	5	3
Revascularization, males 45-64, rate per 1000 per year								
Estonia	26	10	20	27	20	24	27	26
Finland	11	10	11	12	11	11	11	9
Israel	12	10	8	3	10	6	3	2
Stroke, females over 65. rate per 1000 per year								
Estonia	25	31	21	16	27	26	27	31
Finland	23	28	21	23	16	19	20	21
Israel	2	3	3	5	6	6	5	2
Proportion of patients using insulin at the end of year								
Estonia	14%	15%	17%	21%	24%	27%	31%	32%
Finland	15%	14%	16%	18%	21%	25%	28%	31%
Israel	9%	7%	8%	9%	11%	14%	16%	19%
Proportion of patients using statins at the end of year								
Estonia	6%	7%	9%	11%	13%	16%	20%	23%
Finland	32%	37%	41%	44%	48%	51%	54%	55%
Israel	53%	57%	63%	68%	71%	73%	74%	75%

4.0 Conclusions

In this chapter, we have described a register-based approach for the evaluation of health system performance. As the examples show, the approach can lead to valuable information that can be produced more or less routinely from the available data. Doing this requires careful planning, suitable standardization and pre-processing of raw data. This is especially true in the case of international comparisons, where – without careful adjustments – small (or large) differences in seemingly similar data sources may lead to erroneous conclusions. Collaboration between experts from different fields is needed to find suitable compromises for the definitions. Enough time must be preserved for the pre-processing of data to a standardized form, and analyses have to be planned so that privacy regulations will not create problems.

Although performance indicators calculated from registry data do not always directly reflect the specific concept of efficiency, there is great potential going forward. Better cost accounting data that capture individual-level patient care costs would make a major contribution to determining the most efficient allocation of patients between care pathways. In the interim, more work could be done to compare patterns of care and identify those pathways that are relatively less resource intensive but which produce favourable health outcomes for patients.

Because they are produced from secondary data, registry-based performance indicators cannot be optimal for all possible purposes. For example, episodes of care are constructed only for one disease or disorder at a time so that the adjusted indicators reflect the health system-specific component of variation in the outputs. Still, carefully produced information based on register data can be extremely useful – for example, in Finland, the current clinical guidelines for the treatment of hip fractures have been partially evaluated using register-based indicators (Sund et al., 2011). Such use gives some perspective for the quality of the information produced. It truly reflects what is going on in ordinary everyday practice and can reveal important differences between providers or countries.

As data sources are gradually improving in many countries, it is only a matter of time when register-based monitoring systems will be a part of routine reporting and follow-up of the performance, effectiveness and efficiency of providers.

References

Ash AS, Schwartz M, Peköz EA (2003). Comparing outcomes across providers. In: Iezzoni LI, ed. *Risk adjustment for measuring health care outcomes*. 3rd edn. Chicago, IL, Health Administration Press.

Cashin C et al., eds. (2014). *Paying for performance in health care. Implications for health system performance and accountability*. Maidenhead, Open University Press.

EuroHOPE study group (2014). Summary of the findings of the EuroHope project (http://www.eurohope.info/, accessed 15 September 2016).

Geue C et al. (2012). Spoilt for choice: implications of using alternative methods of costing hospital episode statistics. *Health Economics*, 21(10):1201–1216.

Häkkinen U (2011). The PERFECT project: measuring performance of health care episodes. *Annals of Medicine*, 43(Suppl. 1):S1–S3.

Häkkinen U, Joumard I (2007). Cross-country analysis of efficiency in OECD health care sectors: options for research. Economics Department Working Papers, No. 554. Paris, OECD Publishing.

Häkkinen U et al. (2013). Health care performance comparison using a disease-based approach: the EuroHOPE project. *Health Policy*, 112(1–2):100–109.

Häkkinen U et al. (2014). Quality, cost, and their trade-off in treating AMI and stroke patients in European hospitals. *Health Policy*, 117(1):15–27.

Häkkinen U et al. (2015a). Towards explaining international differences in health care performance: Results of the EuroHOPE Project. *Health Economics*, 24(Suppl. S2): 1–4.

Häkkinen U et al. (2015b). Outcome, use of resources and their relationship in the treatment of AMI, stroke and hip fracture at European hospitals. *Health Economics*, 24(Suppl. S2):116–139.

Iversen T et al. (2015). Comparative analysis of treatment costs in EuroHOPE. *Health Economics*, 24(Suppl. S2):5–22.

Kiivet R et al. (2013). Methodological challenges in international performance measurement using patient-level administrative data. *Health Policy*,112(1–2):110–121.

Moger TA, Peltola M (2014). Risk adjustment of health-care performance measures in a multinational register-based study: a pragmatic approach to a complicated topic. *SAGE Open Medicine*, 2: 2050312114526589.

OECD (2013). Strengthening health information infrastructure for health care quality governance. *Good practices, new opportunities and data privacy protection challenges*. Paris, OECD Publishing.

OECD (2015). Health data governance. Privacy, monitoring and research. OECD Health Policy Studies. Paris, OECD Publishing.

Peltola M et al. (2011). A methodological approach for register-based evaluation of cost and outcomes in health care. *Annals of Medicine*, 43(Suppl. 1):S4–S13.

Shani M (2000). The impact of information on medical thinking and health care policy. *International Journal of Medical Informatics*, 58–59:3–10.

Sund R (2003). Utilisation of administrative registers using scientific knowledge discovery. *Intelligent Data Analysis*, 7(6):501–519.

Sund R (2010). Modeling the volume-effectiveness relationship in the case of hip fracture treatment in Finland. *BMC Health Services Research*, 10:238.

Sund R et al. (2011). Monitoring the performance of hip fracture treatment in Finland. *Annals of Medicine*, 43(Suppl. 1):S39 –S46.

Sund R et al. (2014). Use of health registers. In: Ahrens W, Pigeot I, eds. *Handbook of epidemiology*. 2nd edn. Berlin, Springer-Verlag.

Chapter 4

Management accounting and efficiency in health services: the foundational role of cost analysis

Christopher S. Chapman, Anja Kern, Aziza Laguecir and Wilm Quentin

4.1 Introduction

Efficiency measurement is concerned with measuring and analysing inputs in relation to outputs or vice versa. Management accounting offers a broad set of tools and techniques for measuring and managing many aspects of this challenge. Rising health care costs, driven by population growth, demographic shifts and advances in medical technology, put the focus on cost analysis and management because cost information underpins decisions on resource allocation and effectiveness at system and organizational levels for providers, purchasers and regulators globally. In this chapter, we focus on costing because cost information feeds into many other common management accounting practices, such as tariff setting, targeted cost improvement plans, benchmarking, budgeting, service redesign and performance management.

The peculiarities of the nature of health care as an area of activity have very specific implications for the scope and nature of cost accounting. First, health care in most countries is a heavily regulated sector, and this regulation has a direct impact on definitions of costing, that is, how costing is carried out, including the calculation itself, but also linked concepts such as the kind of cost object that becomes a focus for analysis. For example, regulations on payment of hospitals on the basis of DRGs has made the DRG the major cost object in the acute sector, in turn having an impact on the costing calculation and medical practice (Chapman, Kern & Laguecir, 2014).

A second impact of the nature of health care on costing practice derives from the fact that treatment must often be adjusted for each patient; therefore, patient-level costing should account for differences between patients. However, the share of total cost that can be directly attributed to patients is relatively small. Studies suggest that the direct variable costs that can be directly influenced by physicians are around 42% (Taheri, Butz & Greenfield, 2000) with 58% of fixed and indirect costs[1] being out of reach of physicians' responsibility. Similarly, studies on hospital cost structure have emphasized the high proportion of fixed costs in this setting, reaching 65%, thus making it difficult for front-line staff to actually manage costs (or more precisely, short-run cash flows) at patient level (Roberts et al., 1999). A volume-based allocation of indirect costs is not appropriate for supporting cost management at the patient-level, which instead requires an activity-based approach. An activity-based approach also allows linking costs with health outcomes in a meaningful way (Kaplan & Porter, 2011).

A third impact arises from the fact that there is high pressure to improve the efficiency of health care services while keeping quality at the same level, the aim being the generation of more benefits from the current levels of spending. As a result, the number of users for costing data has increased, now ranging from government and regulators at national or regional level, to health care professions, insurers, health care providers, patients and the general public. This unusually wide range of users makes it difficult to adjust the nature of calculations to the potentially different purposes and interests of these users (Smith et al., 2008).

Perhaps this diversity helps to explain why, despite a growth in the reach and complexity of costing in recent years, progress has been hampered by a tendency towards a lack of conceptual clarity over the costing methodologies appropriate to particular kinds of purposes and decision-making objectives (Chapman, Kern & Laguecir, 2014). Recent developments have shown far greater attention to the detailed task of costing. Costing has been recognized by policymakers as the key for improving the quality of evaluation of health care services. The kind of costing in place does not only directly influence the accuracy of the tariff, but also how health care can be managed (Monitor, 2014a). The rapid development of patient-level information and costing systems also shows the recognition that cost data must sit alongside other patient information (including comorbidities and outcomes). Making this link helps raise the stakes of analysis to include effectiveness beyond efficiency (Kaplan & Porter, 2011).

However, before costing can live up to such expectations, we must first address the widely noted concern over the variability and quality of existing cost information (Busse, Schreyögg & Smith, 2008; Busse et al., 2011; Chapman et al., 2013; Monitor, 2006, 2013; Northcott & Llewellyn 2004). In fact, many countries find it difficult to produce high-quality costing data (Busse, Schreyögg & Smith, 2008; Busse et al., 2011). Analysis of health care costs across countries has revealed that the cost structure behind a certain procedure or treatment varies significantly from one country to another and between providers within countries.

---

1 In this article the terms indirect costs and overhead costs are used interchangeably. We argue that it is not the location where costs are incurred (e.g. medical or administrative areas) that is decisive for cost system design, but rather their relation to cost objects. The relation of costs to the cost object determines if costs are direct or indirect costs.

Table 4.1 shows the analysis of costs for a single procedure (AMI) across countries as analysed by Tiemann and colleagues (2008). Particularly notable variances are ward costs, which vary between 9.76% in Denmark and 74.55% in the Netherlands, with corresponding changes to the level of overheads reported in each of these countries. While variations in medical practices across countries can be at the origin of differences, there are significant differences caused by variations in costing methods and conventions as to what is classed in which category of cost.

Poor-quality cost data – whether in terms of unexplained sources of variance or inappropriate disguising of variance through excessive reliance on averages – are a threat to the delivery of efficient and effective health care. Poor-quality data will not be used in decision-making (or will not be effective if used) while resources will be consumed in producing it. Towards the end of the chapter we offer a detailed discussion of the kinds of efficiency decisions that high-quality cost data might inform. However, given the centrality of cost system design to the production of data that can be used in decision-making, we will address this crucial issue first.

Table 4.1 *Costs in different cost categories for AMI*

	England	France	Germany	Hungary	Italy	Netherlands	Poland	Spain	Denmark[a]
Diagnostic procedures	€345.74	€446.79	€296.84	€70.43	€316.97	€349.71	€138.19	€349.52	€349.52
As % of total costs	6.90%	7.55%	10.36%	17.79%	4.25%	6.25%	13.47%	18.78%	7.53%
Normal ward/catheter lab									
As % of total costs	31.40%	46.45%	58.63%	35.34%	41.48%	74.66%	48.14%	53.67%	9.76%
Physician	€217.20	€614.43	€356.80	€67.95	€406.04	€316.86	€212.46	€167.67	€76.79
Nursing	€644.79	€683.56	€782.29	€71.98	€375.10	€2121.49	€210.42	€831.09	€117.67
Others	€90.51	€136.77	€50.32	[b]	€22.18	€209.02	€70.92	[b]	€34.54
Materials	€621.65	€1313.46	€491.26	[b]	€2286.91	€1533.33	[b]	[b]	€224.17
Drugs	€1556.36	€1347.82	€164.97	€89.20	€696.36	€424.28	€189.26	€29.83	€10.78
As % of total costs	31.04%	22.78%	5.76%	22.53%	9.35%	7.58%	18.45%	1.60%	0.23%
Overheads	€1537.39	€1373.62	€723.89	€96.40	€3346.66	€644.61	€204.52	€482.91	€3829.73
As % of total costs	30.66%	23.22%	25.25%	24.35%	44.92%	11.51%	19.94%	25.95%	82.48%
Total cost	**€5013.64**	**€5916.45**	**€2866.36**	**€395.97**	**€7450.22**	**€5599.30**	**€1025.76**	**€1861.02**	**€4643.20**
Total costs (PPP-adjusted)	**€4646.51**	**€5507.93**	**€2723.07**	**€657.14**	**€7251.03**	**€5322.83**	**€1863.61**	**€2050.18**	**€3455.00**
Reimbursement	**€4351.00**	**€5731.06**	**€3113.96**	**€808.86**	**€7574.58**	**€8722.00**	**€932.50**	[c]	[c]
Profit	-€662.64	-€185.39	€247.60	€412.89	€124.36	€3122.70	-€93.26	[c]	[c]
Profit margin	-13.22%	-3.13%	8.64%	104.27%	1.67%	55.77%	-9.09%	[c]	[c]

Sources: Table II in Tiemann (2008).
Notes: [a]Partly subsumed in overhead costs. [b]Subsumed in overhead costs. [c]No data available. AMI = acute myocardial infarction; PPP = purchasing power parity.

4.2 Analysing the challenge of cost system design

In thinking about the fundamental steps required in attaching the elements of organizational cost to a particular cost object (such as a patient), there are three basic analytical steps that must be taken:

1. The costing system needs to identify and group together the costs of the various types of resources that the organization has (for example, clinical staff, drugs, premises).
2. Resource costs need to be grouped into cost pools (based around departments or other managerial cost centres, or activities) for which choices are made as to the cost driver for the cost pool.
3. Costs have to be linked (showing more or less variability depending on the choices made) to the chosen cost object (for example, the patient, the service line, and so on).

Choices must be made as to the level of granularity in each of these three steps and there is no single universally best approach to making these choices. Partly this is a result of the many different purposes towards which cost data might be put (for example, price setting, cost management, resource allocation). Partly this is a result of the trade-off to be struck between rising costs as granularity increases set against the possibility of better decisions such granularity may or may not offer. In considering this, it is vital to understand that granularity is not simply a function of the granularity of the cost object (step 3), but also of granularity choices made in the first two steps. Also, while we have separated these steps for the purposes of conceptual clarity, in practice many of these decisions are interdependent and taken simultaneously.

4.2.1 Step 1: determining the granularity of costs at resource level

Based on the chart of accounts (that is, a listing of the accounts found in the general ledger of an organization), costs are most typically grouped according to the kind of costs they represent, such as salaries or materials. The way the chart of accounts is constructed significantly influences the detail that is available for costing. For example, instead of simply dealing with salaries as an overarching category, there can be a detailed breakdown of the salaries of nurses, clinicians, technicians, administrative staff, and so on. In addition, the chart of accounts may allow for the separation of salaries for certain grade levels.

The structure of the chart of accounts and its details therefore greatly influence the detail and nature of costs that are readily available for the costing calculation undertaken in steps 2 and 3. Further detail can always be added to that made available through the chart of accounts if detailed ad hoc analysis is undertaken, but this is costly to produce and maintain accurately, and so cost system design relies heavily on the structure of the chart of accounts. This is not always to its benefit given that often the chart of accounts is structured with external financial reporting in mind (Johnson & Kaplan, 1987).

With this concern in mind, it is quite common for the chart of accounts to introduce relevant notions of cost behaviour in terms of differentiating between fixed (costs that do not change with the level of output) and variable (costs that change with the level of output) costs in relation to specific resources being mapped. This kind of distinction can feed into ad hoc analysis of marginal cost changes in relation to service redesign decisions and the application of a set of basic management accounting techniques comprising cost–volume–profit analysis. The strength of this framing of cost behaviour is that it quickly and easily allows the modelling of short-run cash flows, something that is both important and intuitively appealing as a matter of concern to a wide range of stakeholders.

The limitations of a fixed and variable framing of cost behaviour are particularly pressing in areas such as health care where a large proportion of cost is fixed. Such a framing can help bring about a relative inattention to fixed costs, even creating a sense that such costs are inevitable. However, even when attention is directed towards fixed costs, under such a framing the approach offers little support for capacity planning and management. Both of these factors can easily lead to a lack of control of fixed costs and inefficient use of them.

Management accounting offers the distinction between direct (costs that can be logically linked to a cost object) and indirect (costs that cannot) costs to address these limitations. In relation to fixed and variable costs, a variable cost is in principle direct. A fixed cost may or may not be. The fixed cash flow cost of a clinician's salary can still be direct in relation to the time spent with different patients, for example. However, the fixed cash flow cost of premises is indirect.

DRG tariff structures are often based on the full cost of specific treatments. Full cost is made up of the direct costs of the treatment and an appropriate share of indirect costs, such that ultimately if all reported treatment costs are added up, the total is the total cost of the provider organization. The central choice to be made is how to determine what an appropriate share of indirect costs is. There are two main alternatives here: volume-based allocation and an activity-based approach.

Traditional volume-based absorption costing assumes that indirect costs are fixed and can be allocated identically to each service delivered. However, since an indirect cost cannot logically be linked to a cost object, volume-based allocation is inherently arbitrary and in principle incorrect. In terms of monitoring short-run cash flows, this is not so damaging because the fixed cash flows are assumed to be largely unaffected by different output choices.

The problem with volume-related allocation (which an activity-based approach is designed to remedy) is that while the indirect costs are not related to volume, they are related to *something*. If the costing system does not reflect these actual relationships, then in the medium term there is a risk of promoting behaviours that will inadvertently increase overheads and short-run fixed cash flows. The central argument of activity-based costing is that traditional volume-based allocations systematically overvalue high-volume simple processes and systematically undervalue low-volume complex ones. As a result, such systems encourage more low-volume complex activities that in turn require greater overhead investments to handle the increased complexity. Thus, the risk with volume-related systems is that indirect costs will rise faster than the volume of services (Kaplan & Cooper, 1998).

While the choice between volume-based and activity-based analysis is most commonly thought of in relation to the next step (step 2), it is important to bear in mind that the relative ease of analysing activity costs depends on the structure and granularity of the chart of accounts.

4.2.2 Step 2: determining the granularity of cost pools and cost drivers

This step involves two related choices. The first choice involves the aggregation of resources identified in the chart of accounts into cost pools that form the basic structure of analysis in cost systems. The second choice involves the selection of a cost driver for the resulting cost pools that allows costs to be linked to the chosen cost object (step 3).

The conceptual challenge in terms of direct costs is not great, although capturing the necessary data can be more difficult. The difficulties arise when dealing with indirect costs. In the health care sector, a distinction is often made between indirect costs linked to medical processes (for example, manager of the operating theatre) and overhead costs linked to the indirect costs of the administration (for example, chief executive officer of the hospital or central departments such as accounting, legal department, and so on). When we use the word indirect cost in this chapter, we refer to all non-direct costs because the choices for their treatment are conceptually the same in terms of the visibility of cost behaviour.

Take, for example, a figure for the overall cost of the finance department. This is an indirect cost in the sense that it is a cost whose behaviour we do not easily understand at the patient level and so we are challenged when it comes to choosing an appropriate cost driver. This difficulty arises because the costs of the finance department are an aggregation of many different resource costs (for example, payroll costs of accounting staff, office costs to house them, utilities such as electricity, but also consumables such as paper and computers), which rise and fall in relation to many different factors. Such department-based aggregations are often a matter of practical convenience. As a department, there will likely be an annual budget that groups together all of these resource costs. In terms of authorizing spending, this is useful; however, this aggregation is not helpful for understanding cost behaviour.

By virtue of aggregating so many different kinds of costs into a single figure, there is no single cost driver that offers a clear reflection of what accounts for costs in the finance department. The volume of services offers an intuitive but noisy basis for analysis. At an aggregate level, it is plausible that more patients will to some extent lead to more finance department costs. As soon as we consider individual patients, however, it seems likely that individual patient consumption of finance department resources might vary considerably depending on many different factors, some of which will have nothing to do with patient behaviour.

The alternative to a volume-related allocation is an activity-based costing approach. This would reanalyse departmental costs, breaking them down into cost pools reflecting specific activities (for example, running the payroll, credit control). Once analysed in terms of activities, it becomes possible to understand what drives costs. For example, payroll costs likely depend more on the number of clinical staff than the number of patients (because staff/patient ratios might vary considerably across specialities) suggesting the need for a two-stage approach attributing payroll costs to clinicians first and then to patients. Credit control costs may also display significant differences between specialities depending on particular financing arrangements that may again have very little to do with patient numbers.

Credit control is another high-level activity. Depending on the nature of decisions to be taken, it might be appropriate to break it down into subactivities and to map resources yet in more detail. When it comes to the nature of the cost driver, again choices must be made about granularity. For example, we must decide whether it is sufficient to assume that credit control costs are driven by patient numbers in particular specialities, or whether a more granular analysis of hours spent on particular patient cases is appropriate as a cost driver.

As always, these decisions are a trade-off between the cost of collecting and analysing more granular data over the possibilities for making better decisions in light of it. The distinction between direct and indirect costs is not purely linked to the nature of costs, but also depends on this trade-off between the cost of understanding indirect cost behaviours such that they may be considered direct costs and the benefit of having such direct costs inform decision-making. For example, drugs are in principle a direct cost, in that specific patients consume them. However, depending on the cost of a drug, the cost system may treat it as a direct or indirect cost. If the cost of a drug is relatively high (for example, a high-cost cancer treatment), it may be beneficial to attribute this cost directly to the particular patient. However, if a drug is less expensive (for example, a standard cancer treatment), its cost may be treated effectively as an indirect cost if the cost of analysis outweighs the possibilities of making better decisions on the basis of more refined information. The same choice must be made for staff costs (that is, should they be treated as direct or effectively indirect costs) and at what level of granularity.

In summary, activity-based costing is an approach to attribute resource costs (step 1) to cost objects (step 3), where careful choices are made to link indirect costs to the specific activities that drive them. Activity-based costing is an alternative to volume-related allocation of indirect costs to cost objects (for example, dividing costs across patient numbers). Volume-related allocation sacrifices precision for the sake of simplicity and reduced cost of measurement. In deciding how best to account for indirect costs, it is important to always consider the costs and benefits associated with collecting such data. The question to ask is: Does the effort to transform a particular block of overheads into direct costs through an analysis of activity pay back with regard to the decision-making benefits obtained from such efforts?

4.2.3 Step 3: determining the granularity of the chosen cost object

A costing system can always produce an estimate of the cost of a particular cost object (for example, patient episode, patient, service line, trust). However, depending on the approach taken in the previous steps, this estimate may more or less reflect reality. As such, this final step is potentially the least informative in terms of giving a useful indication of the granularity of a costing system, which in practice derives much more from choices made in the preceding two steps. A key matter in terms of granularity at this level arises more from the degree to which a particular cost represents an average across a particular level of cost object, or shows reliable variability between costs at that level.

This issue is often discussed with regard to top-down and bottom-up costing. Dividing total operating theatre costs by the number of patients to identify a cost attributable to an individual patient is a top-down approach. Aggregating the per-theatre minute costs to arrive at a total per-patient cost is a bottom-up approach that allows visibility of cost variation between patients. To rephrase this distinction, with words that make it more obvious how and why these distinctions matter: a top-down approach is a cheap way to produce average costs.

A bottom-up figure helps to reflect variability of resource consumption across particular cost objects, but it is more expensive to produce.[2]

The development of time-driven activity-based costing (TDABC) (Kaplan & Anderson, 2004) represents a development that can reduce the costs of more flexible and granular analysis using a bottom-up, activity-based approach. The first step is to work out the total cost of relevant resources required by a cost object and determine the level of practical capacity of the resources to provide services. Time in TDABC reflects the observation that for a surprisingly wide range of resources, this is an appropriate unit of capacity. The second step is to charge cost objects with their consumption of capacity at the per-unit cost of capacity worked out in the first step.

An advantage of TDABC is that it simplifies step 2 as undertaken in earlier activity-based costing systems. So, for example, an early activity-based costing system might have aggregated clinical staff costs as a resource (step 1). This would then be split across inpatient and outpatient activities based on consultant job plans (step 2). These costs would then be driven to patients in the inpatient and outpatient areas (step 3). A TDABC approach avoids the need to make a priori assumptions about the split in step 2. When dealing with the activity of people, this is particularly useful since their split across many activities can significantly and frequently vary. TDABC instead works out a per-minute cost of clinical staff time and then builds costs up from the assignment of that cost to minutes spent with inpatients and outpatients. Granularity at step 3 can then be easily adjusted by doing this using estimates, or standard minute rates per activity, or direct measurement depending on the importance of the information in terms of its capacity to inform useful decisions.

4.3 Demonstrating cost system design choices with two detailed examples

To place the various choices and distinctions discussed in the previous section within a more concrete context, next we analyse how these choices play out using two detailed examples chosen for their impact in terms of clinical and financial importance. First, we discuss how these cost system design choices impact on the analysis of costs in the operating theatre, and second how they have an impact on the analysis of property costs. The examples are based on observations of costing practices and national costing guidelines Germany and the United Kingdom.

---

2 Here, we use the terms volume-based and activity-based costing to distinguish two different kinds of treatments of indirect costs. In the literature, other distinctions that are often used synonymously can be found, for example, micro costing and bottom-up costing. These are used synonymously for activity-based costing and macro costing, while top-down costing is often used as synonym for the volume-based allocation of costs.

4.3.1 Tracing operating theatre costs to patients

The operating theatre in an acute care hospital represents a highly significant resource and location of clinical activity. As such, the way in which cost is traced to patients receiving treatment in operating theatres is a matter of considerable importance. As documented in Chapman & Kern (2010) and based on research in the United Kingdom, there is considerable variability to be found in terms of the sophistication of cost system design relating to activity in operating theatres.

The least granular level of cost modelling observed consisted of a single cost pool that assembled all resources assigned to the operating theatres (for example, space costs, clinical staff costs, consumables costs, and so on) with minutes in theatre as a cost driver applied to a single cost pool. This has been mapped out in Table 4.2, which shows this very simple costing approach to operating theatres with resources on the horizontal axis (columns), activities on the vertical axis (rows), and the chosen cost driver at the intersection.

Table 4.2 *A very simple costing approach for operating theatre activity*

	RESOURCES	All costs
ACTIVITIES		
All operating theatres		Per-minute cost

This system gives a per-minute cost rate based on total cost and total minutes across all patients as applied to the minutes of a particular patient on the operating theatre register. The cost driver *minutes* seems activity-based and the cost object is the patient, so this may lead to the belief that this is a patient-level, activity-based approach to costing. However, the problem is that the choice of cost pools is *not* activity-based and there is a minimum possible granularity with regard to activity and resource analysis (although the cost driver shows at least more granularity than simply patient numbers would have given). Hence this cost calculation is closer to a volume-based then an activity-based approach.

At the next level of sophistication, we encountered an intermediate level of cost model granularity. This arose when providers had multiple operating theatres, and we found that individual theatres were often used for particular clinical specialities. This allowed for the construction of individual operating theatre cost pools that collected the various costs of the procedures undertaken in each particular theatre. As a result, the system could reflect the potentially very different costs for staff (for example, because of very different staffing levels for particular kinds of procedures) within different specialities resulting in different per-minute costs for the different operating theatres. We have mapped this approach in Table 4.3.

Table 4.3 *An elaboration of the very simple costing approach for operating theatre activity*

ACTIVITIES	RESOURCES	All costs for theatre 1	All costs for theatre 2	All costs for theatre 3
Operating theatre for speciality 1		Per-minute cost		
Operating theatre for speciality 2			Per-minute cost	
Operating theatre for speciality 3				Per-minute cost

As in the simple model, the cost object is the patient, and again there is little granularity at the resource level where all kinds of resources are grouped together. It is more granular than that seen in the previous model (Table 4.2) given that there is a cost centre-based grouping of resource costs. The lack of resource granularity makes it difficult to differentiate between resources like clinician time and nurse time, however. As such, when it comes to developing a more granular set of cost pools to map the resources onto, there is little to go on. And so we find a cost system that produces three separate cost-per-minute rates that can be traced to patients in the three different specialities. Overall however, the level of granularity is still very low.

At the most sophisticated level we encountered a cost system that distinguished resources and activities at a far more granular level. Such an approach also mirrors the detail of the costing approach to be found in the InEK Kalkulationshandbuch (DKG, 2007) used in Germany. We map an example of this approach in Table 4.4.

This properly reflects an activity-based approach because it shifts from treating the operating theatre as a single, departmental-based cost pool to one in which the operating theatre is understood as a location where many different (and separately costed) activities take place, each of which draws on particular subsets of resources. As discussed in Section 4.2, once these activities are identified, the next step is to understand what drives the cost incurred in carrying them out.

Table 4.4 shows how for each activity a relationship between the activity and the consumed resources is established, depending on the practicalities of data collection. In some cases, this leads to charging a standard rate, for example, for preparing the theatre. In other cases, the consumed resources are related to an activity on the basis of a cost driver, such as time. Anaesthetic drugs, for example, are charged on the basis of the length of time the patient is anaesthetized. The data for the time when anaesthetized are available in the system and can be retrieved easily. Costs for nurses take into account the number of nurses present, which can also be captured in the system. However, as it is too complicated to include the actual staff cost for each particular nurse, a standard charge rate is applied for each nurse. For senior clinicians, the actual staff cost is assigned to the session, while for juniors it is again a standard charge rate.

In this last model, the cost objects are again patients. In contrast to the simple and intermediate costing models, however, this activity-based model identifies the activities in the operating theatre and cost drivers for each activity with considerably more granularity. Therefore, it produces more accurate costs than the simple and intermediate model. This is important, for example, when setting tariffs and represents a significant improvement in accuracy when using actual patient costs to do DRG costing. Another equally, if not more, important benefit is in terms of the enhanced opportunities this kind of granular information offers for managers who are considering the efficiency and effectiveness of clinical activities.

Table 4.4 *Much more granular costing of operating theatre activity*

	RESOURCES Nurses	Clinicians	Technicians	Drugs	Transplants	Other consumables
ACTIVITIES						
Preparing the operating theatre	Cost per minute (standard rate)	Cost per minute	Costs per minute			Itemized list of consumables
Anaesthetic activity	Cost per minute of nurse time	Cost per minute		Amount of drugs consumed		Itemized list of consumables
Operation	Skin-to-knife time (standard rate)	Cost per minute based on skin-to-knife time	Cost per minute based on skin-to-knife time	Amount of drugs consumed	Costs for specific transplant	Itemized list of consumables
Clean up after theatre use	Cost per minute (standard rate)					Itemized list of consumables
Recovery of the patient	Cost per minute (standard rate)					Itemized list of consumables

Source: Based on DKG (2007), p. 239.
Note: Empty cells reflect an activity for which a resource is not used.

4.3.2 Tracing estate costs through to patients

In the preceding discussion, we largely focused on a range of resources and activities that were relatively easily linked to patient activity. A significant portion of organizational costs is made up of indirect costs (overheads, support, infrastructure), which are more complicated to link to patients. In this section, we present the additional challenges of dealing with these kinds of costs in terms of granularity of cost system design taking the example of estate or property costs.

Perhaps the simplest way to deal with estate costs would be to adopt a minimum granularity, a top-down, volume-based approach. Such an approach would divide the total estate costs across the number of departments (service lines, points of delivery), and then from there allocate costs onto patients within each of those service lines. This is not likely to be particularly accurate, but the costs of such an approach to costing are low. The most obvious cost driver here, and what is mandated in many jurisdictions in their costing guidance, is to use a space measure, such as square metres of space occupied, as the basis to attribute estate costs to cost centres/service lines.

However, there is considerable variability in the level of guidance in different jurisdictions with regard to the level of granularity with which this broad approach is to be applied. As a result, the treatment of property costs across organizations can be irregular. The model shown in Table 4.5 would be the simplest possible that is still consistent with the regulation.

Table 4.5 *A very simple costing approach for property overheads*

DEPARTMENTS	RESOURCES	All costs
All departments		Square metres

A more granular approach is shown in Table 4.6; here, variation that is cost driven by different space use starts to become apparent.

Table 4.6 *Beginning to distinguish cost behaviour in more detail*

DEPARTMENTS	RESOURCES	Rent / light / heating	Cleaning / infection control
Medical		Square metres	Square metres
Administrative		Square metres	Square metres

The question remains, however, of how to link property costs to actual patients. If estate costs at the cost centre or service line level (for example, in the operating theatre) are divided by the number of operations or patients, it will correspond to a top-down, volume-based costing approach. Even if the first step was a bottom-up, activity-based costing approach, through this second step, the calculation turns into a top-down, volume-based calculation. If, however, property costs are attributed to patients based on minutes spent in the operating theatre, it remains a bottom-up, activity-based costing.

Table 4.7 shows the bottom-up, activity-based approach used to account for estate costs in the German costing standards. As a first step, estate costs are accounted for on a specified indirect cost centre (department). Then, the costs for services between cost centres are calculated. Property costs are attributed to cost centres according to square metres of used surface. Then, estate costs are allocated in a last step from direct cost centres to patients on the basis of activity cost drivers. Through these activity cost drivers, a kind of cause-and-effect relationship between estate costs and patient is established. The level of granularity underpinning this calculation (for example, separating clinical estate costs from administrative estate costs and disaggregating estate costs according to each clinical area) affects the ability to accurately explain variations in patient costs.

Table 4.7 *List of cost drivers to link estate costs with patients in the German costing standards for providers informing the tariff*

DEPARTMENT PROCESSES	RESOURCES Property costs traced to department
Ward	Days of care
ICU	Hours of intensive care
Dialysis	Weighted dialysis according to different kinds of dialysis
Operating theatre	Knife-to-skin time with set-up time
Anaesthesia	Time of anaesthesia: taking over of the patient with set-up
Delivery room	Time of the patient in delivery room
Endoscopic diagnostics	Time of intervention (points according to the service catalogue)
Radiology	Points according to the service catalogue
Laboratory	Points according to the service catalogue
Other diagnostic and therapeutic areas	Points according to the service catalogue

Source: Based on DKG (2007), p. 239.
Note: ICU = intensive care unit.

4.3.3 Hybrid cost systems in practice

Given the variety of costing methods and the wide range of possible levels of granularity discussed, the question arises as to what best practice of costing in health care is. This question can be answered by considering the ultimate objective of clinical costing from a management point of view: to make costs transparent. While in principle this objective can be obtained with all methods, variations in patient costs are more easily and accurately identified using an activity-based costing approach. Further, activity-based, patient-level information allows for more appropriate links between cost and health outcomes, which are essential for evaluating services in health care (Kaplan & Witkowski, 2014). However, the difficulties (and costs) of achieving activity-based costing are greater than for volume-based allocation.

In practice, costing approaches are dominated by regulatory requirements for DRGs as a basis for tariff setting; this is subject to widely varied sophistication, detail and constancy of guidance internationally. However, given the trade-off between the cost of cost analysis and the quality of cost information, it is not surprising that, in practice, costing standards and systems usually consist of a mixture of different methods (that is, activity- and volume-based).

Based on our analysis, we suggest that rather than label a costing system or standards as a whole in terms of being activity-based or volume-based, one could calculate the percentage of costs that follow each costing methods. Costing standards in the United Kingdom recognize that different costing methods exist within costing systems; at the provider level, materiality and quality scores (MAQS) are used to rate the quality of cost information based on the choice of cost drivers. The closer the cost calculation is to actual resource consumption, the higher the score; the choice of cost driver is rated as bronze, silver or gold. This enables providers to better understand how their costing system functions in a more useful way and to evaluate the quality of their cost information.

That said, currently, MAQS primarily focus on the nature of the cost driver, devoting far less attention to the construction of the cost pool to which the cost driver is applied. As discussed in relation to property costs, there are many important choices to be made in this regard, and these significantly affect the ability of costing systems to show actual costs, regardless of which cost driver is chosen. Given this focus on cost drivers, the MAQS score is currently well placed to indicate through a low score that there might be room for improvement in the quality of costing data. At higher scores, however, the approach loses the ability to discriminate between costing systems that have good cost drivers and good cost pools, and those that have good cost drivers but deficiencies in cost pool structure.

4.4 The role of cost data in delivering efficient health care

Much of the emphasis in this chapter has been placed on the importance of the technical characteristics of costing system design. When designing a costing system, it is important to maintain a clear understanding of the decisions and objectives that the system is there to support. In this section, we review in more detail the various ways in which cost data can act as a vital input into efforts to measure and manage efficiency at both provider and health care system levels.

4.4.1 The role of cost data in system-wide resource allocation systems

At the health care system level, cost data feed into major resource allocation exercises through tariff systems, and also as the basis of negotiations around block contracts and the setting of budget levels between providers and purchasers. However, tariff setting within DRG financing systems is often the dominating purpose of costing across countries (Chapman, Kern & Laguecir, 2014).

Countries with DRG-based financing systems use costing data from providers to inform tariff setting, comparisons across providers and efficiency and performance assessment at the system level. In contrast to many other industries, detailed product or service costing is regulated, collected by government and sometimes publicly reported. This raises questions about the process of collecting and using such costing data at the system level. In particular, there are important questions regarding the stewardship responsibilities of governments and regulators in terms of the costing approach (Smith et al., 2008).

Development of a clear conceptual framework and a clear vision of the purpose of the costing approach are needed. Part of such a framework must be the link of costing with practices that are informed by costing, such as DRG development, tariff setting, cost–effectiveness calculations and links with financial accounting and IT. The guidance must specify the design of the cost systems, including, for example, the structure of cost pools and the cost drivers.

Detailed guidance then allows the standardization of cost data across providers, which is a major stewardship responsibility. In fact, standardization is a condition for tariff setting or comparisons across providers. Further, the question of which body or institution designs the guidance and collects the data needs to be addressed, as does the organization of the data collection process. In terms of data collection, we need to consider whether data are collected from all providers or whether a sampling approach should be chosen. The question of costs, but also of the representativeness of the costing data, plays a role in this later consideration. Another crucial question that needs to be answered is how to handle information governance (Smith et al., 2008). Costing data need to be audited and data quality needs to be checked. The quality of the information produced using costing data depends on the quality of the raw cost data. Audits and quality checks are therefore essential to ensure public trust in information and to ensure a well-informed public debate.

Cross-country research suggests that considerable variability remains (Chapman et. al., 2013). A growing number of countries that initially opted for a volume-based allocation model for tariff setting are now moving towards activity-based costing. For example, both Ireland and the United Kingdom are currently developing an activity-based approach to costing at the provider level (Chapman et al., 2013). The reason is that while volume-based allocation enables the relatively quick calculation of a tariff, the tariff itself and the underlying costs are not considered relevant or reliable enough (Monitor, 2014b). The perceived inaccuracy of volume-based overheads allocation at clinical unit levels can even lead clinicians to reject the tariff. Ultimately, volume-based costing is most problematic because it limits the potential for cost data to meaningfully inform clinical and managerial decision-making.

These limitations become apparent once we shift our attention beyond the tariff rates to examine the detail of the various cost elements making up the tariff figures. If calculation of these cost elements is based on a volume-based allocation, the result is the reporting of averages, with no variation in costs across patients. However, if the calculation is based on an activity-based approach, costs across patients will vary. Table 4.8 shows the detailed costs for the German DRG for the revision or replacement of hip joints as an example of the level of detail.

What becomes important as the emphasis shifts from tariff setting to informing clinical and managerial decision-making, however, is the costing approach adopted in arriving at these various cost elements. In the case of volume-based allocations, patients are attributed an average cost for each cost category (for example, physician, nurse, ward and overhead costs). This means that there is very little variation in reported costs at the patient level. The difference in reported patient costs may be explained by just a couple of key drivers, such as variation in length of stay or variation in time in the operating theatre, for example, with many other sources of variation of actual costs left unknown. This becomes problematic when seeking to link costs with health outcomes and using costs to make decisions on service redesign, as discussed further on.

Table 4.8 *Tariff in the German DRG for revision or replacement of hip joint*

German DRG catalogue — I47B — Revision or replacement of hip joint without complicating diagnosis, arthrodesis or major CC, age >15 years

Cost-centre groups	Labour			Material					Infrastructure		
	1 Physicians	2 Nursing	3 Medical/technical staff	4a General drugs	4b Individual drugs	5 Implants and grafts	6a Material (without drugs, implants and grafts)	6b Individual material (actual consumption, without drugs, implants/grafts)	7 Medical infrastructure	8 Non-medical infrastructure	Total
1: Normal ward	345.04	863.19	46.95	75.72	4.87	–	72.41	7.16	171.25	806.71	2393.30
2: Intensive care unit	35.53	94.54	6.07	12.60	0.61	0.00	15.93	0.71	11.22	44.36	221.56
3: Dialysis unit	0.00	0.00	0.00	0.00	0.00	–	0.00	0.00	0.00	0.00	0.00
4: Operating theatre	351.15	–	224.70	15.86	6.36	1363.53	174.88	62.48	136.39	205.65	2541.01
5: Anaesthesia	204.47	–	130.68	18.55	0.63	–	47.91	1.80	24.18	67.11	495.32
6: Maternity room	0.00	–	0.00	0.00	0.00	–	0.00	0.00	0.00	0.00	0.00
7: Cardiac diagnostics/therapy	0.17	–	0.16	0.00	0.00	0.03	0.04	0.06	0.03	0.09	0.58
8: Endoscopic diagnostics/therapy	0.43	–	0.53	0.02	0.00	0.00	0.19	0.01	0.19	0.36	1.74
9: Radiology	17.41	–	35.12	0.45	0.02	0.01	8.49	13.89	10.07	24.99	110.45
10: Laboratories	5.81	–	44.89	3.18	40.38	0.00	33.63	20.79	4.65	21.14	174.47
11: Other diagnostics and therapies	16.42	2.06	150.58	1.85	0.01	0.01	10.82	7.40	7.15	68.31	264.60
Total	976.43	959.79	639.68	128.23	52.88	1363.58	364.30	114.30	365.13	1238.72	6203.03

Source: InEK (2010).
Note: DRG = diagnosis-related group.

Activity-based costing of overheads enables reporting of costs at the patient level that take into account a wide range of differences in resource consumption (for example, the specific size of clinical teams for different procedures, rather than an average cost per minute across many procedures). This provides more useful information for clinical and managerial decision-making, as variations between patients can be captured in terms of their actual resource consumption. The resulting tariff may then be a fairer basis for resource allocation. Accurate data are crucial, as these funding mechanisms are used by regulators and purchasers to incentivize reforms in health care practice and delivery at both provider and system levels.

4.5 Cost data and support of local clinical and managerial decision-making

The effectiveness of incentives to enhance the efficiency of health care services depends on the quality of the cost data. This, in turn, is dependent on a constructive engagement between costing and clinicians. Providers will not make the necessary investments to obtain quality cost data if the data do not play a role in clinicians' day-to-day decision-making. Furthermore, quality cost information in health care is difficult to achieve without active engagement of clinicians in the design of the cost system, since they are the ones with the granular knowledge of activities that is required to produce robust and reliable cost data in the first place. This then sets up a potentially vicious or virtuous circle. If things go badly, then poor-quality cost data are largely ignored by clinicians to the extent they can manage to do so. If things go well, however, then data on cost variations can become an important tool to identify areas for clinical improvements.

Importantly, the process of developing the quality of cost information can prompt clinical deliberations and decisions over what represents cost-effective health care. The point of costing is not simply to reflect what is going on; more ambitiously, it can play a role in thinking about better ways to do things so that clinicians can play an active role in generating the maximum health benefits for their patients within the resources available to them. Clinicians engage with costing information through a range of common management accounting practices. We discuss the main ones in the following sections.

4.5.1 Targeted cost improvement plans

Cost reduction targets are often initially formulated at national or political levels. They then cascade downwards through providers with the production of targeted cost improvement plans derived for individual clinical units and departments. The capabilities of clinical units to respond effectively to such targets depend crucially on the nature and quality of the cost information available. As discussed earlier, volume-based allocations tend to lead to average reported costs, showing variation only in relation to drivers such as length of stay. Based on this, information can relatively easily be produced to highlight some of the variance in actual patient costs, for example, showing average highs and lows. The challenge is that without an activity-based analysis of cost, such variation acts as a largely hypothetical promise that overall costs can be reduced if more patients were as cheap as the cheapest. Unfortunately, a volume-based costing system offers little insight or support in terms of how to effectively and safely achieve this.

An activity-based approach to costing enables cost improvement plans that take into account the impact of indirect costs on activities. Certain types of overheads may be more linked with certain service lines than with others. Rather than advising to cut costs by 10% across all activities, cost management can better focus on the specific costs and the specific activities that cause excessive costs. Analysed at the patient level, this information can then be compared with the health outcomes achieved to inform analysis of both efficiency and effectiveness.

An important caveat to the ongoing relevance of targeted cost improvement plans is that in the face of continued growth in demand for health care services, it seems likely that more attention will need to be given to generating more health from existing spending rather than hoping to make significant reductions in current spending. This agenda suggests greater attention to the following management accounting practices.

4.5.2 Benchmarking

Once cost data are activity-based and linked to health outcomes, benchmarking is a powerful way to engage clinicians in exactly the kind of analysis that cost improvement plans require. Effective benchmarking builds from discussions with physicians about the reasons that costs are higher or lower than those of other providers. Discussions between costing experts and clinicians are also essential to ensure that cost data appropriately reflect physicians' practice and resource consumption decisions.

Such discussions aim to explain the variation in cost between clinicians and patients. In some cases, higher costs are justified by patients requiring more complex care. In other cases, differences in costs are caused by differences in medical practice. A difference could be caused, for example, by the use of different drugs or other consumables, but also by different surgical techniques. Such differences, once visible, form the basis of discussions among clinicians aimed at confirming a shared understanding of when variation is appropriate, and align diverse clinical practice where evidence shows a clinically determined balance of health outcomes and cost.

Discussions around comparisons of costs between the service lines of different hospitals can also reveal differences in resource consumption for indirect costs. If activity-based costing is in place, decision-makers can then spot more easily the origin of such differences and potentially make services more efficient. While activity-based costing has been shown to reduce overall costs (see, for example, Pizzini, 2006), its main advantage may actually lie in using the existing resources more effectively. This is particularly important in a context of coping with rising demand without increasing the available resources.

4.5.3 Budgeting

Building on these kinds of analyses, activity-based costing data can go on to inform more appropriate budgetary processes as part of the ongoing management of providers. When there are no costing data at the patient level, the danger is that budgets are set based on past arrangements, power and interests rather than clinical needs, practices and outcomes. Activity-based costs at the patient level allow for more accurate estimates of costs at the service line-level based on the number and type of patients expected. The budget process becomes more objective and fair-based on clearly specified modelling of resource consumption and less on power and local interests.

Activity-based costing has two main advantages here. It enables the construction of the budget in a bottom-up way, enabling the budget holder and operational staff to participate in the budget process while having a better understanding of the impact of their work processes on the costs entailed. This is supported by the use of language that directly speaks to clinical activities as opposed to technical accounting terminology. Staff can understand when constructing the budget how the costs of work processes, for example, are linked to certain overhead costs. Further, it enables a breakdown of the responsibility of budget holders to activity levels (that is, budget holders for the different activities can be defined). In administrative areas, this can allow a more effective definition of responsibilities and cost management.

4.5.4 Service redesign

As has been discussed, activity-based cost information informs a variety of conversations that can inform robust decisions regarding the nature of how health care services might be more effectively arranged. At its bluntest, redesign can take the form of product/service selection decisions, whereby procedures or clinical areas might be dropped altogether, or more optimistically, improved on.

This kind of decision has become important in many countries at the health care system level also, where providers face a restructuring, as there are too many providers per patient in certain catchment areas, such as central London. Providers are then asked to focus on certain services representing their strengths, while competitors may take over those services that are considered a weakness. A common tool recommended by Monitor in the United Kingdom, for making decisions in such cases, is the portfolio matrix. The portfolio matrix calculates the profit/loss per service line and the relative size of the service line for the provider (Monitor, 2006). A more sophisticated approach over and above such service selection decisions, however, is to use activity-based cost information to inform redesign activities so that services become more clinically and economically beneficial.

4.5.5 Performance management

A popular metric for measuring efficiency is the average length of stay in hospital. This offers a simple way to reduce the potentially vast complexity of individual patient resource consumption patterns to an easily observed driver of overhead costs. However, studies have shown that the length of a hospital stay has limited influence on the total costs of a patient stay (Taheri, Butz & Greenfield, 2000). Taheri, Butz & Greenfield showed that reducing length of stay by 1 day decreases total costs of care by only 3%. They concluded that staff should instead focus on process changes and better use of capacity when seeking to improve efficiency. This requires delving into the complexities of resource consumption and resource spending that measures such as length of stay simplify away from.

More advanced approaches to performance management include the use of costing data, activity data and clinical data from a service line, for example, taking into account the number of patients treated in a service, costs for certain DRGs in that service line and other relevant indicators. Some providers have introduced performance indicators based on the balanced scorecard system (Kaplan & Norton, 1996). For example, Monitor recommends the use of a balanced scorecard at provider and service line levels in the United Kingdom. This system is designed to link strategy and performance indicators, by choosing those performance indicators that are instrumental for achieving strategic goals.

State-of-the-art performance management systems in health care go a step further. They seek to link both economic and clinical performance (Kaplan & Porter, 2011). For example, the Healthcare Costing for Value Institute in the United Kingdom aims to improve the quality of the costing information in health care, but also to further develop links between costs and outcomes to measure values. This again is only meaningful at a patient-level of disaggregation, and requires both outcome and cost data to demonstrate value (Kaplan & Witkowski, 2014).

4.6 Conclusions

In this chapter, we have reviewed the technical characteristics that underlie good-quality cost data, and some of the ways in which such data can inform efforts to measure and enhance the efficiency of health care services. We have argued that the main questions for the design of a costing system relate to matters of granularity at each of the three steps in costing system design: granularity of the resources, granularity of cost pools and granularity of cost objects. It is only when resources and cost pools are defined in a sufficiently granular way that an activity-based costing approach can be achieved. Shifting away from volume-based methods is essential if cost information is to accurately reflect resource use and play a more direct role in health care management.

Activity-based costing enables the management of indirect costs by virtue of its reorganization of cost pools away from traditional (often financial reporting-driven) structures towards analysis of activities with defined cost drivers. Realizing the decision-making benefits of these data also requires that cost pools be mapped onto areas of decision-making responsibility. In general, the misalignment of cost analysis and decision-making structures risks inhibiting efforts at service redesign in the first instance. Such misalignment runs the risk that any savings from service redesigns are unlikely to ultimately translate into changes in resource spending. While activity-based costing cannot directly inform reductions in overall spending, particularly in a setting with a high percentage of fixed costs, it can contribute to greater efficiency by indicating where slack exists and thereby contribute to increases in outputs. This seems particularly pertinent in health care settings where there is likely to be increased demand for services and thus expectations of reduced spending seem unrealistic.

Our emphasis in this chapter arises from our sense that cost information is fundamental to a wide range of efficiency-oriented practices. Past efforts to clearly and consistently conceptualize costing in the health care sector have not been strong enough to bring about widespread production and use of costing data that can support evidence-based decision-making. We argue that regulators should play an essential role in ensuring that resources set aside for the development of costing systems are not spent reinventing the wheel. It is essential that costing guidance be sufficiently detailed so that costing in practice can deliver on the promise to enhance the efficiency of health care provision.

References

Busse R, Schreyögg J, Smith PC (2008). Variability in healthcare treatment costs amongst nine EU countries: results from the HealthBASKET project. *Health Economics*, 17(Suppl. S1):S1–S8.

Busse R et al., eds. (2011). *Diagnosis-related groups in Europe: moving towards transparency, efficiency and quality in hospitals*. European Observatory on Health Systems and Policies Series. Maidenhead, Open University Press (http://www.euro.who.int/__data/assets/pdf_file/0004/162265/e96538.pdf, accessed 24 July 2016).

Chapman CS, Kern A (2010). Costing in the National Health Service: from reporting to managing. London, Chartered Institute of Management Accountants (http://www.cimaglobal.com/Documents/Thought_leadership_docs/R226%20Costing%20in%20the%20National%20UPDATED%20%20(PDF).pdf, accessed 22 July 2016).

Chapman CS, Kern A, Laguecir A (2014). Costing practices in healthcare. *Accounting Horizons*, 28(2):353–364.

Chapman CS et al. (2013). *International approaches to clinical costing*. Bristol: Healthcare Financial Management Association.

Deutsche Krankenhausgesellschaft (DKG) (2007). Kalkulation von Fallkosten: Handbuch zur Anwendung in Krankenhäusern. Düsseldorf, DKG (https://www.gkv-spitzenverband.de/media/dokumente/krankenversicherung_1/krankenhaeuser/drg/drg_entwicklung__kalkulation__falldaten/kalkulation/KH_DRG_Kalkulationshandbuch_Version_3_2007_09_18.pdf, accessed 22 July 2016).

Institut für das Entgeltsystem im Krankenhaus (InEK) (2010). G-DRG V2008/2010 HA-Report-Browser. Siegburg, InEK (http://www.g-drg.de/cms/content/view/full/2553, accessed 22 July 2016).

Johnson HT, Kaplan RS (1987). *Relevance lost: the rise and fall of management accounting*. Boston, MA, Harvard Business School Press.

Kaplan RS, Anderson SR (2004). Time-driven activity-based costing. *Harvard Business Review*, 82(11):131–138.

Kaplan RS, Cooper R (1998). *Cost and effect: using integrated cost systems to drive profitability and performance*. Boston, MA, Harvard Business School Press.

Kaplan RS, Norton DP (1996). *The balanced scorecard: translating strategy into action*. Boston, MA, Harvard Business Review Press.

Kaplan RS, Porter ME (2011). How to solve the cost crisis in health care. *Harvard Business Review*, 89(9):46–52.

Kaplan RS, Witkowski ML (2014). Better accounting transforms health care delivery. *Accounting Horizons*, 28(2):365–383.

Monitor (2006). How service-line reporting can improve the productivity and performance of NHS foundation trusts. London, Monitor.

Monitor (2013). Approved costing guidance. London, Monitor.

Monitor (2014a). Long-term reform of the NHS payment system. London, Monitor.

Monitor (2014b). Improving the costing of NHS services: proposals for 2015–2021. London, Monitor (https://www.gov.uk/government/uploads/system/uploads/attachment_data/file/381990/Improving_the_costing_of_NHS_services_-_final.pdf, accessed 22 July 2016).

Northcott D, Llewellyn S (2004). *Cost variability in health care*. London, Chartered Institute of Management Accountants.

Pizzini MJ (2006). The relation between cost-system design, manager's evaluations of the relevance and usefulness of cost data, and financial performance: an empirical study of US hospitals. *Accounting, Organizations and Society*, 31(2):179–210.

Roberts RR et al. (1999). Distribution of variable vs fixed costs of hospital care. *JAMA*, 281(7):644–649.

Smith PC et al. (2008). *Performance measurement for health system improvement: experiences, challenges, and prospects*. Cambridge, CUP.

Taheri PA, Butz DA, Greenfield L J (2000). Length of stay has minimal impact on the cost of hospital admission. *Journal of the American College of Surgeons*, 191(2):123–130.

Tiemann O (2008). Variations in hospitalisation costs for acute myocardial infarction: a comparison across Europe. *Health Economics*, 17(Suppl. S1): S33–S45.

Chapter 5

Health system efficiency: measurement and policy[*]

Bruce Hollingsworth

5.1 Introduction: data envelopment analysis and stochastic frontier analysis

There are many indicators available to assess whether scarce resources for health are used in the most efficient manner, ranging from measures that compare activity (see Chapters 2 and 3), to measures that compare costs (see Chapter 4). Performance indicators, league tables and cost ratios have all been used, but these have been criticized for having no conceptual bases and for disregarding the actual needs of health service staff who might need to use them. If measures are constructed and weighted in such a way that does not reflect activities accurately, or which do not benchmark effectively, this will give misleading impressions and may create perverse incentives. High-level summary indicators that are not transparent are often underused for similar reasons (Hollingsworth & Parkin, 2003).

Methods based on sound economic concepts can provide transparent and potentially useful information on efficiency comparisons. Data envelopment analysis (DEA) and stochastic frontier analysis (SFA) are two of the most common methods used to estimate the efficiency of health services. Over 400 published applications have used these methods within health care settings over the past 30 years (Hollingsworth, 2003, 2008, 2012).

Both methods see efficiency as essentially a simple relationship between health care inputs and the outputs they produce, and assess how effectively a unit of production, such as a hospital, uses its own inputs, such as staff and drugs, to produce outputs, such as patients treated. To measure the efficiency of these processes, comparison is made against other units undertaking similar activities. DEA has been used a great deal more than SFA, making up the majority of applications in health care settings (>90%) and can account for multiple inputs and outputs, varying weights and returns to scale.

---

[*] Permission has been granted by Elsevier, Springer, and John Wiley & Sons Ltd, respectively, to reproduce some of the content of this chapter.

This chapter describes how we can measure the relationship between inputs and outputs using these methodological tools, and how we can provide information that improves the efficiency of how health services are delivered. The relative merits of each method, how useful they have been, and how useful they really could become are discussed by following a set of simple guidelines.

5.2 Efficiency measurement methods

As explained in Chapter 1, technical efficiency (TE) indicates that the organization is minimizing the use of inputs in producing its chosen outputs, regardless of the value placed on those outputs. An alternative but equivalent formulation is to say that it is maximizing its outputs given its chosen level of inputs. In contrast, allocative efficiency (AE) indicates whether the value of the chosen outputs creates the maximum value to society (or alternatively, the costs of the chosen inputs are the minimum feasible).

These are illustrated with reference to Figure 5.1, where we have a hospital using its combination of labour and capital to produce output at point C. We can see that this point is not on the efficiency curve, which is constructed from the other hospitals in the sample based on how they would use their combinations of labour and capital to produce the same level of output as the hospital at point C. To get to the efficient frontier, this hospital must use less labour and capital. We could measure this hospital's TE as a ratio:

$$(1) \quad TE = OA/OC$$

where TE must take a value >0 and ≤1. If TE = 1, the hospital is technically efficient and is operating on the efficient frontier. If TE is <1, the hospital is technically inefficient and we can measure how inefficient by the distance the hospital is from the frontier.

AE can be measured by:

$$(2) \quad AE = OB/OA$$

where similarly AE must take a value >0 and ≤1. AE can be interpreted as a measure of excess costs arising from using inputs in inappropriate proportions.

If producing at Q in Figure 5.1, the hospital would be technically and allocatively efficient; otherwise, there may be some trade-off between the two.

How can we measure these concepts and distances in applied terms that would produce information of use to those who have to deliver services? There are two main frontier-based methods: DEA and SFA.

Figure 5.1 *Hospital efficiency frontier*

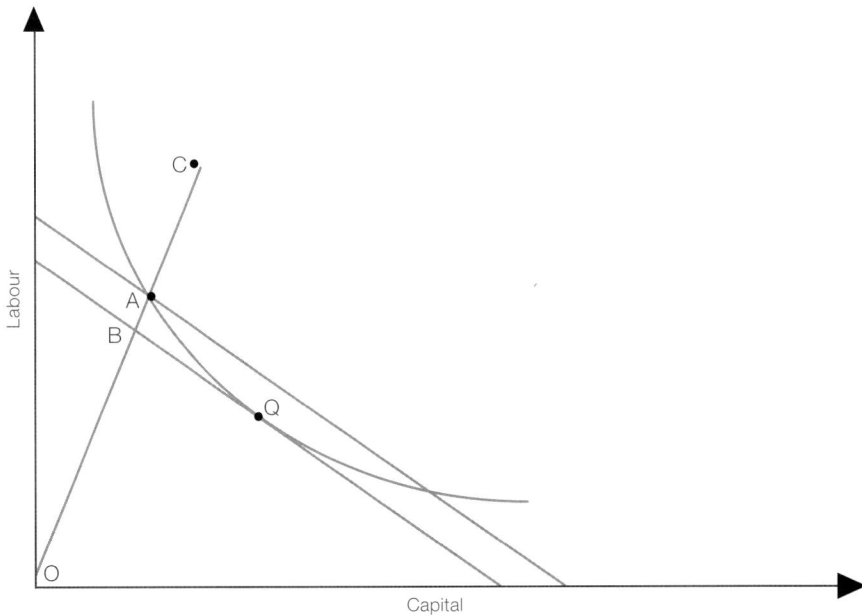

5.2.1 Data envelopment analysis

DEA is by far the most common method for analysing efficiency in health care. It has now been applied over 400 times within health care settings. DEA makes use of linear programming methods to place weights on the inputs and outputs to show the hospital in the best possible light relative to how the other hospitals in the sample are using their inputs and outputs. In the simple case of a single output/single input firm, a measure of TE[3] can be defined as:

$$(1) \quad TE = \text{outputs/inputs}$$

The greater this ratio, the greater the quantity of output for a certain amount of input. For a multiple output/multiple input firm, like a hospital treating different types of cases using staff of different types, various equipment, and so on, an overall measure of a hospital's TE requires summing these different inputs and outputs in some way. The problem with this is that inputs and outputs cannot be simply summed as they usually measure very different things, for example, the number of doctors and operating theatres. Rather, we must give weights to each of the inputs and outputs. The weights are chosen so that TE lies between 0 and 1. If the weights are fully flexible, TE is defined for each firm as the ratio of a weighted sum of its outputs relative to a weighted sum of its inputs.

---

3   Other forms of efficiency can be measured using DEA, including, as noted earlier, allocative efficiency (for example, by comparing firms using identical weights); here we concentrate on TE for ease of exposition.

Important here is that the weights are unknown a priori; they must be calcu-lated. Of all of the possible sets of weights (conditional on a set of constraints), the linear program optimizes the ones that give the most favourable view of the firm. This is the highest efficiency score, which shows the firm in the best pos-sible light. The efficiency of any firm or unit, say a hospital (or nursing home, GP practice, and so on), is assessed relative to other firms within a peer group that form the efficiency frontier (that is, the firms that are deemed efficient).

Most areas of the economy, and in turn the health sector, are not linear in terms of the relationship between input use and outputs produced. So it is useful to account for possible increasing or decreasing returns to the inputs used. Figure 5.2 illustrates the DEA frontiers under constant returns to scale (CRS) and under variable returns to scale (VRS).

The AB section of the VRS frontier exhibits increasing returns to scale (output increases proportionately more than inputs), BC exhibits CRS and CD decreasing

Figure 5.2 *Constant and VRS under DEA*

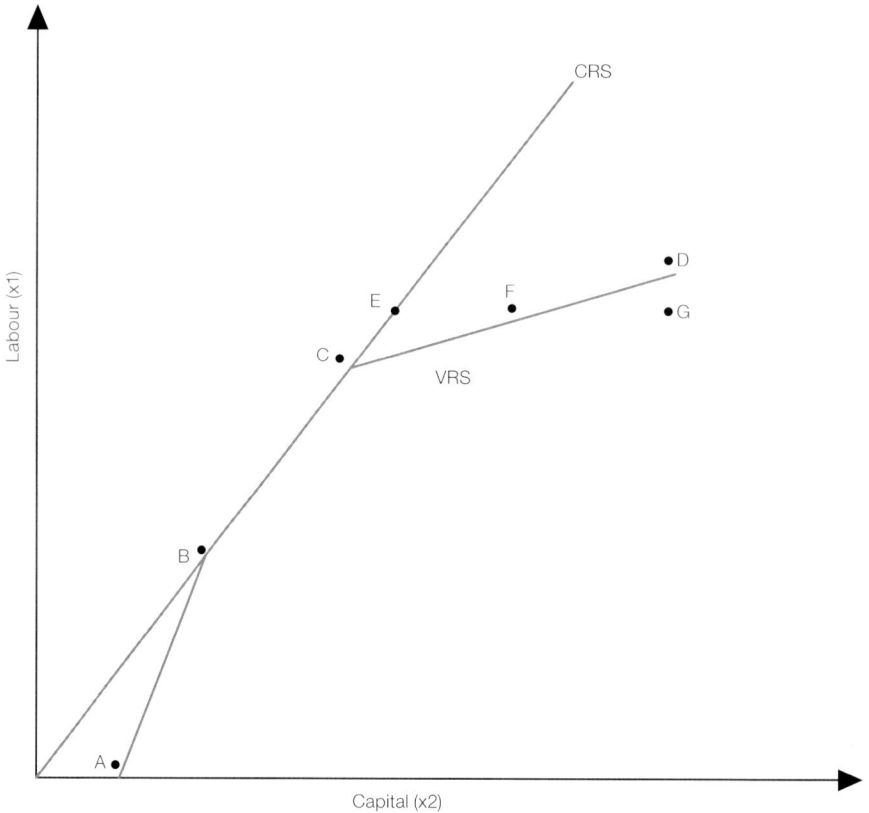

Note: CRS = constant returns to scale; DEA = data envelopment analysis; VRS = variable returns to scale.

returns to scale (output changes proportionately less than the change in inputs). For a given hospital (G), the distance EF measures the effects of economies of scale in production, and FG measures pure inefficiency.

Thus, results under CRS (where returns to scale are part of the inefficiency) or VRS can be very different. The VRS frontier draws in more hospitals to the frontier, so more are given a score as efficient. Often, this means both CRS and VRS are useful to conduct – the latter showing the tendencies related to returns to scale, the former being more discriminatory as to efficiency differences. These techniques can be very sensitive to the assumptions made, so the models and relationships being considered need to be very carefully thought through — something returned to when looking at the guidelines for their use.

In analyses of this type, it is important to account for influences of the distribution of medical case complexity (case mix) on producer efficiency in the production of health care. One approach to modelling the effects of case mix is to include an aggregated measure of patient characteristics at each hospital as a type of input in the production frontier. However, patients are not inputs that are transformed to make the final product (which in this case is health care interventions). Instead, patients consume treatments to (hopefully) produce improvements in their health status.

The characteristics of patients and their illness (or illnesses) will influence the production of health. DEA models can incorporate patient case mix by first adjusting outputs to reflect variations in case severity (see Chapter 2). Not accounting for the mix of cases in some way would produce results that may not be useful comparisons – however, the method of adjustment needs careful consideration. For example, it is now common to incorporate DRG weights into output measures (for example, case mix-adjusted inpatient admissions) in developed countries, where such data are often collected for payment systems. However, it is less common to have such accurate case mix adjustments for outpatients or primary care. This often makes comparisons of efficiency a lot cruder in these areas.

Another method to account for such characteristics involves adding a second stage of analysis to the DEA approach. The first stage involves running a DEA model based on inputs and outputs to yield efficiency scores for units (say hospitals again), as shown earlier. The second stage then takes these efficiency scores and statistically regresses them against hospital-level case mix variables to assess the impact of the patients' sociodemographic and clinical characteristics on the production process and efficiency. This allows the inclusion of variables that do not fall neatly into the input–output analysis to potentially see if they have a significant impact on the efficiency scores obtained in the first stage, but there are many statistical issues with undertaking such second-stage analysis (see Simar & Wilson, 2008 for further reading).

5.2.2 Limitations of DEA

Before proceeding, it is important to note that DEA has several major limitations that require some care on the part of those constructing models and others interpreting the results. There are statistical issues to account for. The technique is deterministic and outlying observations can be important in determining the frontier (which is made up of the most efficient units). Closer investigation of these outliers is often warranted to ensure the sample is actually uniform in nature, that is, you really are comparing like-with-like.

Care must be taken in interpreting the results, as the DEA efficiency frontier may be influenced by stochastic variation, measurement error or unobserved heterogeneity in the data. DEA makes the strong and non-testable assumption of no measurement error or random variation in output. Small random variation for inefficient hospitals will affect the magnitude of the inefficiency estimate for that hospital. Larger random variation may move the frontier itself, thereby affecting efficiency estimates for a range of hospitals.

DEA is sensitive to the number of input and output variables used in the analysis. Overestimates of efficiency scores can occur if the number of units relative to the number of variables used is small. A general rule of thumb is that the number of units used should be at least three times the combined number of input and output variables.

DEA only provides a measure of relative efficiency in the sense that a hospital which is deemed efficient by DEA is only efficient given the observed practices in the sample which is being analysed. Therefore, it is possible that greater efficiency than that observed could be achieved in the sample.

DEA can be used to measure efficiency changes over time (often referred to as a Malmquist Index). Measuring changes over time, rather than a snapshot of efficiency, gives a more accurate picture of what is really happening in efficiency terms. The interested reader is referred to Thannasoulis, Portela & Despić (2008) for a much more technical explanation of these methods.

5.2.3 Stochastic frontier analysis

SFA has been used in a much smaller number of efficiency analyses in health care than DEA, but the number of papers is increasing. SFA uses statistical regression analysis rather than mathematical programming to do basically the same thing as DEA in terms of measuring the distance a hospital is from a calculated efficient frontier. In SFA, the usual statistical error term in such regression equations is split into inefficiency and error. Some researchers see this as a more precise measure of efficiency, as it accounts for statistical noise, which DEA does not do. However, other researchers recommend using both techniques and looking at the direction both point in (for example, Varabyova & Schreyögg, 2013). If both methods indicate inefficiency in a hospital, then a closer investigation is perhaps warranted.

The use of SFA in the production of health care has received increasing attention in recent years. This is partly because of greater interest in efficiency measurement in general in health and health care, but also because of advances in modelling techniques and increased computing capabilities. As with DEA, there are several limitations. Estimation of an SFA production frontier requires that all outputs can be meaningfully aggregated into a single measure. This assumption is questionable within the health context. To allow multiple outputs to be modelled (as outputs in health care are typically heterogeneous) researchers often estimate costs rather than production frontiers. Costs can be easily aggregated into a single measure using common monetary units such as dollars.

The inclusion of variables capturing case mix and producer characteristics in the model allows statistical testing of hypotheses concerning the relationship between these factors and producer efficiency. Assumptions concerning the error term in SFA may also be important. In technical terms, if an assumption of normality in the error term does not hold, and its distribution is skewed, inefficiency may be under- or overestimated. Also, the functional form of such models is a source of potential error. (The interested reader is pointed to Greene, 2008 for further and more technical reasoning.)

5.3 The application of DEA

Illustrative use is made here of an example from a hospital setting in the United Kingdom. The sample in this study is relatively small, 44 United Kingdom hospitals over two years. The full study has been published (Hollingsworth & Parkin, 2003), and the interested reader is referred to that article for more detail.

When undertaking any applied empirical work, it is useful to first specify a model based on the data and variables available. This involves choices, as rarely are data so comprehensive that they represent perfectly any theoretical model. There are few criteria for choosing between different efficiency models (Parkin & Hollingsworth, 1997; Smith, 1997), but there are some practical considerations. For example, the greater the number of variables in the model, the more information produced on which variables impact on efficiency. However, the more variables, the greater the number of efficient hospitals on the frontier; a balance must then be struck.

In the case illustrated here, sensitivity analyses of different models with different variables was undertaken using correlation analyses to test the robustness of results to changes in the models. They were all based on the same theoretical model, but aggregated in different ways to test for information trade-offs. The final model arrived at is shown in Table 5.1.

Table 5.1 *Inputs and outputs in a DEA model*

	Model
Inputs	Medical and dental staff numbers
	Nursing and midwifery staff numbers
	All other staff numbers
	Capital charge
	All other costs
Outputs	Mental illness and learning disability episodes
	Maternity episodes
	Total general and acute episodes
	General, acute and maternity outpatient first attends
	Accident & emergency (A&E) attends

Note: A&E = accident and emergency department.

DEA was used with an input orientation – that is the analysis shows the minimum level of inputs that could feasibly be used given a hospital's chosen outputs. Of course, the equivalent output-oriented model could also be estimated. The results obtained are shown in Table 5.2.

Table 5.2 *Results from DEA example*

Hospital type	Sample size	Minimum score	Mean score	SD
Acute 1994–1995	16	53.90	86.32	13.90
Acute 1995–1996	16	72.64	90.73	11.02
Priority 1994–1995	15	9.41	85.81	23.80
Priority 1995–1996	15	14.60	83.79	26.36
Combined 1994–1995	13	14.18	89.93	23.39
Combined 1995–1996	13	3.57	83.04	33.74
All hospitals 1994–1995	44	21.30	85.13	17.00
All hospitals 1995–1996	44	23.68	86.15	17.60

Notes: Combined hospitals undertake both acute and priority activities. SD = standard deviation.

The overall results for all hospitals and by group of hospital are shown. The minimum score is useful, as it demonstrates the range of results (the range from 3.57 to 100% efficient for those hospitals on the frontier). Overall, the hospitals were operating on average with more that 10% inefficiency.

We can illustrate these results in many ways. Figure 5.3 contains the ranked scores by hospital.

Figure 5.3 *Hospital DEA ranking*

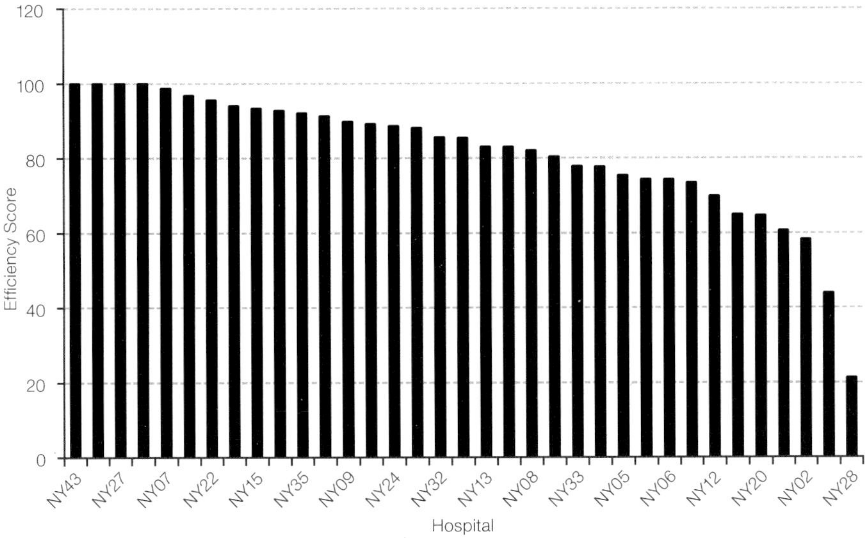

Note: DEA = data envelopment analysis.

Figure 5.4 *Changes in DEA efficiency scores from 1994–1995 to 1995–1996, shown by hospital*

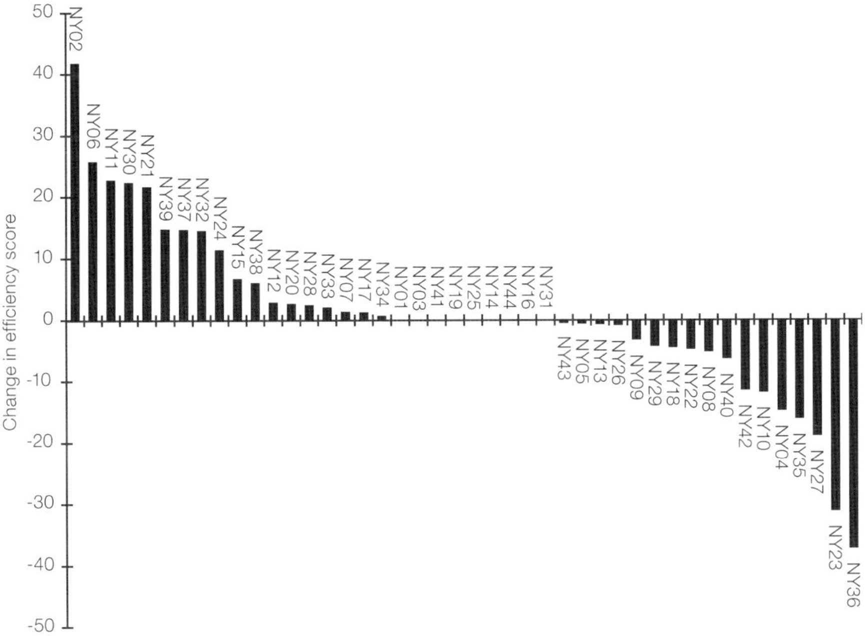

Note: DEA = data envelopment analysis.

Figure 5.4 looks at the changes in scores from one year to the next. Information of this nature demonstrates which hospitals are outliers, which have potential for efficiency gains and which are most useful as benchmarking units.

Information can also be fed back to each inefficient hospital on the improvements that could be made to increase efficiency. This is done by calculating the reduced level of resources that would be used if the hospital was on the efficient frontier calculated by the DEA for its chosen level of outputs. Figure 5.5 contains an example for one such hospital (anonymized as NY11 here – but a real hospital in this real data set) in terms of reducing input use to get to the efficiency frontier. (Any one overall reduction, or a combination of lesser reductions, could result in a move to the frontier.)

Based on Figure 5.5, this hospital can see that in 1994–1995 it was using its medical staff inefficiently in terms of using a lot more staff to produce the same outputs as its comparator units (those similar in input/output mix and size). However, in the following year, we can see this hospital did a much better job of using its medical staff (and in fact most other inputs) in producing outputs. This is reflected in its overall efficiency score, which improved dramatically by more than 20%. One area of concern that remains is that this hospital appears to have high other costs (in this example, these include all non-staff and capital costs) relative to similar hospitals that are more efficient. Policymakers may find it useful to go to hospital NY11 and ask their management just how they changed procedures on staff use, or how capital spending was changed over this time period, so that other hospitals can learn in benchmarking terms from this best practice.

Figure 5.5 *Input reduction targets to improve efficiency in hospital NY11*

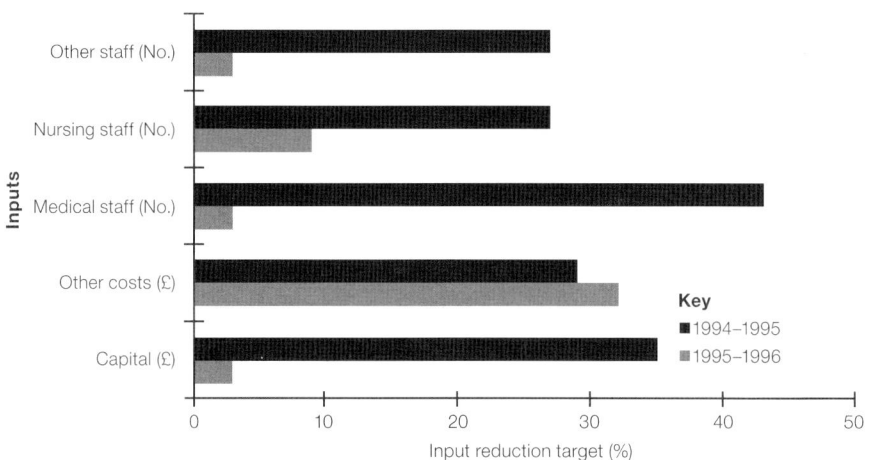

This particular project used results similar to these to feed back to these hospitals, with great success. Hospital managers and those commissioning care found the results to be of great interest. On occasion, they could explain the results in terms of data deficiencies, but there were also efficiency gains to be made by looking at benchmark examples of best practice. All of the participants found the results useful based on the amount of detail that could be presented in a practical manner. They were all made aware of the limitations of the work, and that often it is not the exact scores that are relevant, but rather, the areas pointed out for potential improvement and the comparators available as benchmarks.

5.4 Setting out the protocol

Given all that has been said above, how can we make these methods even more useful? There are published guidelines for the application of the DEA and SFA techniques. A slightly modified version of these guidelines is reproduced here. They set out clearly how these methods can be of use to those who need to undertake such analyses (that is, suppliers), and, perhaps most importantly, those who need to interpret and make use of the results generated (that is, demanders).

5.4.1 Suppliers

Suppliers should consider how to make their studies more effective. In other words, are there specific criteria or guidelines, which would make efficiency measurement more user-friendly, for example, to those involved in using such information to make policy choices? Here, we establish some initial non-exhaustive criteria as a starting-point, in both macro and micro terms. By macro, we mean the overall process of undertaking the study in terms of set-up and management, in a way to help ensure that the information provided will be of use in policy terms. By micro, we mean the actual production of the efficiency scores.

Macro issues include the following:

1. Applied research needs to be placed within a policy context. One important element of any efficiency analysis is to get potential end users involved early on. This helps ownership of the research from the users' perspective and keeps the researcher on track. This may initially involve finding the right person or group of people. (Having a number of people involved reduces risks, for example, staff moving positions.) Meetings held to feed back results at the various stages and to different levels of users (for example, hospital managers, health

department staff, those involved with policy development) will help make sure information is provided to those who want to use it. An advisory group featuring such participants to initially help set up the model specification may be useful.

2. Hospital managers may have concerns about health authorities using efficiency measures as *big sticks* and are generally interested in more detailed information within their specific unit; health authority staff tend to be more interested in comparisons between hospitals; government policymakers may be more interested in the overall picture of how care is delivered in different sectors, perhaps primary compared to secondary care. The researcher has to balance these views; providing all of the information to everyone may help. Also, it is important to ask what information would be useful that the data/modelling is not already providing. Analysts should try and accommodate this, or suggest means (for example, extra data) that could help. It is essential to identify what value is being added to the way efficiency is already being measured.

3. End users should be given the information that was intended. Surveying end users may help in refining measures. Results should also be disseminated as widely as possible. Users should know the limitations of efficiency measures: they are *a* useful policy tool, not *the* useful policy tool. Results can be manipulated so full provision of information to all may be helpful.

Micro issues include the following:

1. Are the right questions being asked?
2. What is the underlying economic theory of production or cost? Do duality theory and the requirement for cost minimization as an objective really apply?
3. Is the model specified correctly? Has extensive sensitivity analysis been undertaken? An advisory group can point out if there are any obvious omitted variables.
4. Are the data really good enough to answer the questions, particularly the output data?
5. Are there any data on quality? What will results using just quantity (throughput) data really show? Will any inefficiency be just made up of omitted quality data?
6. If there are quality data, how will they be weighted relative to quantity data to avoid being swamped by relatively large numbers of throughput information? Unless carefully weighted, potentially vital information on quality may have little impact on results.

7. Is the sample inclusive enough, comparing like-with-like? Exploratory analyses are useful; even if all hospitals in the sample have the same categorization, there may be a rogue specialist unit or teaching hospital which will confound the results, as frontier techniques are very susceptible to outliers. Sample size is also an issue.

8. What techniques should be used: parametric, non-parametric or both? If there are multiple inputs/outputs, non-parametric techniques have an advantage (when comparing DEA and SFA) in terms of disaggregation.[4] They provide more detailed information on specific areas of inefficiency. Panel data techniques will also provide more information, not only on what happens between units, but what happens over time. Looking at trends over time is more useful than a snap shot.

9. Is it useful to do two-stage analyses, and if so, how can any statistical problems to be accounted for (see Simar & Wilson, 2007)?

10. Is it necessary to generate confidence intervals? Unless the sample is all-inclusive, it may be prudent to account for sampling variation.[5]

5.4.2 Demanders

Table 5.3 contains a checklist for assessing if an efficiency analysis is useful. This is a starting-point, based on the list by Drummond et al. (2005) for assessing economic evaluations. Suppliers of efficiency studies may also wish to take note of these points.[6] The two assessment questions asked by Drummond et al. (see Chapter 3 of their book) are also pertinent here: is the methodology appropriate and are the results valid; and if the answer to this is yes, do the results apply to the setting being evaluated? As Drummond et al. acknowledge, it is unlikely every study can fulfil every criterion, but criteria are useful as screening devices to identify the strengths and weaknesses of studies, and of course to identify the value added by comprehensive extra analysis of this nature.

From a policymaker's perspective, the same questions should be asked, but some will be more useful than others in assessing how useful a particular study will be if looking at the bigger picture. For example, under checklist item 1, what is the perspective of the study – if it is to look at efficiency within a single hospital, this may be of interest to a local authority policymaker, but not someone at the WHO wanting to make comparisons between hospitals funded in different ways in different countries. Again, when looking at the samples used, is a policymaker

---

4   A single output stochastic production frontier can be adapted to the multiple output case, making use of distance functions. There is a growing technical literature in the area of multiple output distance functions, see, for example, Kumbhakar & Knox Lovell (2000) or Coelli et al. (2005).

5   See Coelli et al. (2005: pp 202–203) for a discussion about concerns with sampling distributions, that is, DEA is measuring the frontier when all the hospitals in a country are in the sample, but it is estimating the frontier if not.

6   This refers to applied efficiency measurement. See Hollingsworth & Street (2006) for a discussion of this.

interested in teaching hospitals, hospitals that have merged, hospitals that are over a certain size, and so on? This is information that should be clearly provided by those undertaking the study to make its impact as useful as possible. Whether analyses should be undertaken over time is another key question policymakers may find useful – a snapshot of efficiency may be useful at a certain level, but looking at how previous policy changes have impacted on efficient production of health care over time in a similar setting, with a similar sample, may be very informative to planning processes.

Table 5.3 *A checklist for assessing efficiency measurement studies*[7]

1. Is the question well defined and answerable?
• Are the inputs and outputs clear?
• Is a particular viewpoint stated (whose objectives are accounted for – managers, government policymakers, patients)?
• Is any decision-making context established?
2. Is a comprehensive description of the sample given?
• Can you tell if any relevant comparator units are excluded?
• Are the samples strictly comparable, are there potential outliers?
3. Are the quality and quantity output data clear and comprehensive?
• Where do the data come from, who collected them and why?
• Are quantity data case mix-adjusted?
• Are quality data useful? For example, can individual patients be followed through the system?
4. Are all the relevant inputs and outputs included?
• Is the range wide enough to answer the research question?
• Do they cover all relevant viewpoints? (For example, hospital mortality may be of interest to patients, scale of operation to policymakers and range of services to managers.)
• Are there measures of physical quantities of inputs as well as costs (although, in a number of contexts, costs alone may be appropriate)?
5. Are inputs and outputs measured accurately in appropriate units?
• Are all resources used relevant to the analysis accounted for?
• Are any data omitted? If so what is the justification?
• Are there any special circumstances that make measurement difficult, for example, joint use of staff? Were these circumstances handled appropriately?
6. Were inputs and outputs (or objectives) valued (or weighted) correctly?
• Were the sources of all values clearly identified? For example, market prices for inputs, case mix weights?
• Was the value of the outputs appropriate? Were the right weights placed on the relationship between the quantities (and qualities) of outputs?
7. Were analyses over time undertaken?
• Were values (and outputs) adjusted to present value?
• How are the specific techniques justified, for example, are random or fixed-effects models used, how is scale accounted for, how is efficiency decomposed?
8. Do techniques add incremental value?
• For example, is DEA used? Or SFA? Which cross-sectional or panel data (over time) techniques are used?
• Are the techniques used clearly justified, for example, what incremental value do they add beyond how efficiency is currently measured?

---

7   This checklist relies heavily on Box 3.1 in Drummond et al. (2005).

9. Was allowance made for uncertainty?

- Were appropriate statistical analyses undertaken?
- Were sensitivity analyses performed? Which dimensions were tested?
- Were the results sensitive to the statistical/sensitivity analysis?

10. Did the presentation and discussion of the study results include all issues of concern to users?

- Were the conclusions based on an overall measure or individual comparisons of efficiency?
- Were the results compared with those of others who have investigated the same question?
- Did the study discuss the generalizability of the results to other settings?
- Did the study allude to other important factors in the decision or choice under consideration, for example, ethical issues, or access issues or equity?
- Did the study discuss issues of implementation, such as the feasibility of adopting efficiency changes, given existing operational constraints, and whether freed resources could be redeployed to other more efficient programmes?

5.5 Conclusions

There are important lessons to be learnt from prior experiences using frontier-based methods to measure efficiency in health care, particularly with regard to how best to implement and interpret such measures. Frontier-based metrics are clearly useful when based on sound data, robust and valid models, and when the limitations of the methods are well understood. In many cases, it makes the most sense to try a mix of both DEA and SFA model specifications, with the hope of finding consistent results.

Additionally, these metrics are most relevant when the results are presented in a manner that is easily understood by those tasked with making changes in policy or service delivery. The use of guidelines is one way forward to ensure that the data produced and presented are pertinent to these end users. Guidelines have made a huge difference to the quality of economic evaluation, and could do the same in terms of efficiency measurement, both in terms of the provision of better information, and the interpretation of such information by end users.

References

Coelli T et al. (2005). *An introduction to efficiency and productivity analysis*. Springer, New York (http://facweb. knowlton.ohio-state.edu/pviton/courses/crp394/coelli_Intro_effic.pdf, accessed 22 July 2016).

Drummond M et al. (2005). *Methods for the economic evaluation of health care programmes*. Oxford, Oxford University Press.

Greene WH (2008). The econometric approach to efficiency analysis. In: Fried HO, Knox Lovell CA, Schmidt SS, eds. *The measurement of productive efficiency and productivity growth*. Oxford, Oxford University Press.

Hollingsworth B (2003). Non-parametric and parametric applications measuring efficiency in health care. *Health Care Management Science*, 6(4):203–218.

Hollingsworth B (2008). The measurement of efficiency and productivity of health care delivery. *Health Economics*, 17(10):1107–1128.

Hollingsworth B (2012). Revolution, evolution, or status quo? Guidelines for efficiency measurement in health care. *Journal of Productivity Analysis*, 37(1):1–5.

Hollingsworth B, Parkin D (2003). Efficiency and productivity change in the English National Health Service: can data envelopment analysis provide a robust and useful measure? *Journal of Health Services Research & Policy*, 8(4):230–236.

Hollingsworth B, Peacock S (2008). *Efficiency measurement in health and health care*. London, Routledge.

Hollingsworth B, Street A (2006). The market for efficiency analysis of health care organisations. *Health Economics*, 15(10):1055–1059.

Kumbhakar S, Knox Lovell CA (2000). *Stochastic frontier analysis.* Cambridge, CUP.

Parkin D, Hollingsworth B (1997). Measuring production efficiency of acute hospitals in Scotland, 1991–1994: validity issues in data envelopment analysis. *Applied Economics*, 29(11):1425–1434.

Simar L, Wilson PW (2008). Statistical inference in non parametric frontier models: recent developments and perspectives. In: Fried HO, Knox Lovell CA, Schmidt SS, eds. *The measurement of productive efficiency and productivity growth*. Oxford, Oxford University Press.

Smith P (1997). Model misspecification in data envelopment analysis. *Annals of Operations Research*, 73:233–252.

Thanassoulis E, Portela MCS, Despić O (2008). Data envelopment analysis: the mathematical programming approach to efficiency analysis. In: Fried HO, Knox Lovell CA, Schmidt SS, eds. *The measurement of productive efficiency and productivity growth*. Oxford, Oxford University Press.

Varabyova Y, Schreyögg J (2013). International comparisons of the TE of the hospital sector: panel data analysis of OECD countries using parametric and non-parametric approaches. *Health Policy*, 112(1–2):70–79.

Chapter 6

Cost–effectiveness analysis

Ranjeeta Thomas and Kalipso Chalkidou

6.1 Introduction

Most health systems are faced with high demand but have a limited budget with which to provide the necessary services. A fundamental objective in health systems is to determine the best use of the limited funds available to promote health and provide health care. The underlying principle in this case can be seen as maximizing value for money by selecting the optimal mix of services subject to the constraints faced by the system. The conventional approach to resource allocation is to assume that a decision-maker chooses to maximize efficiency subject to the budget constraint facing the health system. This has led to the development of an extensive suite of techniques usually referred to as cost–effectiveness analysis (CEA) in helping to set priorities, which have had widespread impact, as seen in the United Kingdom's National Institute for Health and Care Excellence (NICE) and other institutions. However, in certain situations the conventional assumptions are too simplistic to offer meaningful information to facilitate efficient resource allocation.

This chapter discusses the potential use of CEA to achieve allocative efficiency (AE) at the health care organization (meso) and health system (macro) level. It begins with an overview of CEA as currently applied at the micro level (for example, the decisions of individual clinicians and choices between treatment options) and highlights its strengths and weaknesses. It then identifies key policy priorities that could be addressed using the tools of CEA. Given the progress in most advanced health systems in assessing and implementing AE at the micro level using CEA, this chapter looks at methodological and informational challenges to adapting these approaches to higher levels of analysis. It concludes with current applications of CEA in policymaking and potential future applications for prospective and retrospective measurement of AE.

6.2 Cost–effectiveness analysis: an overview of its strengths and weaknesses

Countries all over the world place a high priority on the health of their people. Collectively funded health systems in particular usually seek to maximize health outcomes through the provision of health service inputs. Measurement of efficiency in such systems is important in determining whether resources are being used to get the best value for money. AE involves examining the extent to which available resources are allocated across and between health services so as to maximize health outcomes. It is thus concerned with more than the relationship between health inputs and outcomes (Drummond, 2005); it is also concerned with the distribution of resources.[8] This societal perspective on distribution distinguishes AE from other aspects of health system efficiencies (such as technical efficiency (TE)[9]). Outputs, in the case of AE, must be representative of societal utility from alternative investments.

For example, let us assume that there are two alternative uses of health care resources, one for a health care service that extends life and the other for a service that improves functional ability, both with outcomes measured in terms of utility (Figure 6.1). Following Wagstaff (1991), the utility possibilities frontier can be represented by PP'. With an assumption of diminishing utility and returns to inputs in the production of a service that extends life and one that improves functional ability, this curve is downward sloping. If society wished to maximize utility from health outcomes given a pool of resources,[10] then the societal utility function can be represented by the 45-degree line SS'. The tangency between SS' and PP' at point A represents the Pareto-optimal point. AE through an optimal product mix occurs where the marginal rate of transformation (opportunity cost) between a service that extends life and one that improves functional ability = –1, that is, resources are reallocated between services up to the point at which the marginal (social) utilities are equal. AE thus suggests there is a unique point of the production possibilities frontier that maximizes societal values relative to all other attainable sets.

In a competitive market, the allocation that maximizes societal welfare will be determined by market forces of demand and supply of health technologies, and price will be indicative of the value society places on different inputs. However, health care is characterized by the absence of perfectly competitive markets (Arrow, 1963) and information asymmetry between health care providers and patients on the suitability and value of services being provided. In such a scenario, any market-driven allocation is likely to be inefficient.

---

8   This differs from the distribution of health outcomes across populations.
9   TE involves maximizing health benefits from a given allocation of health care resources.
10 This assumes the value of a health outcome is the same irrespective of who receives it.

Figure 6.1 *Trade-offs in utility from alternative uses of health care resources*

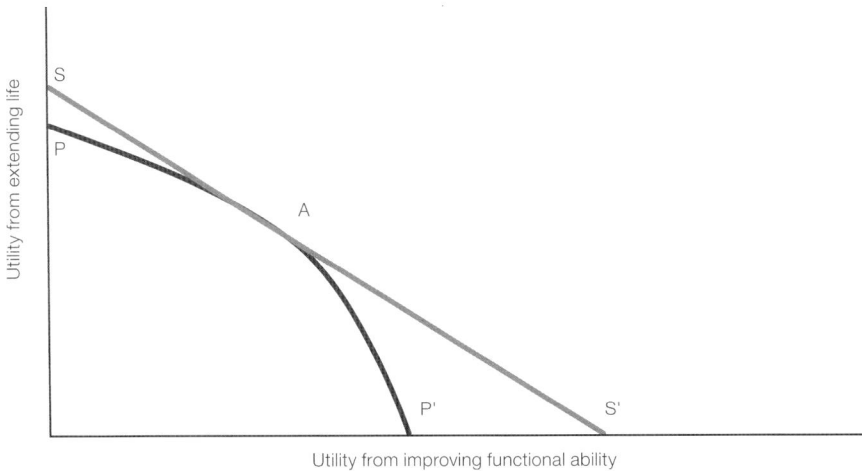

Utility from improving functional ability

This analysis of AE can be applied to different levels of the health care system, for example, at the micro (choice of treatments for specific health conditions), meso organizational (selecting the optimal mix of services for hospitals) or macro (primary versus secondary care) levels. However, as described earlier, measuring AE requires valuing health system outputs from a societal perspective. This involves an aggregation of individual utility functions and preferences to construct a societal welfare function. An allocation that maximizes this societal welfare function can be seen as allocatively efficient. In practice, however, it is not feasible to construct such a societal welfare function and the absence of perfectly competitive markets in health care necessitates the use of a tool that facilitates efficiency in allocation by determining the rationing of limited resources to unlimited demand. Methods of economic evaluation have been developed to facilitate efficient resource allocation. Economic evaluation can be defined as "the comparative analysis of alternative courses of action in terms of both their costs and consequences" (Drummond, 2005, p. 4).

CEA is one form of economic evaluation that has become a central policy tool in many health care systems (Tam & Smith, 2008). It was developed to help decision-makers with fixed resources to compare programmes that produce different outcomes. For a particular level of health care resources, the goal is to choose from among all possible combinations of programmes a set that maximizes the total health benefits produced. In keeping with the earlier discussion on AE, it uses a common unit of measure that captures utility of outcomes – QALYs. This measure allows CEA to simultaneously incorporate the increase in quantity and quality of life (Weinstein, Torrance & McGuire, 2009). Thus, in theory, it is consistent with welfare economics by allowing efficiency in production and product mix. In practice, however, the type of efficiency that can be achieved by applications of CEA is dependent on the decision rules applied. This is discussed in further detail later in this chapter.

CEA has been widely applied to health policy in Europe and other publically funded health systems such as those in Australia and Canada. In these countries, it is an important tool in informing coverage decisions. In other health systems, such as the USA, the use of CEA has played a limited role in rationing care but has influenced the use of interventions that are found to make good use of resources. These include major preventive interventions, such as HIV testing, cervical smears and influenza vaccinations. The principles of cost–effectiveness are applicable in many different contexts. Meltzer & Smith (2011) provide some examples: a private insurer can use CEA to determine the package of covered benefits that will maximize profits; or a social insurer can apply the principle to obtain the maximum health gain with a given budget.

The applications of CEA in these health systems have focused on incremental analysis. Typically, CEA describes a medical technology or health intervention in terms of the ratio of incremental costs per unit of incremental health benefit, the incremental cost–effectiveness ratio (ICER). This captures the difference in effects between the new technology under consideration and the current technology for a given population (incremental benefits), and the difference in costs between the two technologies (incremental costs).

The simplicity of the underlying principle of maximizing health gains subject to a fixed budget makes CEA applicable in many other contexts. For example, in countries looking to establish a package of treatments that could be publically funded, decision-makers would estimate the cost–effectiveness of a range of treatments, rank them in increasing order of cost–effectiveness and accept treatments until the available budget is exhausted.

In all the applications mentioned here, the focus has been on micro level resource allocation decisions. For example, in the United Kingdom, NICE identifies cost-effective technologies and makes recommendations for their use in the National Health System (NHS). NICE has developed a reference case to standardize the way economic evaluations are carried out, that "specifies the methods considered by the institute to be the most appropriate for the Appraisal Committee's purpose … with an NHS objective of maximizing heath gain from limited resources"(NICE, 2013). NICE uses CEA to inform decisions relating to new medicines and diagnostic appraisals, as well as clinical guidelines and public health, staffing levels and service delivery guidance (NICE, 2013). More recently, NICE International under its Methods for Economic Evaluation Project developed a reference case to support health economic evaluations funded by the Bill & Melinda Gates Foundation (NICE International & Bill and Melinda

Gates Foundation, 2014). NICE's reference case provides methodological guidance to be used in the analysis, including the perspective of the analysis, the comparator on which the incremental analysis is based and the discount rate to be applied. However, each of these methodological areas has controversies, which are discussed in the following sections.

6.3 Methodological issues in the use of economic evaluations at the micro level

The objective of a health system to improve health outcomes requires a measure of population health. Within a health system, several categories of measures are available including epidemiological (mortality rates), biomedical (for example, high blood pressure), behavioural (smoking, alcohol consumption) or psychosocial (health-related quality of life) (Cookson & Culyer, 2010). In all these instances the objective is to determine the impact of interventions in improving these outcomes. QALYs were developed by economists as an overall measure of population heath that combines many of the individual categories of health outcomes (Williams, 1995). It represents one year of life, adjusted for the health-related quality of that year of life. QALYs thus enable a quantitative assessment of several aspects of health and account for improvements in length as well as quality of life (Williams, 1985). As an overall measure, it is applicable to many different kinds of interventions and is particularly useful in improving efficiency by eliminating the difficulty of comparing interventions with diverse measures of health outcomes.

6.3.1 Equity considerations

Most cost–effectiveness analyses value health benefits in terms of QALYs, which represent both the quality and quantity of life in a consolidated single value. By focusing on cost per QALY as its basis for achieving efficiency in allocation, CEA incorporates assumptions on equity that imply the value of QALY is the same irrespective of the beneficiary. Such an assumption can be considered egalitarian in that it is not influenced by the characteristics of the recipient of the intervention (age or economic status). However, if the objective is efficiency in allocation then arguments can be made in favour of more QALYs for those who have greater productivity and contribute more to society. In contrast, a vertical equity[11] argument would imply that a QALY is weighted more in the case of those who are likely to have lower benefits without the treatment (such as the poor) than those whose health outcomes are likely to be higher in the absence of the treatment (the rich). Alternatively, in favour of the idea of a fair innings

---

11 Horizontal equity arguments imply persons with equal need should be treated the same (Culyer & Wagstaff, 1993).

(Williams, 1997), it may be considered better to allocate resources to improve the health of the younger individuals in society (who have not enjoyed much health during their current lifetime) as opposed to older individuals who are ill and have had the opportunity of a fair innings. Efficiency- and equity-based QALY weights have thus far seen few applications in the CEA. Dolan & Tsuchiya (2006) provide a detailed discussion of these issues. More recently, Cookson et al. (2016) have proposed an extension of the QALY to include adjustments for income and consumption of goods and services.

6.3.2 Decision rules in cost–effectiveness analysis

The objective of the decision-maker is to maximize health benefits or QALYs generated subject to the available budget constraints. Birch & Gafni (1992) present the following combinations of incremental benefits and incremental costs, which are also represented in the cost–effectiveness plane (Figure 6.2):

1. Incremental costs are positive and incremental benefits are negative (quadrant II in Figure 6.2): This situation is clear in terms of a decision not to adopt the new technology.
2. Incremental costs are negative and incremental benefits are positive (quadrant IV in Figure 6.2): The benefits of the new technology outweigh the costs and hence justify adoption.
3. Both incremental costs and benefits are higher/lower (quadrants I and III in Figure 6.2): Where the sign is the same, it provides a trickier situation in CEA and requires decision rules to facilitate a choice.

Figure 6.2 *Cost–effectiveness plane*

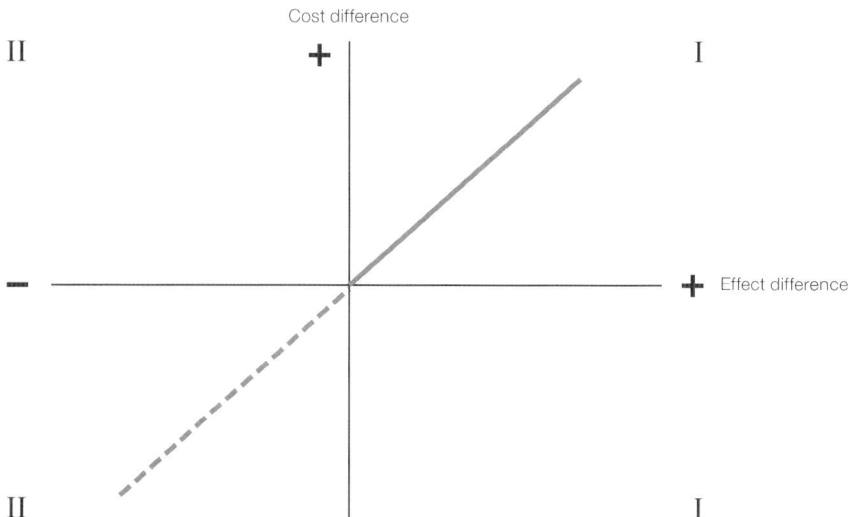

The decision rules of CEA allow a policymaker to make choices in situations such as statement 3 with the aim of producing maximum health gain from the available resources. Two main types of types of decision problems have been addressed using CEA at the micro level. The first is the allocation of resources on interventions across multiple diseases. The second decision problem involves choices between different medical technologies for a particular disease.

The nature of policy questions that can be addressed using CEA at the micro level go beyond these two decision problems and can be classified according to Murray, Kreuser & Whang (1994) into three categories:

1. Ground zero: given a fixed health budget and infrastructure, what allocation of non-fixed resources would result in maximizing health outcomes (or reduce disease burden)? This problem is typical of the policy question most publically funded health systems in Europe face.
2. Marginal expansion: given a current allocation that cannot be changed and a fixed infrastructure, what is the optimal allocation for a marginal increase in the budget?
3. Ground zero with political constraints: with fixed infrastructure and certain services that must be protected from budgetary reallocation for political or other reasons, given a fixed budget, how best can resources be allocated so as to maximize health outcomes without reducing resource allocation to the protected services?

The main rules used in resource allocation decisions (Weinstein & Zeckhauser, 1973) through CEA are:

1. The league table rule: programmes are selected in ascending order of their ICERs until the total available budget is exhausted.
2. ICER threshold rule: programmes with an ICER less than or equal to a defined threshold are selected.

These two decision rules can be applied to the three policy questions listed earlier. If we knew the ICERs of all the interventions, then the league table approach can be applied in all three cases. However, it is rarely the case that the ICERs of all the interventions are available and hence the threshold rule provides an alternative solution to the resource allocation problem.

The ICER threshold rule has been the most applied in policy, for example, in Australia (Commonwealth Department of Heath and Ageing, 2002), the United Kingdom (NICE, 2008) and Canada (Ontario Ministry of Health, 1994). Devlin (2002) and Birch & Gafni (2003) have suggested that the former is not easily applicable given that ICERs are not available for all programmes to create a comprehensive league table.

Both of the decision rules are based on two critical assumptions, first that programmes are perfectly divisible (that is, that a programme can be delivered to specific proportions of the population) and second, that programmes have constant returns to scale (CRS), meaning the QALYs generated do not vary by the size of the programme (Drummond, 2005). In practice, these assumptions are unlikely to hold. Birch & Gafni (1993) have suggested that this makes CEA methods unreliable. In making choices between multiple programmes, decision-makers have to decide between programmes of varying sizes. By using ICERs to compare across programmes, the decision is based on the average cost per QALY. This means that programmes of different sizes and varying opportunity costs are compared on a single statistic. On the other hand, relaxing these assumptions implies decision-making without a specified amount of resources. In contrast, Johannesson & Weinstein (1993) have argued that CEA methods provide an acceptable approximation that can guide efficient resource allocations.

Interpreting whether the ICER of a given programme makes it acceptable requires a cost–effectiveness threshold value against which it can be compared. The specification of a threshold value has generated a lot research in the field. The threshold represents the opportunity cost of the marginal programmes funded from the available resources (Weisnstein & Zeckhauser, 1973). For example, when NICE issues positive guidance that allows the adoption of a new intervention, it increases the amount of resources required to allow for this new intervention (Gafni & Birch, 1993). However, the health budget is typically fixed and the resources to deliver the new intervention must come from displacing other interventions or services (Williams, 2004). In theory, two approaches can be applied to determine the threshold value; the first involves solving the maximization problem (of allocations resulting in the highest benefits) subject to the available resources, the second is the league table approach. In either case information on the ICERs of all possible combinations of programmes must be known, making it difficult to estimate the threshold (Gafni & Birch, 2006). In a recent report Claxton et al. (2013) developed and demonstrated methods that can be applied to estimate the cost–effectiveness threshold for the NHS by relying on routine data. They presented the best estimate of the cost–effectiveness threshold given the existing data and provided recommendations for future data collections efforts that will allow more precision in threshold estimates.

6.3.3 Discounting costs and benefits

The application of CEA to medical technologies often involves measuring benefits and costs generated in the future. While there is generally agreement on the inclusion of future costs and benefits, a major area of controversy has revolved around the rate at which these costs and benefits must be discounted, with a higher discount rate implying lower value to future costs and benefits. The importance of discount rates is particularly obvious in the case of prevention programmes, where benefits from avoiding illness and future treatment costs all occur in the future. In economic theory, discounting reflects the value consumers (in this case of health care) assign to future benefits and costs. The debate has also included differential rates of discounting for costs and benefits. In practice, different countries apply different rates based on the recommendations of the guidelines. In the United Kingdom, until 2004 NICE recommended that costs be discounted at 6% and benefits at 3.5%. Since then, a uniform discount rate has been applied to both costs and benefits. This decision has led to a lot of debate, as captured in Claxton et al. (2011) and Gravelle et al. (2007).

6.4 Cost–effectiveness analysis as a measure of organizational and system efficiency

6.4.1 Allocative efficiency at the organization and system level

This section moves beyond micro level efficiency to consider the scope and priorities for AE gains at the meso and macro levels of the health system. The promotion of efficiency is of interest to policymakers, taxpayers and consumers of health care. AE implies that the best mix (that maximizes health outcomes) of health services is being provided for the given budget. At the meso level this could, for example, reflect the AE of hospitals in the services they provide. At the health system level, it could represent how services can be provided across primary and secondary care or how funds are allocated between different welfare sectors, such as education, health or infrastructure. We next present two examples where CEA can be applied to assessing AE at higher levels of the health system.

Integrated long-term care

A major challenge facing most European health systems is an ageing population and longer length of life. By 2050, it is estimated that the number of individuals >65 years in the WHO European Region will have risen from 129 to 224 million. While many people live long and healthy lives, growing numbers of individuals are now affected with chronic and long-term conditions, such as dementia. The ageing population will increasingly require a package of long-term care that integrates health and social care. Such new models of care must focus on a shift in resources from acute hospitals to prevention and care closer to people's homes, with the aim of improving health outcomes and patient experiences. They must also be comprehensive in the range of services provided to the target population (Ham et al., 2011). CEA can be used to assess new integrated models of long-term care and guide resource allocation towards models that maximize health outcomes at best cost compared to other alternatives. These models could consider integration at many different levels. For example, at the meso level this could mean merger or integration of actual service provision across organizations or virtual integration by developing better networks of care providers to coordinate and enhance the quality of care provided.

Formation of clinical commissioning groups in the English NHS

As the role of primary care in the English NHS grows, the traditional boundaries between primary and secondary care are no longer distinct. With more focus shifting to prevention and community-based care, the role of the general practitioner (GP) and other components of the primary care service are expanding. The establishment of clinical commissioning groups (CCGs) in 2013 with the objective of integrating primary, secondary and social care has meant significant restructuring of the NHS, particularly primary care services (Naylor et al., 2013). Under this reform, all general practices in England are legally required to join a CCG. The objective of this reform is to encourage clinicians to have a greater role in deciding how funds are spent. A CCG has two distinct roles: to commission secondary and social care for their local population; and to support quality improvement in general practice. CCGs also have full responsibility for actual budgets in their areas. CEA of CCGs compared with its predecessor (practice-based commissioning) and other methods of commissioning care are vital to understanding the effects of this health system reform. It can assess the extent to which integration of services and resource reallocation from secondary to primary care leads to changes in health outcomes.

CEA offers a compelling mechanism for ensuring that decisions are evidence-based and transparent. The widespread use of CEA is reflective of the simplicity it provides in maximizing health gains subject to budget constraints. However, such simplicity can be a limiting factor when considering the complexities of entire organizations or health systems. These limiting factors do not make CEA irrelevant because it still provides vital information. But for greater accuracy in more complex interventions and programmes of care, current approaches to CEA may need to be enhanced to include constraints and objectives that are reflective of the scenario at hand.

6.5 Methodological and informational challenges

This section reviews the potential application of the fundamentals of CEA to meso/macro level resource reallocation decisions. As in the case of micro level decisions, measurement of AE at higher levels of the health system has two aspects:

1. to estimate deviation of current allocations from an optimal allocation; and
2. to reallocate resources towards an allocatively efficient mix.

To achieve an estimate of the optimal mix must be known before any deviation can be estimated. At the macro level this means potentially that all programmes of care must be compared against one another; additionally, the opportunity costs of public funds used in the health system that can be invested in other sectors must be considered. At the meso organizational level, all services an organization can potentially provide must be compared against one another. At both these levels such an exercise is likely to be unfeasible given the variety and breadth of services and programmes that constitute a health system. Knowing all inputs and outputs of each programme and service is not possible. At the micro level, even with a more constrained set of options, it would be impossible to estimate an optimal mix from which current deviations can be compared (for example, this might require knowing all the health technologies in an Essential Medicines list). Epstein et al. (2007) highlighted this problem at the micro/individual treatment level. They proposed a more limited way of approaching this issue by focusing on the technologies currently recommended by NICE in the United Kingdom based on CEA. Their objective was to determine the optimal mix within the recommended list that maximized the gross benefit subject to the available budget constraints.

In principle, the approach of Epstein et al. (2007) can be applied to all levels of the health system. However, the primary limitation is information. To make comparisons, the value of all health system outputs at each level must be known. But even before values can be assigned to outputs, a clear definition of outputs for different organizations, services and programmes is necessary. Once these outputs are determined, their value must be ascertained. This requires a uniform measure of benefits, such as the QALYs currently used at the micro level. Such a measure must be a relevant mechanism that applies to all the services and outputs in the health system. It must also be able to capture non-health outcomes, such as patient experience and improvements in productivity both for patients and care providers. But as in the debate on QALYs used at the micro level, there are additional concerns beyond relevance that revolve around the measurement of preferences. These include whose preferences for the optimal mix should be considered and whether it is possible to aggregate these utilities. This brings into question the applicability of CEA instruments currently used for eliciting societal values of outcomes such as the EQ-5D, SF-36, visual analogue scales, and so on. Even if an appropriate instrument for measuring societal values for meso and macro level services is developed, there remains the difficulty of generating values for all services and programmes of care. This discussion has shown that informational weaknesses prevent estimation of an optimal mix from which deviations in current allocations can be estimated. In reality, the informational requirements for comprehensive monitoring of AE are enormous and policymakers must make decisions in the absence of certain information.

Applications of CEA to micro level resource allocation decisions (see Box 6.1) have often focused on achieving the maximum health for a given budget.[12] This implies that the main constraint in the decision process is the available budget. However, in reality there are several other constraints, such as transition costs, infrastructure capacity and personnel redundancies that must be included in evaluations of reforms at higher levels of the health system. For example, at the meso level, if a hospital was to consider altering its current mix of services by removing certain services currently being provided and expanding other services, it must consider the ability of its personnel to adapt to these changes and the implications for health care staff no longer being employed by this hospital because of its narrowing of speciality areas. In addition, patient outcomes for those currently in care but no longer likely to be treated at the hospital must be considered, including availability and access to suitable alternative facilities. This implies that even at the meso level a decision-maker cannot simply focus on budgetary constraints in altering the mix of services but must consider other resource and adaptability constraints.[13] A decision-maker may also need to consider externalities generated by a package of services beyond those reflected directly in health outcomes. Conventional cost–effectiveness ratios do not reflect gains beyond direct outcomes. For example, in considering altering the current mix of services, a decision-maker might be comparing the outcomes from a service being considered for exclusion with those of a new service to be included. One possibility is similar benefits are observed when only direct outcomes are compared. However, they may vary significantly in positive externalities generated that could result in a decision that runs contrary to those implied by cost–effectiveness ratios alone. As a result of these constraints, governments may choose to focus on achieving a certain acceptable level of benefits rather than maximizing them as required by CEA, and they may choose gradual changes to service mixes using criteria that are not standard to conventional cost–effectiveness models. For example, marginal changes may prioritize those with low transition costs and minimum negative externalities. Thus, approaches to resource allocation must maximize health objectives subject to a wider set of constraints.

---

12 There are some instances at the micro level when decision rules favouring, for example, severe conditions or younger patients or certain subgroups (for example, workers with mesothelioma) allow for the maximization of a health assumption/objective to be relaxed even at the micro level.

13 Such constraints also exist at the micro level; for example, in relation to rolling out a new surgical procedure, trained personnel may not be available immediately. However, such constraints are more pronounced at organizational or systems levels.

Box 6.1 *Micro level applications: surgery versus conservative management*

CEA has been widely applied in evaluating individual treatments options. One area of extensive use has been in comparing surgical intervention with conservative treatment/management of a disease. This is particularly important for diseases that might have spontaneous exacerbations and remissions. This uncertainty means that, for certain patients, surgery is likely to be unnecessary.

Surgery versus pharmacotherapy for benign prostatic hyperplasia

One such disease with uncertain outcomes (exacerbations or remissions) and increasing prevalence in ageing men is benign prostatic hyperplasia (BPH). Approximately half of all men are likely to have some evidence of BPH by the age of 60 years. Lowe (1995) used a decision analytical model to compare the outcomes and costs (for an initial two years) of three treatment options: prostate surgery, or treatment with finasteride or terazosin. They concluded that as a primary intervention for patients, all three approaches were equal in terms of months of successful treatment. However, surgery was much more expensive and accompanied by a greater number of productive days lost.

Prioritizing health care services through efficient allocations is at the core of option 2 (to reallocate resources towards an allocatively efficient mix) mentioned earlier. In the absence of adequate information to estimate the optimal mix against which current allocations can be compared, option (2) provides the next best alternative. Reallocations from the current mix of services essentially involve displacing a service or sector currently being funded. To estimate whether such a reallocation is more efficient than the current mix means examining the effects of altering the balance of expenditure between programmes. This is defined as marginal analysis, where any improvement in health benefits is a result of a change in the service or programme mix rather than an increase in expenditure. "Marginal analysis takes the current expenditure allocation as the starting-point (rather than an 'optimal allocation') and examines the effect of small changes to that pattern"(Cohen, 1994). It thus focuses on the marginal gains from expanding a programme and marginal losses (opportunity cost) from removing or contracting a service or programme of care.

In the health sector, applications of marginal analysis have most often been combined with programme budgeting exercises and hence been termed programme budgeting and marginal analysis (PBMA) (Mitton & Donaldson, 2001). Donaldson & Mooney (1991) described how these methods can be applied by health authorities. In principle, PBMA involves first dividing the health services provided at any level, that is, health system, organization or clinical unit into a set of programmes. The divisions are based on specific objectives such as target populations or disease groups. For each, programme costs and outputs are quantified. This is followed by the marginal analysis stage where shifts of resources from one programme to another are analysed in terms of benefits generated or losses incurred. For example, if a hospital shifted £500 000 from speciality care in a disease area to more general outpatient services, what benefits would be lost from speciality care and what gains would be made in outpatient care? While this approach is in principle applicable to all levels of the health system, it also faces the same drawback of CEA in that all benefits must be measured in the same units of health gains so that comparisons can be made across programmes of care. This is evidenced by the current applications of PBMA, which have primarily focused on, for example, grouping areas of clinical activity and estimating the effects of increasing or reducing spending in some areas.

This implies that improving AE at higher levels can be a complex process when compared with the incremental comparison of competing technologies as in conventional CEA. Applications to sectoral comparisons or programmes of care would require generating optimal mixes under different configurations, with the inclusion of a range of constraints and sometimes differing objectives from health benefit maximization.

As discussed in an earlier section, a major equity assumption that underlies CEA is that the value of a QALY is the same irrespective of the beneficiary. Some of the issues relating to this assumption at the micro level were discussed earlier. In the case of reallocations at higher levels of the health system, such an assumption of equality in value of outcomes is almost impossible to justify. For example, one of the primary reasons for reallocation may be to improve equity in health outcomes or to improve access of poorer populations. Such a reason for reallocation in itself moves away from pure AE. A decision-maker must therefore first define an equity objective and an outcome measure that collectively reflect individual viewpoints on the notion of fairness. Consider a national decision-maker applying CEA to assess whether reallocation of some resources from secondary care to primary care would improve efficiency from the current allocation. Such a reallocation assumes that less access to secondary care affects all individuals in the same way. But the influence of limited secondary care could vary greatly depending on, for example, socioeconomic backgrounds. A concern with equity of outcomes implies a need to weight benefits differently depending on the population groups being considered. Alternatively, if the focus is on equity of access, then the need to adjust costs arises. For instance, costs of securing access of certain services among some groups of the population may be higher than among others. Thus, the expected costs of some services within programmes of care must we weighted differentially. CEA can incorporate these equity considerations,[14] however, implementing these weights or adjustments in a cost–effectiveness model is demanding in

---

14   There is emerging literature on incorporating equity concerns in cost–effectiveness analysis. See, for example, Asaria et al. (2013).

terms of information and data requirements (for example, baseline information on the current distribution, and societal valuation of changes to the current distribution, is difficult to obtain).

The applicability of current approaches of CEA to questions of AE is also constrained by the relevance of its assumptions on scope and scale. As discussed earlier, the decision rules of CEA are based on the assumptions of indivisibility of programmes and CRS. This means that comparisons are made on long run average costs of individual treatments. Hospitals by design provide a range of services that draw on the economies of scale of providing different forms of care using an underlying infrastructure base. Decisions of reallocation for efficiency gains cannot focus on comparisons of average costs of individual services but must take into account bundles of the services being provided and the implications of shifting resources and redefining packages, and the corresponding losses or gains because of changes in scale and scope of the packages.

6.6 Cost–effectiveness analysis in policy: present and future

CEA in health care has a long-standing tradition in many high-income countries. This section begins with a discussion of current applications of CEA in health policy. The scope of CEA varies widely across regions and countries. In Europe, policymakers responded to financial pressures and growing public demand for improved quality by setting up HTA agencies, such as the Institute for Quality and Efficiency in Health Care in Germany or NICE in the United Kingdom. Across the EU, technology appraisals are used in policies for pricing, health care provider reimbursements and guiding clinical practice. For example, in the United Kingdom, NICE produces clinical guidelines (NICE, 2008) for the NHS and is required to make recommendations on the basis of both effectiveness and cost–effectiveness.

While CEA is an essential part of the evaluation process in many European countries, there is diversity in how final resource allocation decisions are made. For example, unlike the United Kingdom, which compares the cost–effectiveness ratio of a new intervention against a threshold value, Germany applies an efficiency frontier approach that compares the ICER of the new interventions with the next most cost-effective intervention, which essentially represents the prevailing efficiency level (Klingler et al., 2013). However, since the German parliament passed the Act on the Reform of the Market for Medicinal Products in 2010 there has been debate on whether the efficiency frontier approach is consistent with the law. Since then no decisions on coverage have been made using this approach.

Expenditure on pharmaceuticals is the fastest growing health care cost category in high-income countries (CIHI, 2007; Duerden et al., 2004). CEA has been used extensively in managing expenditure on pharmaceuticals in Australia, Canada and the United Kingdom (Clement, 2009). In Canada, the Common Drug Review provides recommendations for new drug listings for the 18 publically funded drug plans (Tierney & Manns, 2008). The recommendations are based on clinical efficacy as well as cost–effectiveness. In a similar manner, Australia's Pharmaceutical Benefits Advisory Committee gives cost–effectiveness-based advice on which drugs should be funded under the Pharmaceutical Benefits Scheme.

More recently, CEA is being extended to the development of complete care pathways. Thus far, the role of cost–effectiveness in clinical guidelines has been piecemeal and selective. In some cases, CEA is applied independently at different points in the care pathway with assumptions that may not be consistent across the pathway (Lord et al., 2013). In other cases, the lack of time to build new models means cost–effectiveness estimates may not be available when resource allocation decisions are made. The risk with this selective approach is that sometimes, adequate evidence does not exist to make an informed decision. For example, in a systematic review of the United Kingdom care pathway for colorectal cancer, Tappenden et al. (2009) found no relevant United Kingdom cost–effectiveness estimates for large segments of the pathway. The Modelling Algorithm Pathways in Guidelines project (Lord et al., 2013) was developed to evaluate the feasibility and relevance of modelling complete care pathways for the NICE clinical guidelines. The rationale for such an approach (Tappenden et al. (2012) refer to this approach as whole disease modelling) is that a model that captures a full guideline should allow CEA of a range of different scenarios. By using a common framework and similar assumptions throughout the care pathway, the accuracy and consistency of the estimates would be improved (Box 6.2).

Provider reimbursement schemes play a critical role in improving productivity and efficiency in health systems. In England, GP payments include a pay-for-performance (P4P) scheme known as the Quality and Outcomes Framework (QOF). The scheme rewards performance in four areas: clinical; organizational; patient experience; and other services. Walker et al. (2010) evaluated the cost–effectiveness of a subset of nine QOF indicators with direct clinical impact. The authors found that QOF incentive payments are likely to be cost-effective even if the actual improvement in care outcomes is modest. However, the study did not include the costs of administering the QOF scheme in the analysis. We now consider the potential to develop a framework for extending CEA to studying AE at the health system level (see Box 6.3).

The discussion of AE can be considered from either an *ex ante* perspective or an *ex post* perspective. In the *ex ante* case, the focus is on prospective assessments of the health system. The role of AE in this case is to guide decisions on the purchase of health care. For example, this could mean whether a new intervention should be adopted or whether a reallocation of resources to a new service mix achieves greater AE. The *ex ante* case is of particular importance to countries that are looking to establish publically funded health systems. Such an exercise is key to the WHO's move to promote universal health coverage in developing countries (WHO, 2010). The objective of AE in this case is to establish a package of health care services that maximizes the health outcomes of the population in the country and is made available free to all individuals at the point of access.

Box 6.2 *Meso level applications: redesigning care pathways*

Care Pathway Simulator

The Care Pathway Simulator (CPS) (Dodd, 2005) allows the design and comparison of different configurations of services to assess benefits and resource needs. Users can specify different care pathway models to determine parameters of interest including resource usage and patterns of care for each scenario. The simulation, which is based on discrete event modelling, allows predictions of capacity constraints in restructuring care pathways and mapping of performance to resource needs. The CPS has been used to redesign an outpatient clinic for vascular surgery in Good Hope Hospital, United Kingdom. In this application, the model used three inputs: patient lists to represent demand at the clinic; the care pathway or sequence; and the resources required to carry out the necessary care. The model was then applied to predict performance under different clinic process designs. CPS has also been used to analyse A&E care pathways and redesign day case surgery units.

For further information: http://mashnet.info/casestudy/care-pathway-simulator-cps/ (accessed 22 July 2016).

Redesign of emergency stroke pathways to maximize thrombolysis rates

In this application, the Peninsula Collaboration for Health Operational Research and Development collaborated with the acute stroke team at the Royal Devon and Exeter Hospital, United Kingdom to evaluate and adjust the emergency stroke care pathway. The objective was to simulate improvements that would result in the uptake and provision of thrombolysis leading to fewer disabilities. The simulations allowed the calculation of benefits (measured as patients free of disability) from alternate designs of the care pathway. The recommendations from the study were implemented in 2011 and 2012. An evaluation following the changes showed thrombolysis increasing throughout 2012 and arrival times to treatment were halved during the period.

For further information: http://mashnet.info/casestudy/redesigning-emergency-stroke-pathways-to-maximise-thrombolysis-rates/ (accessed 22 July 2016).

Box 6.3 *Macro level applications: a research agenda*

Cost–effectiveness at the health system level: the optimal mix of health care sectors

AE at the macro level is about the optimal balance of broad services at the health care system level. The macro level may include questions such as whether policymakers ought to be investing more in primary care vis-à-vis hospitals, including aspects such as workforce training and infrastructure investment. Once the balance of investment across the various tiers of the system has been addressed, the question of whether those new resources are being used properly becomes a lower, meso or micro level question, as discussed earlier. In addition to horizontal allocation between sectors such as primary and secondary care, vertical allocation between different disease programmes is another macro/system level question.

However, there is little analytical work done on how economic evaluation, and cost–effectiveness analysis in particular, can be applied to this kind of macro level question. More research is needed to address such big policy questions faced increasingly by countries moving towards universal health care coverage, including the development of a methodological framework that allows the micro and meso levels effectively to interface with macro level decisions.

On the other hand, there is a strong case for also measuring AE in *ex post* analyses. For example, in low to middle income countries looking to improve AE in their health systems, *ex post* analyses can establish a baseline to identify the potential for efficiency savings. The retrospective approach to measuring value for money is particularly applicable in established publically funded systems such as the ones in Europe, Australia or Canada. In this case the focus is more on improving efficiency through changes in the current mix of services provided by different levels of the health system. Take, for example, the case of a publically funded health system, where the government allocates resources to services based on perceived societal valuations of those services. It may then be relevant to ensure that providers are making available services that are consistent with the societal valuations rather than diverting resources to other service areas. For example, at the hospital level retrospective analysis might identify excessive capacity or investment in specialities or services not consistent with the needs of society. It may also mean divergence from prescribed clinical guidelines that reflect cost–effectiveness. Deviations from the preferred options can reflect inefficiency and therefore a reduction in the value for money.

Measuring allocative inefficiency at the organizational level can offer insights into the performance of the different organizations that comprise a health system. There have been several metrics developed to achieve this objective (Hollingsworth, 2003). However, health care organizations, particularly hospitals, are complex structures providing a range of services to heterogeneous populations. Thus, any such metrics of deviation and inefficiency must be scrutinized to ensure that they indeed reflect allocative inefficiency rather than being caused by constraints faced by the organization in servicing its population. For example, observed variations in AE must be conditional on adjustments for the case mix in hospitals (see Chapter 2).[15] They must also reflect the policy constraints, environmental factors and determinants of demand for services that are likely to influence performance. For example, the use and take-up of services offered by a hospital depend on the demand for its services and the elasticity of this demand with respect to substitute and complementary services. The elasticity of demand for any of its services varies to different extents by price, distance and convenience.

Scrutinizing the accuracy of metrics of inefficiency becomes even more important at the health system level which by design might preclude flexibilities that allow adherence to an allocatively efficient mix. Such constraints might include the structure of physical capital and administrative arrangements, financial constraints including long-term commitments to certain groups of patients, and at least in the short-term, workforce constraints. In addition, there may be governance constraints including the absence of effective accountability mechanisms that prevent health systems from maximizing performance.

Retrospective analyses of AE can also be applied by international donors to evaluate the value for money received on their external aid to developing countries. Teerawattananon et al. (2013) described the potential applications of CEA for monitoring and evaluating the performance of the Global Fund to Fight AIDS, Tuberculosis and Malaria. They emphasized the importance of retrospective CEA being included as part of final reports submitted by grant recipients. Such analyses not only facilitate an understanding of the value for money achieved by Global Fund grants, but equally they provide important information to recipient countries on the interventions that are cost-effective in their settings and therefore worthy of long-term finance. Thus, *ex post* cost–effectiveness evaluations provide opportunities to inform decision-makers in developing countries of the implications of potentially sustaining or rolling out programmes initially funded by external donors. An example of *ex post* CEA in the case of HIV prevention is presented in Tosanguang et al. (2012). The programme aimed to expand HIV preventive services among high-risk populations in Thailand. Concern over the long-term sustainability of the programme beyond the initial five-year international funding led to a retrospective CEA. The analysis indicated that the programme had a much higher cost per person in Thailand than similar programmes in other

15 DRGs we originally developed to allow cost comparisons after adjusting for the case mix of patients (Fetter, 1991).

countries, such as India and Bangladesh, and did not perform as well. These examples illustrate the importance of incorporating CEA in decision-making at international organizations and global health initiatives to ensure allocatively efficient resource allocation.

6.7 Conclusion

The final part of this chapter highlights potential areas for future research that will enable the application of CEA to meso and macro level efficiency analysis, both in retrospective assessment of past performance, and as a tool for guiding future allocation decisions.

There is growing awareness that the design and performance of national health systems has large implications for other sectors within a country. This focus has been particularly accentuated with the stagnation of health budgets in most European countries and with the recognition of the importance of maximizing health outcomes given the constraints. Health system level analyses of AE offer a powerful tool for identifying potential gains that can be made with the given resources. The currently widely applied tool of CEA provides an important framework within which assessments of AE can be made and offers a framework for both prospective purchasing decisions and retrospective evaluations. In the absence of information on all possible health care interventions and services, marginal analysis offers an opportunity to improve AE. However, several challenges must be addressed before efficiency is evaluated at the meso or macro levels of the health system.

First, research is required into the appropriateness of existing measures of preference valuation for higher levels of evaluation. The second challenge relates to finding and allowing for one or more equity criteria that influences policymaker decisions in allocating resources across and within health sectors. Current applications of equity-adjusted CEA are limited. Some examples from the emerging literature that allow for broader objectives in the CEA objective function include the evaluation of the impact of policies across multiple domains using extended CEA (Verguet, Laxminarayan & Jamison, 2015); allowing for distributional concerns (Asaria et al., 2013); and financial concerns (Smith, 2013). But at higher levels of the health system these criteria can be major determinants of allocations. Third, factors beyond the budget constraints present challenges to adopting an optimal mix of services. These might include human resources constraints, transition costs of either eliminating or incorporating new services or even the dynamic aspect of the health system. Thus, current methodologies for incorporating equity considerations and other non-financial constraints in conventional CEA must be explored. It is important to acknowledge that many health outcomes currently observed are the results of decisions taken in earlier time periods and that often changes may not reflect in the outcomes for a long time. Finally, decision-making tools such as CEA must also allow for externalities and system-wide effects in estimating the gains and losses from changing the current mix of services or in moving resources between sectors.

References

Arrow KJ (1963). Uncertainty and the welfare economics of medical care. *American Economic Review*, 53(5):941–973.

Asaria M et al. (2013). Distributional cost–effectiveness analysis of health care programmes. CHE Research Paper 91. York, Centre for Health Economics (https://www.york.ac.uk/media/che/documents/papers/researchpapers/CHERP91_distributional_CEA_healthcare.pdf, accessed 22 July 2016)

Birch S, Gafni A (1992). Cost effectiveness/utility analyses: do current decision rules lead us to where we want to be? *Journal of Health Economics*, 11(3):279–296.

Birch S, Gafni A (1993). Changing the problem to fit the solution: Johannesson and Weinstein's (mis) application of economics to real world problems. *Journal of Health Economics*, 12(4):469–476.

Birch S, Gafni A (2003). Economics and the evaluation of health care programmes: generalisability of methods and implications for generalisability of results. *Health Policy*, 64(2):207–219.

Canadian Institute for Health Information (CIHI) (2007). Drug expenditure in Canada, 1985 to 2006. Ottawa, ON, CIHI.

Claxton K et al. (2011). Discounting and decision making in the economic evaluation of health-care technologies. *Health Economics*, 20(1):2–15.

Claxton K et al. (2013). Methods for the estimation of the NICE cost effectiveness threshold. York, University of York.

Clement FM (2009). Using effectiveness and cost–effectiveness to make drug coverage decisions: a comparison of Britain, Australia, and Canada. *JAMA*, 302(13):1437–1443.

Cohen D (1994). Marginal analysis in practice: an alternative to needs assessment for contracting health care. *BMJ*, 309(6957):781–784.

Commonwealth Department of Health and Ageing (2002). Guidelines for the pharmaceutical industry on preparation of submissions to the Pharmaceutical Benefits Advisory Committee. Including major submissions involving economic analyses. Canberra, Australia: Commonwealth of Australia.

Cookson R, Culyer A (2010). Measuring overall population health: the use and abuse of QALYs. In: Killoran A, Kelly MP, eds. *Evidence-based public health: effectiveness and efficiency*. Oxford, Oxford University Press.

Cookson R et al. (2016). Years of good life based on income and health: Re-engineering cost-benefit analysis to examine policy impacts on wellbeing and distributive justice. CHE Research paper 132. York, Centre for Health Economics (https://www.york.ac.uk/media/che/documents/papers/researchpapers/CHERP132_income_health_CBA_wellbeing_justice.pdf, accessed 19 September 2016).

Culyer AJ, Wagstaff A (1993). Equity and equality in health and health care. *Journal of Health Economics*, 12(4):431–457.

Devlin N (2002). An introduction to the use of cost–effectiveness thresholds in decision-making: what are the issues? In: Towse A, Pritchard C, Devlin N, eds. *Cost effectiveness thresholds: economic and ethical issues*. London, King's Fund and Office of Health Economics.

Dodd S (2005). Designing improved healthcare processes using discrete event simulation. *British Journal of Healthcare Computing & Information Management*, 22(5):14–16.

Dolan P, Tsuchiya A (2006). The elicitation of distributional judgements in the context of economic evaluation. In: Jones AM, ed. *The Elgar companion to health economics*. Cheltenham, Edward Elgar Publishing.

Donaldson C, Mooney G (1991). Needs assessment, priority setting, and contracts for health care: an economic view. *BMJ*, 303(6816):1529–1530.

Drummond M (2005). *Methods for the economic evaluation of health care programmes*. 3rd edn. Oxford, Oxford University Press.

Duerden M et al. (2004). Current national initiatives and policies to control drug costs in Europe: UK perspective. *Journal of Ambulatory Care Management*, 27(2):132–138.

Epstein DM et al. (2007). Efficiency, equity, and budgetary policies: informing decisions using mathematical programming. *Medical Decision Making*, 27(2):128–137.

Fetter RB (1991). Diagnosis related groups: understanding hospital performance. *Interfaces*, 21(1):6–26.

Gafni A, Birch S (1993). Guidelines for the adoption of new technologies: a prescription for uncontrolled growth in expenditures and how to avoid the problem. *CMAJ*, 148(6):913–917.

Gafni A, Birch S (2006). Incremental cost–effectiveness ratios (ICERs): the silence of the lambda. *Social Science & Medicine*, 62(9):2091–2100.

Gravelle H et al. (2007). Discounting in economic evaluations: stepping forward towards optimal decision rules. *Health Economics*, 16(3):307–317.

Ham C et al. (2011). Where next for the NHS reforms? The case for integrated care. London: The King's Fund (http://www.kingsfund.org.uk/sites/files/kf/where-next-nhs-reforms-case-for-integrated-care-ham-imison-goodwin-dixon-south-kings-fund-may-2011.pdf, accessed 22 July 2016).

Hollingsworth B (2003). Non-parametric and parametric applications measuring efficiency in health care. *Health Care Management Science*, 6(4):203–218.

Johannesson M, Weinstein MC (1993). On the decision rules of cost–effectiveness analysis. *Journal of Health Economics*, 12(4):459–467.

Klingler C et al. (2013). Regulatory space and the contextual mediation of common functional pressures: analyzing the factors that led to the German Efficiency Frontier approach. *Health Policy*, 109(3):270–280.

Lord J et al. (2013). Economic modelling of diagnostic and treatment pathways in National Institute for Health and Care Excellence clinical guidelines: the Modelling Algorithm Pathways in Guidelines (MAPGuide) project. *Health Technology Assessment*, 17(58):v–vi, 1–192.

Lowe FC (1995). Economic modeling to assess the costs of treatment with finasteride, terazosin, and transurethral resection of the prostate for men with moderate to severe symptoms of benign prostatic hyperplasia. *Urology*, 46(4):477–483.

Meltzer DO, Smith PC (2011). Theoretical issues relevant to the economic evaluation of health technologies. In: Pauly MV, McGuire TG, Barros PP, eds. *Handbook of health economics*. Volume 2. Amsterdam, Elsevier.

Mitton C, Donaldson C (2001). Twenty-five years of programme budgeting and marginal analysis in the health sector, 1974–1999. *Journal of Health Services Research & Policy*, 6(4):239–248.

Murray CJ, Kreuser J, Whang W (1994). Cost–effectiveness analysis and policy choices: investing in health systems. *Bulletin of the World Health Organization*, 72(4):663–674.

Naylor C et al. (2013). *Clinical commissioning groups: supporting improvement in general practice?* London, The Kings Fund (http://www.kingsfund.org.uk/sites/files/kf/field/field_publication_file/clinical-commissioning-groups-report-ings-fund-nuffield-jul13.pdf, accessed 22 July 2016).

National Institute for Health and Care Excellence (NICE) (2008). Social value judgements: principles for the development of NICE guidance. London, NICE.

NICE (2013). Guide to the methods of technology appraisal 2013. London, NICE (https://www.nice.org.uk/process/pmg9/chapter/1-foreword, accessed 22 July 2016).

NICE International, Bill and Melinda Gates Foundation (2014). The Gates Reference Case: what it is, why it's important and how to use it. NICE International (https://www.nice.org.uk/Media/Default/About/what-we-do/NICE-International/projects/Gates-Reference-case-what-it-is-how-to-use-it.pdf, accessed 22 July 2016).

Ontario Ministry of Health (1994). *Ontario guidelines for economic analysis of pharmaceutical products*. Toronto, Ministry of Health, Ontario.

Smith PC (2013). Incorporating financial protection into decision rules for publicly financed healthcare treatments. *Health Economics*, 22(2):180–193.

Tam TY, Smith MD (2008). Pharmacoeconomic guidelines around the world. *ISPOR CONNECTIONS*, 10:4–5.

Tappenden P et al. (2009). Systematic review of economic evidence for the detection, diagnosis, treatment, and follow-up of colorectal cancer in the United Kingdom. *International Journal of Technology Assessment in Health Care*, 25(4):470–478.

Tappenden P et al. (2012). Whole disease modeling to inform resource allocation decisions in cancer: a methodological framework. *Value in Health*, 15(8):1127–1136.

Teerawattananon Y et al. (2013). Health technology assessments as a mechanism for increased value for money: recommendations to the Global Fund. *Global Health*, 9:35.

Tierney M, Manns B (2008). Optimizing the use of prescription drugs in Canada through the Common Drug Review. *CMAJ*, 178(4):432–435.

Tosanguang K et al. (2012). Economic evaluation of comprehensive HIV prevention interventions targeting those most at risk of HIV/AIDs in Thailand (CHAMPION). Nonthaburi, Health Intervention and Technology Assessment Program.

Verguet S, Laxminarayan R, Jamison DT (2015). Universal public finance of tuberculosis treatment in India: an extended cost–effectiveness analysis. *Health Economics*, 24(3):318–332.

Wagstaff A (1991). QALYs and the equity-efficiency trade-off. *Journal of Health Economics*, 10(1):21–41.

Walker S et al. (2010). Value for money and the Quality and Outcomes Framework in primary care in the UK NHS. *British Journal of General Practice*, 60(574):e213–e220.

Weinstein MC, Zeckhauser R (1973). Critical ratios and efficient allocation. *Journal of Public Economics*, 2:147–157.

Weinstein MC, Torrance G, McGuire A (2009). QALYs: the basics. *Value in Health*, 12(Suppl. 1):S5–S9.

Williams A (1985). Economics of coronary artery bypass grafting. *British Medical Journal*, 291(6491):326–329.

Williams A (1995). The measurement and valuation of health: a chronicle. Centre for Health Economics Discussion Paper. York, University of York (http://www.york.ac.uk/che/pdf/DP136.pdf, accessed 22 July 2016).

Williams A (1997). Intergenerational equity: an exploration of the 'fair innings' argument. *Health Economics*, 6(2):117–132.

Williams A (2004). What could be nicer than NICE? Office of Health Economics annual lecture. (https://www.ohe.org/publications/what-could-be-nicer-nice, accessed 22 July 2016).

WHO (2010). *Health systems financing: the path to universal coverage*. The World Health Report. Geneva, WHO (http://apps.who.int/iris/bitstream/10665/44371/1/9789241564021_eng.pdf, accessed 22 July 2016).

Chapter 7

Cross-national efficiency comparisons of health systems, subsectors and disease areas

*Jonathan Cylus and Mark Pearson**

7.1 Introduction: the basis for interest in cross-country efficiency comparisons

The notion of health system efficiency, and related concepts such as cost–effectiveness and value for money, are some of the most discussed dimensions of health system performance. Health care financiers including governments, insurers and households are interested in knowing which systems, providers and treatments contribute the largest health gains in relation to the level of resources they consume. This is particularly important given the financial pressures and concerns over long-term financial sustainability, as decision-makers seek to demonstrate and ensure that health care resources are put to good use.

Health system efficiency metrics should be useful for the following purposes: to facilitate the analysis of policies; identify best practices; and detect areas of the health system that are not producing as well as desired and that could potentially benefit from reforms. However, it is challenging to appropriately attribute particular inputs to health outcomes because health is the result of complex processes involving not only medical care but also wealth, education, occupation, housing, the environment and genetics. Likewise, the observed efficiency of a single health system or health care provider may be due to factors unrelated to specific policies or events of interest; for example, variations may occur because of unobserved changes in patient characteristics, the effects of interrelated inputs over long periods of time, issues with data collection and comparability or simply random fluctuations. Without being able to clearly identify the reasons why a health system or provider appears inefficient, it is difficult to develop targeted policy or management levers to improve. In this case, the simplest action may be to just reduce health resources. This is a naive approach unlikely to lead to true efficiency gains and one that may ultimately worsen performance.

---

* The views expressed in this chapter are those of the authors alone, not those of the OECD or its member countries.

To monitor and pinpoint the causes of variability, it can be helpful to compare efficiency within, as well as across countries. Comparative data on health system efficiency across multiple country settings is potentially important, both for benchmarking and to try to gauge whether different types of health care delivery or policies may be successful at realizing efficiency gains or improving health. As a result, the development of metrics that can compare health system efficiency across countries has been on the agenda of researchers and policymakers for some time (Hollingsworth & Wildman, 2003; OECD, 2004; WHO, 2000).

However, in spite of the interest surrounding them, in practice, internationally comparable efficiency indicators are among the most elusive of health system comparative performance metrics. In fact, a 2008 review found that of all health care efficiency studies, only 4% were cross-country analyses (Hollingsworth, 2008). This is partially because of limited availability and comparability of cross-country longitudinal health data, despite recognition that such data are desirable to capture trends in efficiency, to compare changes over time and to identify the causal effects of policies.

In this chapter, we review the availability of internationally comparative health system efficiency data, which we consider to be indicators that assess the relationship between health system inputs (including, but not limited to expenditure, personnel and beds) and health system outputs (including, but not limited to, physician visits and discharges), or health system inputs and health outcomes across countries. The distinction between health outcome-based and health care output-based indicators is important as outcome-based approaches are in theory superior given that what matters to patients is to obtain quality health services that will improve their health; however, in practice, output-based indicators are easier to collect and more widely available. The focus in this chapter is primarily on measures of technical efficiency (TE) – that is, the effectiveness of a given set of inputs to produce a given set of outputs or outcomes – because studies and data sets comparing allocative efficiency (AE) or dynamic efficiency across countries are uncommon.

While there are many different ways to conceptualize and calculate efficiency metrics, estimates do not generally lead to definitive conclusions regarding efficient health systems, providers or practices. Frequently collected metrics are simple, compare entire health systems and are readily available in international databases, but because of their high level of aggregation, these metrics are not particularly useful for identifying determinants of inefficiency or developing appropriate policy responses. Advanced analytical tools are often used to construct more sophisticated, system-level metrics based on data from these same international databases; however, their use of the same, limited data sets raises potential questions on their external validity. Cross-country comparisons of providers or subsectors allow for more detailed analysis and are a promising way forward, but are primarily focused on hospitals, with limited analysis of other types of care settings. Some of the most important gains have been made by disease-based efficiency studies; these studies capture variations in the costs, processes and outcomes associated with treating particular diseases, and can often be linked to registry data containing non-health-based characteristics (for example, income, education, occupation). Longitudinal disease-based studies that take advantage of high-quality patient-level data allow numerous observable non-health-related confounders to be controlled for when comparing the treatment of specific diseases across countries, providing important insight into health production processes. We conclude the chapter by reviewing key future challenges.

7.2 Cross-country databases containing health system efficiency metrics

We begin by reviewing international databases that routinely collect comparable health system efficiency data. Comparable cross-country data on health systems are collected and regularly updated by intergovernmental organizations, such as the WHO, Eurostat and the OECD. Member countries typically supply these organizations with their own national data, which are then reviewed and harmonized to ensure comparability across countries and time. Resources such as the System of Health Accounts (SHA), for example, have made important advances on the input side to ensure that health care expenditure data are collected under a common framework and are comparable across countries (OECD, 2000).

The OECD Health Statistics database provides a comprehensive set of comparable health and health systems data, primarily for high-income countries in the OECD region (OECD, 2013a). The WHO European Health for All Database contains similar data to the OECD Health Statistics database for the 53 European WHO Member States; Eurostat contains similar data for EU countries. Each database is updated annually and covers a wide range of health care inputs (for example, health care expenditure, physician density or hospital beds), outputs (for example, hospital discharges) and outcomes (for example, life expectancy or infant mortality) that can be used to compute efficiency metrics. For the purposes of this chapter and because so many other studies make use of it, we focus primarily on the OECD Health Statistics database.

While many health system efficiency comparison studies use the OECD Health Statistics data to construct efficiency metrics, the database itself contains few ready-made indicators that capture ratios of outputs and inputs, and which might allow efficiency comparisons. One variable that is available for the majority of countries is the common metric average length of stay. This indicator is calcu-lated by dividing the total number of days in hospital for all inpatients in a year by the number of admissions or discharges. The data is available for all hospital stays, as well as by selected diagnostic category. Shorter stays are assumed to indicate greater efficiency, because they are expected to be less costly overall, as they theoretically require fewer inputs to produce a hospital visit. There is some ambiguity though, as short stays could be a result of very intensive, expensive care, which may be costlier. Likewise, very short stays may indicate poor qual-ity of care, which may require readmission to hospital and higher costs for the entire episode of care. Based on data from European countries reporting to the OECD, Finland had the longest length of stay in 2012 (11.2 days) while Turkey had the shortest (4.0 days) (Figure 7.1). A number of factors unrelated to hos-pital efficiency may explain this disparity, including differences in health needs between countries. However, because the data are not adjusted for confounding factors, such as differences in case mix, it is not possible to make an informed statement of whether differences in length of stay are because of more efficient practices or other factors. This case mix issue can be partially accounted for by focusing on the length of stay for specific diagnostic categories, though this still cannot adjust for variations in case severity within a diagnostic category (see Section 7.3 on disease-based indicators for more information).

Figure 7.1 *Average length of stay in hospital for all causes, 2000 and 2012 (or nearest year)*

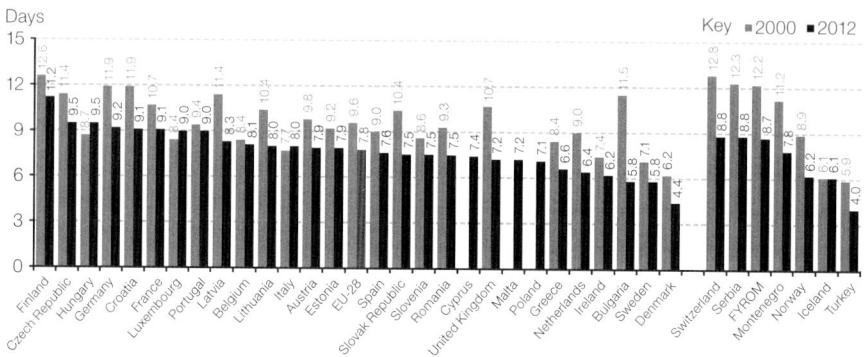

Sources: OECD Health Statistics 2014; Eurostat Statistics database; WHO Europe health for all database.
Note: Netherlands: Data refer to average length of stay for curative (acute) care only (resulting in an underestimation). FYROM = Former Yugoslav Republic of Macedonia.

Another available metric that compares efficiency across countries is the curative care occupancy rate, calculated as the number of curative bed days divided by the number of available beds multiplied by 365 days. The assumption is that, generally, a higher percentage of beds occupied means that resources are being used effectively; in many countries, decreases in hospital beds have coincided with increases in occupancy rates, suggesting efficiency gains. However, very high occupancy rates could indicate an undersupply of beds, or indicate that patients are not moved out of acute care appropriately. The definition of acute care beds also differs across countries, which makes this figure not necessarily comparable; for example, some countries use acute care beds for long-term care services. According to the most recent OECD data, the highest occupancy rates in 2012 were in Israel (96.6%) with the lowest in the Netherlands (45.6%).

Total health spending as a share of gross domestic product (and other similar metrics which relate health spending to available resources) and total per capita health care expenditure adjusted for purchasing power, are also frequently available and could be considered efficiency indicators. In this case, we would have to assume that health outcomes are identical across countries, so that using fewer resources implies greater efficiency. However, outcomes are never identical across countries, and even if they were, it would be very difficult to attribute these differences entirely to the health system. As a result, expenditure-based indicators are not typically suitable for comparing efficiency unless they appear relative to some measure of health system outputs or outcomes.

Despite few efficiency metrics in the OECD Health Statistics database, given the large number of variables in the data set, it is possible to manually calculate simple efficiency indicators. For example, since the number of practising physicians and the number of physician consultations are presented, it would seem logical to calculate the number of visits per physician to examine whether physicians are using their time efficiently. Yet this direct calculation without manual adjustment may produce inaccurate estimates of efficiency for a variety of reasons. For example, there are often inconsistencies between input and output data reported by countries, so that ratios calculated may not fully capture the level of output produced by a given input. Taking the simple ratio of number of consultations per physician as an example, the data reported on the number of consultations are often more limited than the data on the number of doctors, because the reported number of consultations will often not include consultations in hospitals or consultations that are not reimbursed fee-for-service (FFS). Therefore, without manually adjusting the data to reflect these issues, the ratio of consultations per physician could underestimate the level of efficiency. Estimated numbers of consultations per physician that are adjusted to account for these data inconsistencies indicate that the highest numbers of consultations per physician are in Turkey, whereas the lowest are in Cyprus and Sweden (Figure 7.2).

Figure 7.2 *Estimated number of consultations per doctor, 2012 (or nearest year)*

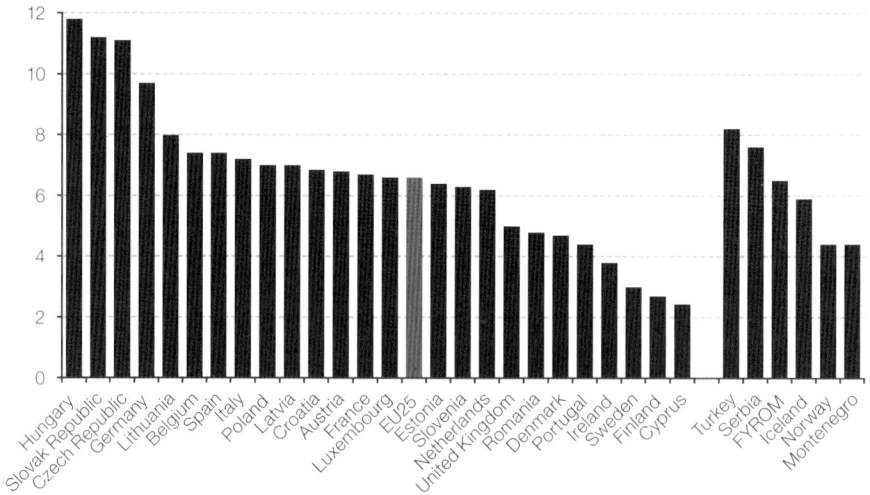

Sources: OECD Health Statistics 2014, Eurostat Statistics database, WHO European Health for All database.
Note: FYROM = Former Yugoslav Republic of Macedonia

Additionally, no information is available on the quality of visits or on the number of hours worked by physicians, so a researcher calculating consultations per physician would have to assume that more visits per physician automatically imply that physicians work more efficiently. This is not necessarily accurate, as physicians who have large numbers of visits may not spend enough time with patients and could be providing poor-quality care. In reality, despite the large number of indicators available in international databases, using these data to calculate ratios of inputs to outputs to infer efficiency can produce misleading findings.

In the same vein, there is great interest among analysts to link readily available health expenditure data to overall health outcome data, such as life expectancy, in an effort to identify whether the health system achieves good value for money overall. For example, a recent report from the International Monetary Fund (IMF) reviewed the Slovenian public sector and concluded that Slovenia's health system was not efficient because its level of per capita expenditure on health did not achieve the life expectancy that might be expected at its level of health spending (IMF, 2015). Using data from a group of countries, the authors manually constructed a production possibilities frontier consisting of outlier countries and considered that those not lying on the frontier were inefficient (Figure 7.3). There are a number of issues with this approach to measuring efficiency. First, life expectancy is not only a result of health spending, so it is not possible to determine how efficiently health care expenditure is producing longer life expectancy without accounting for a long list of other determinants of life expectancy, such as health behaviours, genetics, education and income. Second, many of the countries that form the frontier in Figure 7.3 do not demonstrate that they achieve the longest life expectancy at the minimum cost. For example, Japan and Switzerland both have similar life expectancies but Switzerland spends considerably more on health care per person than Japan, yet both are on or near the efficiency frontier. At the same time, Chile, Mexico and Turkey also spend comparable levels on health care per person, but have drastically different life expectancies.

Figure 7.3 *Health-adjusted life expectancy and health expenditure*

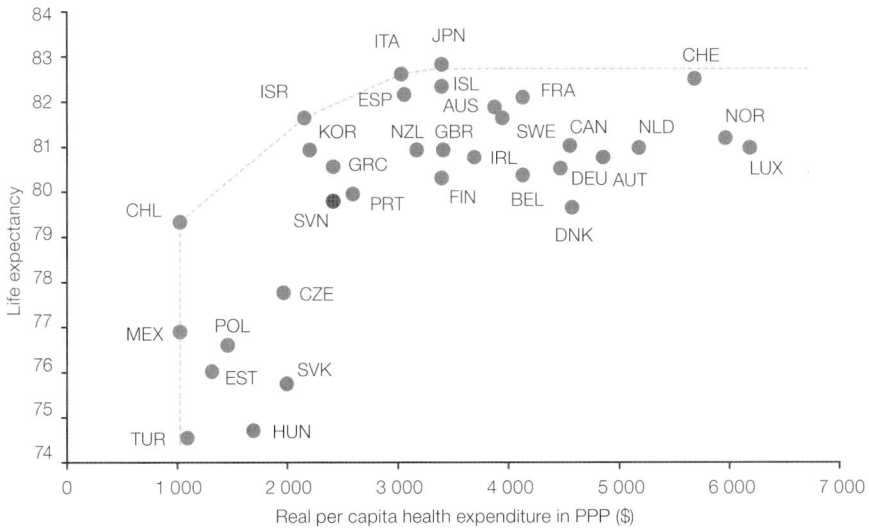

Source: IMF (2015).
Note: Data are from 2010–2012. PPP = purchasing power parity.

An arguably more appropriate approach would be to compare per capita expenditure to amenable mortality rates. Amenable mortality reflects deaths that should not occur in the presence of timely and effective health care; it is more directly attributable to the health system than life expectancy, although it is still a product of more factors than just current expenditure levels. Using this approach, we see a very different picture than when using life expectancy (Figure 7.4). For example, for men and women, Slovenia (highlighted by a red cross in the figure) is located in the bottom left quadrant, indicating that it secures fairly low amenable mortality rates at low cost. Other countries, like Slovakia or Hungary spend only slightly less per person but have much higher amenable mortality rates, whereas countries like the Netherlands spend much more but only have marginally lower amenable mortality rates.

Figure 7.4 *Amenable mortality and health expenditure, 2012*

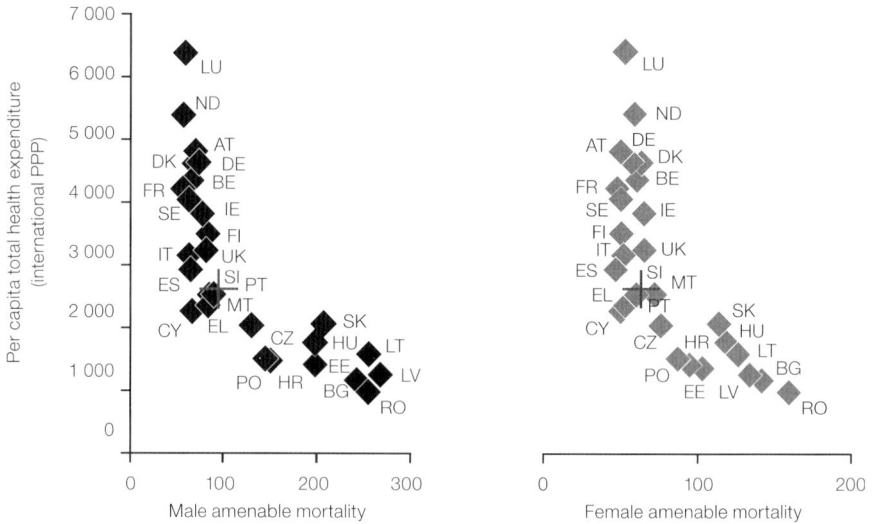

Source: Authors' calculations using the WHO Global Health Expenditure Database and Mortality Databases.
Note: PPP = purchasing power parity

Generally, it is difficult to find health outcome data that are fully attributable to health system inputs. The OECD Health Care Quality Indicators Project has made major strides to collect comparable health care quality data; these data are reported in the annual Health at a Glance report as well as in the OECD Health Statistics database (OECD/EU, 2014). The project collects data regarding avoidable admissions, in-hospital mortality, cancer survival rates, patient safety and patient experiences. However, there are still few input data that can be directly attributable to the quality indicators collected.

Overall, we find that there are few longitudinal, regularly updated databases that compare health system efficiency across countries. Available data are at an aggregated level, making it difficult to directly attribute output or outcome data to input data, or to properly adjust for confounding factors that might influence efficiency. Despite the common use of analytic methods such as DEA or SFA in multicountry efficiency studies (see Section 7.3), we could not identify any regularly updated longitudinal databases that employ these tools in an effort to report efficiency scores that account for multiple inputs and outputs, or that control for factors exogenous to the health system. Current international databases are therefore limited to simple measures, primarily unadjusted ratios of outputs to inputs, to gauge cross-country differences in health care efficiency.

7.3 Multicountry health care efficiency studies at the system, subsector and treatment levels

Although efficiency indicators are scarce in international health databases, there are a number of studies that compare health care efficiency across countries. These studies are often cross-sectional and not regularly reproduced. One characteristic that sets these studies apart from the databases discussed previously is that these studies frequently employ analytic frontier methods to calculate efficiency scores (see Chapter 5). These methodological approaches can address some of the issues that otherwise inhibit comparisons, for example, by accounting for multiple inputs to health production and adjusting for differences in production capabilities at various scales. Many of these studies have also made use of the input and output data included in international health databases, particularly the OECD Health Statistics database, to construct efficiency metrics. Cross-country studies also compare subsectors (often hospitals) using the available data, or use comparative instruments such as vignettes or DRGs to analyse similar patients and similar types of care using micro level data (see Chapter 2). In this section, we present a selection of multicountry health care efficiency studies, distinguishing between whether the studies take a system-level, subsector or disease-based approach.

7.3.1 Health system-based approaches

System-based health care efficiency studies use aggregate country data to construct measures of efficiency. Often, studies have made use of the aforementioned OECD data to conduct these analyses. Many analytic approaches have been taken, with no consensus on the correct methodological approach. The majority of studies use DEA to estimate a production possibilities frontier and incorporate multiple inputs and outputs into the estimate. Studies occasionally take more simplistic approaches; one such study calculated ratios of mortality rate reductions relative to the health care share of gross domestic product for 19 countries (Pritchard & Wallace, 2011). However, this type of analysis is problematic because mortality is not directly attributable to health care spending without efforts to control for factors outside the health system that are also likely to affect mortality rates. Second, in this particular study there was no effort to adjust for differences in scale, for example, even the same health spending as a share of gross domestic product will reflect very different levels of resources dedicated to health depending on the size of the economy.

One of the first large studies to compare the efficiency of health systems is also one of the most well-known and often criticized studies of health system efficiency. An analysis of panel data from 191 countries was conducted by the WHO to compare per capita health expenditure to life expectancy (adjusted to account for disability), after controlling for educational attainment (Evans et al., 2001). The models used country-fixed effects, which take advantage of variations within each country over time to estimate parameters; only one country was deemed to be efficient using this method. An efficiency index was then constructed, where the expected level of health if there was no health care expenditure was compared to the expected level of health if all health systems were as efficient as the best performer. Based on this analysis, Oman was ranked the most efficient country, with Zimbabwe the least efficient.

The WHO efficiency study (Evans et al., 2001) and related study of overall performance in the 2000 World Health Report (WHO, 2000) have been heavily criticized both on methodological and data quality grounds. For example, a study by Hollingsworth & Wildman (2003) uses parametric and non-parametric approaches and found that their results varied from the method used by the WHO. Using DEA and SFA, they demonstrated how the panel data approach used by the WHO did not permit assessment of changes over time, but rather, assumed that efficiency within a country remains constant. They also suggested that analysis in the future should compare similar countries, rather than attempt to estimate efficiency across a range of countries with very different characteristics that cannot be appropriately accounted for using modelling techniques. Other research into the robustness of the WHO methodology has also revealed how sensitive the rankings are to how efficiency is defined and how models are specified (Gravelle et al., 2003). Gravelle et al. suggested that the use of country-fixed effects to estimate the models is inappropriate, particularly because 50 of the 191 countries in the study had only one year of data, and therefore had no variation over time. They found that alternative approaches, including using a model that exploits variation between countries (rather than relying on variation within countries over time), and changing the units of the variables so that they are not logarithmic, changed the results considerably. For example, in a model that used between-country effects instead of country-fixed effects, Oman changes from the most efficient country to being ranked 169th. Following widespread criticism of this analysis, the WHO has not attempted any further performance ranking.

Similar research using DEA and panel data regressions has been prepared using the OECD data (Joumard, André & Nicq, 2010). Joumard, André & Nicq (2010) estimated the contribution of health spending to life expectancy, accounting for lifestyle and socioeconomic determinants. The authors concluded that if health spending in all countries were as efficient as the best performing countries, life expectancy would increase by two years without a need to increase the actual level of spending. In contrast, increasing health expenditure levels in countries where health expenditure is not high-performing to begin with does little to increase life expectancy. The results suggested that Australia, Japan, South Korea and Switzerland are among the countries that make the most efficient use of health care expenditure. The study also found negligible relationships between output measures of efficiency (such as average length of stay) and outcome measures (such as life expectancy). This indicated that countries that most efficiently produce health system outputs might not necessarily also produce actual health gains most efficiently.

Rather than control for lifestyle factors at an aggregate country level, one recent study attempted to compare health system efficiency using data on life expectancy and health care expenditure that are adjusted a priori for individual-level differences in lifestyle factors, such as smoking, alcohol consumption and body mass index (European Commission, 2015). Unsurprisingly, the research concluded that healthier lifestyles would lead to longer life expectancy at per-person curative health care spending levels. However, despite wide variation in health behaviours across the 30 European countries in the study, the lifestyle-adjusted country efficiency estimates did not differ considerably from those that were unadjusted; most countries appeared to be positioned similarly relative to the efficiency frontier in both adjusted and unadjusted analyses. Additionally, the effects of changes in lifestyle were difficult to infer from this analysis, since the estimates were based on cross-sectional data. As noted by the authors, interventions to actually improve health behaviours may themselves be costly, and may also not have short-term health benefits that are comparable in magnitude to those reported.

Using life expectancy as an outcome measure also only tells part of the story. Other studies using OECD data adopted other health outcomes, such as reductions in infant mortality as a measure of health system outcomes. One such study used a DEA approach, where health outcomes, life expectancy and infant mortality are dependent on a number of inputs (Retzlaff-Roberts, Chang & Rubin, 2004). Rather than only focus on health expenditure as an input, this study accounted for health care resources such as the number of beds, MRI units and physicians, as well as social factors such as schooling, the Gini coefficient and tobacco use. For example, using an input oriented model of infant mortality, the authors found that the efficiency frontier is formed by Ireland, Mexico, Sweden and Spain. Based on this, the authors concluded that the USA should be able to reduce its health care inputs by 9.3% and, if it were more efficient, would still be able to maintain its level of infant mortality. However, there is no clear rationale for including all inputs together in the model; including health expenditure in addition to human and capital resources, which are purchased by the health sector, would seem to double count inputs and could invalidate the findings of this study and others that take a similar approach.

Indeed, there is no clear agreement on how to identify appropriate inputs or to control for non-health system factors that influence health. A study that used both OECD and WHO panel data demonstrated how complex the health production process is by considering socioeconomic determinants of health that are outside the health system as inputs to producing life expectancy (Spinks & Hollingsworth, 2009). The authors suggested that using both macro level socioeconomic factors, such as government policies, housing or working conditions, in addition to intermediate-level socioeconomic factors like psychosocial characteristics and health behaviours in the same model could be problematic, as the inputs are inherently interlinked. The study instead used a single measure each for education (school expectancy), employment (total unemployment rate), income (gross domestic product per capita) and health expenditure as inputs to producing either life expectancy or disability-adjusted life expectancy. Using DEA, the authors found that countries have generally moved away from the efficiency frontier over time, implying that on average, efficiency decreased slightly. The countries that formed the efficiency frontier and were deemed efficient for all model specifications were Greece, Japan, Mexico, South Korea, Spain and Turkey.

Other studies have illustrated the complexity of health production and also highlighted that inputs other than medical care play a large role in producing health. One such study used OECD data to investigate the differential effects of health system and non-health system inputs on DEA estimates of efficiency (Hadad, Hadad & Simon-Tuval, 2013). In two separate models, in addition to total per capita health expenditure as an input, the other inputs included either health system characteristics such as beds and physician density, or factors arguably outside the control of the health system such as gross domestic product and consumption of fruits and vegetables; life expectancy and infant survival were the chosen health outcomes. The study found that many countries that were efficient in the model accounting for health system inputs were not efficient when accounting for factors outside the health system. For example, using both models, the Czech Republic, Estonia, Iceland, Japan, Poland, Portugal, Slovenia and South Korea were efficient; Australia, Canada, Israel, Italy, Luxembourg, Spain, Sweden, Switzerland and the United Kingdom were efficient when using health system inputs, but not when using gross domestic product and consumption of healthy food as inputs instead. The authors allowed for super efficiency (where inputs and outputs in each country are weighted to maximize the efficiency score without being constrained to a maximum possible score of 1) to calculate rankings and found that the most efficient country using the health system input model was Iceland, whereas the most efficient country using non-health system inputs was Japan. The study also calculated rankings using cross-efficiency, where all countries shared the same weights; this is a potential measure of AE if we assume that the weights used represent the optimal mix of inputs and outputs. Using the cross-efficiency approach, Canada was the most efficient country using the health system inputs model, while using non-health system inputs, the Czech Republic was most efficient.

An earlier study also used the OECD Health Statistics data and similarly found that features referred to as environmental factors play a large part in observed variations in efficiency estimates (Puig-Junoy, 1998). With male and female life expectancy as the outcomes and five health system inputs (numbers of physicians, non-physician personnel and hospital beds, as well as tobacco and alcohol consumption, all relative to population size), various model specifications found that the most efficient countries are most consistently Canada, Greece, Italy, Japan, Portugal and the USA. The study then employed a two-stage approach, where after DEA was used to calculate country efficiency scores, regression techniques assessed the relationship between observed scores and environmental factors: human capital (that is, average years of schooling), the private share of total health expenditure and the presence of primary care gatekeeping. Nevertheless, much of the variation in efficiency scores remains unexplained by their regression models.

While the majority of studies employ DEA in a traditional sense to assess inputs relative to outputs, one study used DEA in a unique way to construct composite indicators of health system efficiency based on the set of efficiency indicators available from the OECD Health Statistics data (Cylus, Papanicolas & Smith, 2015). In this study, each individual efficiency indicator was treated as an output in a DEA model and inputs were held constant. DEA then attached weights to each efficiency indicator separately for each country so that each country's composite score was maximized, casting it in the best possible light. By combining several efficiency indicators into a single measure, the objective was to see if there was evidence of system-wide efficiency effects. Using all partial efficiency measures as outputs, five countries – Estonia, Hungary, Slovak Republic, Slovenia and the United Kingdom – formed the efficiency frontier. The study found that Hungary was the only country that was efficient in all model specifications presented.

Finally, although most studies used publicly available international databases like the OECD Health Statistics database, the Commonwealth Fund has assessed health system performance based largely on its own International Health Policy Survey (IHPS). This data set differs substantially from the OECD and WHO data, because it is a telephone-based survey of a random sample of individuals from a set of high-income countries, rather than national-level data from official sources. Caution should be exercised as the samples in each country are small, and the data are self-reported and may thus be subject to bias. The survey captures some variables that could be considered as indicative of efficiency, such as whether an individual had a duplicate medical test, rehospitalization and timely access to records, and whether a physician used information technology. In their 2014 report, the Commonwealth Fund assessed health system efficiency based on these data in addition to data on expenditure levels (Davis et al., 2014). The authors found the USA to be the least efficient of the countries analysed – a consistent finding across all waves of their survey. The USA spends high shares of total health spending on administrative costs, and its doctors report that they spend too much time on paperwork, clearly indicating that there are administrative inefficiencies in the USA. Yet, there are important discrepancies in the report that warrant further analysis; overall, the United Kingdom was the most efficient country based on its low level of expenditure and high scores according to the process measures collected in the IHPS. However, the United Kingdom performs second from last in terms of healthy lives, which raises questions of how a health system that fails to achieve good health outcomes can be considered the most efficient.

Overall, many system-level studies have taken advantage of access to international harmonized data sets to compare efficiency, with their added value generally being the use of analytic techniques. Despite efforts to account for other inputs that have an effect on health outcomes, such as lifestyle, education or institutional characteristics, much of the variability in efficiency scores appears to be unexplained by health system characteristics or other factors. It is unclear how successfully confounders can be controlled for. Additionally, most studies took a very narrow perspective on the outputs of health system, with the main products of the health system being life expectancy and infant mortality. Of note, there seems to be little consistency across studies in the countries that are found to perform most efficiently, despite studies frequently relying on the same data sets.

7.3.2 Subsector-based approach

While the aforementioned studies use country-level data to compare health systems, similar international comparisons have been done at the subsector level, the most common being to compare hospital sectors across countries. At this less aggregated level, because patient characteristics are often more homogeneous than population characteristics, variations in outcomes are likely due to unobserved confounding factors to a lesser degree. There are also a number of outputs, such as hospital discharges or physician visits, which can be assessed that are not possible at the health system level. Common frontier-based analytic techniques, DEA and SFA, are also employed.

For example, using the OECD panel data between 2000 and 2009, a recent study employed both DEA and SFA methods to explore efficiency in hospitals, adjusting for differences in case severity and environmental factors (Varabyova & Schreyögg, 2013). Using discharges weighted on the basis of case severity as an activity-based output and in-hospital mortality rates for AMI, haemorrhagic stroke and ischaemic stroke as additional outcome measures, the authors assessed the efficiency of the number of beds and hospital workers, and a number of other factors, such as health care spending, length of stay, education and patient mix. Importantly, the authors found that countries that demonstrated good health outcomes, like Japan, might be technically inefficient based on their use of health care resources. The authors also found that countries with longer length of stay are less technically efficient using their methodology, implying that length of stay may be a reasonable proxy measure for efficiency of the hospital sector.

To more appropriately compare the prices and volumes of health care services across countries, there have been joint efforts by the OECD and Eurostat to develop output-based purchasing power parity (PPP) price indices (Koechlin et al., 2014). This involves estimation of quasi-prices based on the reimbursement levels paid for comparable medical services (for example, payments covering direct, capital and overhead costs), as opposed to being based on the prices of inputs to care (for example, wages), which can be used to compare hospital prices and volumes across countries. This is important for the measurement of health care efficiency, as the input-based PPP price index methodology unrealistically assumes that health care productivity is identical across countries, because hypothetical countries with the same input prices (for example, wages) and health care expenditure would implicitly be assumed to have produced the same volumes of health care goods and services. In addition to improving the estimation of hospital volumes, in an earlier iteration of this study, the methodology was used to calculate novel comparisons of inpatient care productivity through metrics such as the cost of an inpatient care day (Koechlin, Lorenzoni & Schreyer, 2010). Per-day costs in 2007 were highest overall in the USA and lowest in South Korea.

Researchers have also compared efficiency for specific types of care provided within a hospital. A recent study using the OECD data investigated inpatient mental health care, where mental health-specific inputs included the number of psychiatrists, psychiatric beds and length of stay, and the outputs were the discharges per 1000 population (Moran & Jacobs, 2013). Factors external to the health system that could potentially play a role involved alcohol consumption, income, education and unemployment rates, and were included in some of the DEA model specifications presented. Unlike in many other studies using DEA, the authors used a bootstrapping approach that allowed them to calculate confidence intervals so that they could ascertain how certain they were of the rankings. They found that countries with greater efficiency, including Denmark, Hungary, Italy, Poland, Slovenia and South Korea, also had wider confidence intervals, suggesting less certainty; in general, however, the countries deemed efficient in one model were also reasonably efficient in other specifications.

Not all studies review large numbers of countries. Often, international comparisons have been limited to smaller numbers of health systems, which could potentially allow for more detailed comparisons. For example, a study comparing the NHS in England to the Kaiser Permanente integrated managed care consortium in California, a private health maintenance organization that integrates both financing and delivery, concluded that Kaiser Permanente performed more efficiently than the NHS (Feachem et al., 2002). This study informally compared costs to quality of care, showing that per capita costs were roughly the same but that there were notable variations in quality and responsiveness across the two systems. Another study comparing many hospitals in Norway and California used DEA to estimate a production frontier to investigate whether privatization and competition lead to greater efficiency (Mobley & Magnussen, 1998). The authors matched hospitals based on a variety of criteria to ensure that they were comparing similar types of hospitals and concluded that private competition among hospitals in California does not lead to greater efficiency in the long run.

Another study compared hospitals in Germany (Saxony federal state) and Switzerland using DEA, finding in all instances the German hospitals were more efficient. Unlike in most studies, the analysis considered the number of patient days as an input rather than an output (Steinmann et al., 2004). The justification for treating days as an input is that in Saxony, hospital financing is based on pre-approved patient days; hospital managers are incentivized to meet this pre-approved level of patient days by attracting less complex cases. Likewise, in Saxony the number of beds per hospital is fixed so in some analyses beds are not included as an input since they are non-discretionary. This underscores how important it is to understand institutional arrangements within countries before conducting any analysis, as incentive structures or financing mechanisms could potentially drive results. Importantly, the authors tested whether their sample of hospitals was homogeneous and found that it was not, which required that they limited the usable sample substantially. This highlights another important issue: most studies that employ frontier-based analyses do not effectively ensure that the decision-making units (for example, countries or providers) are comparable and exist as part of the same production possibilities frontier.

It is essential to note the large number of studies that have been done in Scandinavian countries because of the wide availability of registry data, which historically has not been readily available in many other countries (see Chapter 3). Using such data, it is easier to make sure that inputs and outputs are well defined and comparable, and to control for confounding factors. For example, a DEA study comparing Finnish and Norwegian hospitals used data on hospital operating costs as inputs and DRG-weighted admissions, and weighted visits and days of care based on National Discharge Registry data (Linna, Häkkinen & Magnussen, 2006). Registry data allowed the authors to cluster cases by NordDRG grouper and use cost weights based on actual patient-level costs. The authors also adjusted input prices based on a hospital-specific input price index comprising hospital-specific wage and operating cost data. The study results were reasonably robust across multiple models and indicated that Finnish hospitals were more efficient than Norwegian hospitals. A more recent analysis of university hospitals in Nordic countries (Denmark, Finland, Norway and Sweden) used similar data and also found Finnish hospitals to be the most efficient. The study also employed a bootstrapping DEA approach that allowed for estimation of confidence intervals (Medin et al., 2011). This gives not only an idea of the range of certainty, but also corrects for bias associated with having only a small number of hospitals.

7.3.3 *Disease-based approaches*

Health system efficiency can also be explored by examining the costs, resources, outputs and outcomes associated with treating specific diseases. The advantage is that patients treated for certain diseases are likely to be more homogeneous. Additionally, it may be possible to more accurately observe the processes leading to differences in efficiency if the data are detailed enough.

For example, the McKinsey health care productivity study examined variations in inputs and outcomes for treating breast cancer, lung cancer, gallstones and diabetes in Germany, the United Kingdom and the USA (Garber, 2003). Data on the levels of inputs, such as physician hours, nursing hours, medications and capital, were used as opposed to the level of spending, because spending could lead to erroneous efficiency estimates because of differences in input costs across countries. These data were linked to outcome measures. Although spending levels in the USA are higher than in Germany or the United Kingdom, the USA was largely found to perform efficiently using this method, suggesting that US providers may use resources efficiently but that their input prices are notably higher.

Additionally, while the OECD Health Statistics database contains primarily aggregate, system-level data, the Health at a Glance report based on these data contains some disease-based efficiency indicators. These data are still aggregated at the country level, but can shed light on the efficiency of treating specific conditions. For example, while Finland and Turkey had the longest and shortest average length of acute care hospital stay in 2012 overall among European countries, the average length of stay for AMI was longest in Germany (10.3 days) and shortest in Denmark (3.9 days). Additionally, there were comparisons of the percentage of cataract surgeries carried out as day cases (Figure 7.5). A higher share is indicative of greater efficiency, as cataract surgeries are a high-volume surgical procedure that can potentially be done using fewer resources as a day case rather than as an inpatient admission. However, caution is advised when comparing across countries for a variety of reasons; for example, some countries do not consider outpatient cases in hospitals or surgeries outside of hospitals when reporting these figures.

Figure 7.5 *Share of cataract surgeries carried out as day cases, 2000 and 2012 (or nearest year)*

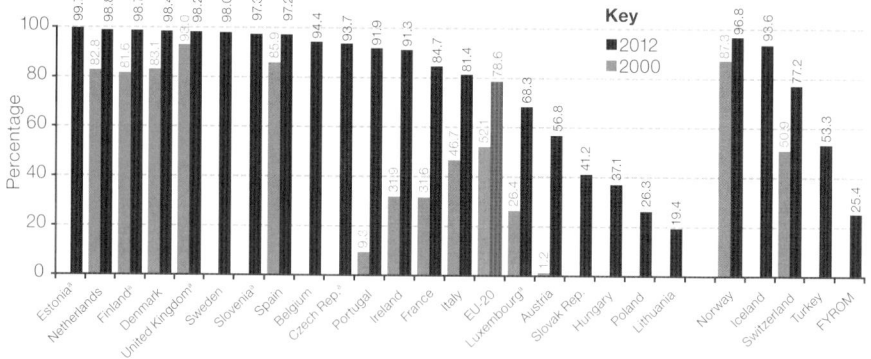

Source: OECD & EU (2014).

Notes: ªData include outpatient cases in hospitals and outside hospital. FYROM = Former Yugoslav Republic of Macedonia.

Other research also compared costs and outcomes for selected diseases. For example, the OECD Ageing-Related Diseases study included some indicators of efficiency, such as length of stay and unit costs of treating diseases including stroke and cancer; however, in many instances data were not available or fully comparable across countries. More recently, the OECD Cancer Care study investigated variations across 35 countries in the resources allocated to cancer care, as well as variations in care delivery and outcomes (OECD, 2013b). For example, the report compares average referral times between GP and specialist visits, finding that referral times are shortest in Denmark (typically only a few days) while they can be a month in Israel or Norway. Comparing waiting time between diagnosis and initial treatment shows even wider variation, from under 3 days on average in Luxembourg to over a month in Poland or the Netherlands. For both of these indicators, in some instances the data are estimates based on expert opinion. In exploratory analysis, the OECD compared resources for cancer care, such as oncologists per million population and use of imaging technology and found a significant association between resources for cancer care and survival. However, the study did not include explicit cross-country comparisons of the efficiency by which cancer care is delivered. Nevertheless, the study suggested that some countries have higher survival rates at given levels of total per capita health spending than others, which could suggest greater efficiency despite per capita health spending being only a weak proxy for health system inputs specific to cancer care. While there appear to be some diminishing returns for cancer survival given greater health spending, Iceland, Israel and Turkey have the highest five-year survival rates for breast cancer relative to their levels of total per capita health spending (Figure 7.6). The OECD has also conducted similar research that links health care quality indicators to expenditure for cardiovascular diseases and diabetes (OECD, 2015).

Figure 7.6 *Relationship between breast cancer survival and total national expenditure on health*

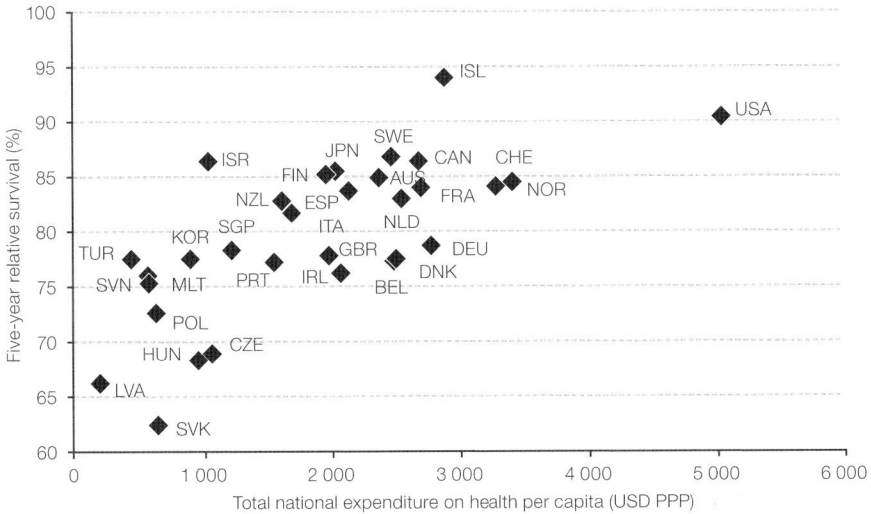

Source: OECD Cancer Care study.
Note: PPP = purchasing power parity; USD = United States dollar.

DRGs and other methods that group similar cases have been used for efficiency measurement, not only to weight discharges and days as described previously, but also to group cases so that similar types of care are compared across health systems (see Chapter 2). Because of their design as patient classification systems that group patients with similar characteristics and resource consumption, they can be effective at ensuring that similar types of patients are matched. Three large studies, the HealthBASKET, EuroDRG and EuroHOPE have made major strides in this domain.

The HealthBASKET project reviewed the costs of care for nine European countries (Busse, Schreyögg & Smith, 2008). Using case vignettes that described particular types of patients (that is, based on age, gender and comorbidities), the study compared and attempted to explain variations in costs within and between countries. The advantage of this approach is that specific services for comparable patients could be costed and compared across countries. Vignettes were developed for inpatient, outpatient, elective and emergency care. Using a sample of providers, the researchers collected information on typical usage patterns and costs. However, despite successfully averting the need to risk adjust by comparing standardized patients, there were limitations. For example, the samples were small and therefore often reflected normative cases rather than actual patient experiences. Additionally, data were not always comparable across countries because providers in some countries do not own their assets.

Likewise, patient outcomes were assumed to be identical, which is not realistic. Nevertheless, the approach revealed how low costs in southern and eastern Europe were largely due to low wages and did not necessarily reveal greater efficiency after adjusting for episode-specific PPPs. Some of the most important reasons for variations in costs were the differences in the types of technologies used to provide care.

EuroDRG used an episode-of-care approach to compare costs across countries (Busse, 2012). This study investigated the classification variables used by different country DRG systems, such as diagnosis, procedure, patient age, length of stay, death and the level of reimbursement for a selection of similarly defined patients based on episodes of care. Examples of the types of care reviewed included child care (Bellanger & Or, 2008), stroke (Epstein, Mason & Manca, 2008) and cataract care (Fattore & Torbica, 2008).

The theory behind the EuroDRG project is based on the fact that most analyses of efficiency cannot properly control for differences in case mix. As a result, the study takes advantage of a different unit of measurement, episodes of care, which are essentially meta-DRGs that are uniformly defined based on a number of diagnosis and procedure codes. Patients are observed from the time of diagnosis until the end of treatment including follow-up. The advantage is that patient characteristics are not standardized, as in the HealthBASKET study, but rather, similar types of patient care are compared. The study subsequently estimated how well the DRG systems could explain variation in resource consumption, particularly how well DRGs explained variations in costs or length of stay for each episode of care (Street et al., 2012). Nevertheless, most of the EuroDRG analyses could not identify variations in quality of care.

A recent paper within the EuroDRG project compared costs and quality (measured as being discharged alive) for AMI and stroke patients in hospitals in Finland, France, Germany, Spain and Sweden (Häkkinen et al., 2014). The study used patient-level data and separate models to predict costs and survival across around 100 hospitals. Though the purpose of the study was to evaluate trade-offs between cost and quality (that is, explicit ratios of survival to cost were not reported) the hospital fixed effects of both equations were plotted against each other to give an idea of whether hospitals that spent more on patients achieved better outcomes, though no conclusive cost–quality relationship was found.

Another recent project, the EuroHOPE, has made important advances in disease-based efficiency comparisons across countries (Häkkinen et al., 2013). This study used linkable patient-level data, which allowed for the measurement of both outcomes (including follow-up) and the use of health care resources (costs, days of care, procedures and drugs) for comparable patient groups. The diseases investigated were AMI, stroke, hip fracture, breast cancer and low birth weight. EuroHOPE could evaluate entire treatment pathways and identify the extent to which a health care system produces better outcomes. Key strengths of the project include: detailed data on patients and their comorbidities; identification of the beginning and end of episodes of care; and reliable data on health care costs; however, such high-quality data is not available for all countries or many types of care.

7.4 Key progress and remaining challenges

Health systems are extremely complex. To evaluate and compare how well health systems function and achieve their goal of improving health outcomes, metrics that allow comparisons across countries are highly valued. Comparative efficiency metrics may be of great interest in principle, but in practice they are not often available, not easily comparable or may produce results that are not consistent across similar analytical approaches (Varabyova & Müller, 2016). As a result, there is no consensus on which countries perform most efficiently, or on how to measure health care efficiency across countries. Some of the reasons for the paucity of efficiency data include data differences and inconsistencies, lack of consensus on appropriate methods and the scope of research, and difficulties directly attributing health outcomes to health care inputs. A summary of the types of indicators reviewed in this chapter as well as their pros and cons are shown in Table 7.1.

7.4.1 Improving data availability and consistency is a key challenge

Differences in data availability and consistency are important challenges to creating comparable health care efficiency indicators. There are few longitudinal efficiency metrics currently in the public domain; while efforts have been made to harmonize data, there are still issues due to differences in definitions, clinical practices and reporting. Additionally, available national-level data allow for only a limited number of efficiency indicators to be constructed manually based on ratios of outcomes or outputs to inputs (for example, consultations per physician). At a subsector level, aggregate national-level data are most readily available to assess resource usage for hospitals, but often not for other types of providers. From a disease-based perspective, conditions for which survival is likely in the presence of timely access to quality health services, such as some types of cancer, are promising areas for efficiency comparison, although episodic data are not always available in many countries.

While international databases like the OECD Health Statistics do not contain many ready-made efficiency comparisons, a large number of the studies reviewed

Table 7.1 *Summary table of international efficiency indicators*

Type	Source/example	Example indicators	Pros	Cons
Cross-country databases	• OECD Health Statistics database • WHO Europe health for all database	• Health expenditure per capita (or as a share of gross domestic product), which is often related to some broad health status measures (for example, life expectancy) • Average LOS • Bed occupancy rates	• Regularly updated time series • Databases contain some ready-made efficiency indicators or can be used to construct efficiency indicators at the system-, subsector- or disease-based level (as described below)	• Links between expenditure, inputs, outputs and outcomes are often weak (or inexistent) • Aggregate (macro) data at the national level (no disaggregation at the provider or patient level) • Limited number of outcome measures
System-level	• OECD efficiency study (Joumard, André & Nicq, 2010) • WHO efficiency study of 191 countries (Evans et al., 2001)	• Efficiency scores, often using analytical methods such as DEA, SFA or other regression-based methods	• Enables comparison of entire systems • Can control to some extent for confounders • Often assesses the entire production process from expenditure to health outcomes (that is, life expectancy)	• Usually cross-sectional • Adjustments for confounders are likely to be imprecise due to aggregation; outputs are not necessarily directly or exclusively attributable to inputs • Results sensitive to model specification and countries chosen for comparison • Often rely on cross-country databases which may inhibit external validity
Subsector-level	• Finnish and Norwegian hospitals (Linna, Häkkinen & Magnussen, 2006) • Swiss and German hospitals (Steinmann et al., 2004)	• Efficiency scores using analytical methods such as DEA, SFA or other regression-based methods	• Can better account for confounders than system-level studies because of patient similarities	• Most research is for hospitals only • Usually cross-sectional • Results sensitive to model specification and countries/facilities chosen for comparison • Often assess health care outputs (for example, discharges) instead of health outcomes
Disease-based	• OECD Cancer Care study • EuroDRG • EuroHOPE	• Waiting time between diagnosis and initial treatment • Comparisons of costs and outcomes for predefined episodes of care	• Often can use patient-level data, which is best at controlling for confounders • Can better identify processes related to health care • Can often follow patients from beginning to end of episode of care	• Limited because of data availability in many countries • Few diseases studied

Note: DEA = data envelopment analysis; DRG = diagnosis-related group; LOS = length of stay; SFA = stochastic frontier analysis.

in this chapter make use of the OECD data to measure efficiency. Yet, there are questions as to whether the use of the OECD panel data is entirely appropriate for calculating efficiency indicators, as the data are sometimes estimates (Spinks & Hollingsworth, 2009). In general, there are inconsistencies in measurement and reporting standards across countries, which researchers have limited capacity to control, in spite of the headway made by resources such as the SHA. Even within the United Kingdom, a National Audit Office report concluded that it was not possible to compare efficiency successfully across the four countries (National Audit Office, 2012), primarily because of a lack of data availability and consistency. For example, differences across the United Kingdom in how countries categorize types of expenditure make spending comparisons nearly impossible.

Therefore, while significant efforts are being made to improve the quality and consistency of expenditure and non-expenditure data, this remains an important challenge to improving efficiency measurement. On the expenditures side, the SHA is an excellent example of the advances that can be made coordinating data reporting across countries. However, efforts are needed to improve the comparability of input data other than expenditure, and particularly, to increase the availability of comparable output and outcome data. While data for many different types of inputs – from expenditure, to beds, to the number of doctors, to drugs – are available, there is also a need to expand the types of outcome data that are available for analysis. Studies that use health outcomes often rely on life expectancy or infant mortality, but these broad indicators of health status are very distant from the activities of health care systems. Outcome data for conditions that are known to be amenable to health care should be more readily available. There is a need to develop more PROMs, following the example of countries such as Sweden and the United Kingdom, to monitor more closely the health outcomes of different health care interventions.

It would be prudent for countries to focus more on harmonizing and improving access to registry or hospital discharge level data. Not only would better micro level data be preferable from a methodological perspective because it would be easier to control for potential confounders such as case severity and compare like-with-like, it could also be more useful to end users, such as hospital managers or policymakers, who require detailed information that allows them to take action. While it is difficult to harmonize registry or discharge data because they are used to meet administrative needs, which often differ across countries, these data are exceedingly useful and allow researchers to determine their own levels of aggregation. Data that allow researchers to follow patients throughout treatment across different providers are essential to understand the efficiency of care pathways. Similarly, longitudinal data need to be available to track changes in efficiency across time.

7.4.2 Researchers should make use of multiple methodological approaches in the absence of the correct methodological approach

There are numerous methodological approaches that can be useful for measuring efficiency, including frontier-based methods like DEA and SFA. Although DEA seems to be preferred based on this chapter's assessment of the international literature, it still remains unclear which methodological approach to use in general for estimating efficiency, regardless of whether comparisons are to be done across countries. While some studies confirm that DEA results are similar to other non-parametric methods (Afonso & St Aubyn, 2005), results are not always the same across methods and can be sensitive to model specification (Gravelle et al., 2003). Even if data are comparable, the question remains of which are the appropriate inputs and outputs to be compared across countries. As demonstrated in this chapter, variations in the selection of these data can lead to very different results. For example, despite high spending and generally poor health outcomes, when input prices are not taken into account, the USA might appear to perform efficiently (Garber, 2003).

As a result, all studies should make use of multiple techniques to ensure robustness and the results of many different studies should be used together to inform conclusions. Likewise, more studies should make use of methods that quantify the level of uncertainty of an estimate, including bootstrapping for DEA to estimate confidence intervals. Ultimately, when deciding which methods to use, researchers must consider the extent to which methods are helpful to policymakers. Given that arbitrary decisions regarding inclusion or exclusion of inputs and outputs can have a significant effect on results, methods like DEA may not be useful for policy purposes (Spinks & Hollingsworth, 2009).

Importantly, methods like DEA and SFA assume that all entities exist in the same production possibilities frontier. A perhaps underappreciated issue with international efficiency comparisons is that this requirement may not be met. Differences in system designs may mean that providers do not have the same production possibilities, leading methods like DEA to inaccurately estimate production frontiers. For example, smaller countries or countries with more geographically dispersed populations may require greater spending on inputs, such as medical imaging technology, to make care available to the entire population. This issue of entity comparability was also elucidated in a study comparing Switzerland and Germany, which found that many hospitals in the two countries were not sufficiently homogeneous to be compared using frontier-based methods (Steinmann et al., 2004).

Other related methodological issues include the need for improved risk-adjustment techniques because of substantial heterogeneity across and within countries. However, to do this well, adjustment needs to be made at the individual level, as national-level risk adjustment does not properly account for variations within population groups. This also supports greater use of patient-level data. Using individual-level data, it is easier to ensure that patients are comparable and to subsequently identify the characteristics of the health system that contribute to differences in efficiency.

7.4.3. More work is needed to properly attribute health outcomes to inputs

One reason why some types of performance metrics are fairly common (for example, population health) while efficiency is not, may also be partially due to the well-known difficulties attributing outcomes and outputs to inputs. The production of health is influenced by many factors that lie outside the health care system. While the challenges associated with attributing health system characteristics to health outcomes do not only apply to international comparisons, it is perhaps an even more salient challenge when comparing across countries because factors that influence health in some countries may vary to such a large extent that they are nearly impossible to control for. For example, factors such as genetic differences, geographical ancestry (Diez Roux, 2011) and cultural lifestyle differences play a role in health. Because the effect of the health system as an input to health is interrelated to and dependent on many country- or context-specific characteristics, it is difficult to accurately isolate the contribution of the health system itself in different country contexts.

Reasons for variations in efficiency across countries or over time, such as changes in the way care is delivered, changes in case mix, economies of scale and determinants outside of the health system are not consistently accounted for, or in many instances, cannot be properly accounted for. Although there have been attempts to include non-health system factors in analyses, it is not precisely clear which are the right ones and whether including all factors makes sense since so many are interrelated. To some extent, all policies and environmental factors are likely to play a role in determining health, making comparisons across dissimilar countries increasingly complex. Likewise, lifestyle behaviours, including healthy eating (Hadad et al., 2013), social class and welfare, or even occupation, may be as important, if not more important than health care in determining population-level health outcomes, highlighting the potential difficulties with attribution across countries. One solution might be to match patients not only based on DRGs or episodes of care, nor on simple characteristics such as age or sex, but also on more detailed observable characteristics including genetics.

On a related front, attribution issues may be one reason why it is difficult to measure efficiency for many subsectors of the health system. For example, there are very few estimates of long-term care efficiency because of the difficulties attributing changes in individual outcomes to care services.

7.5 Conclusion

While there has been considerable progress, much work remains before internationally comparable efficiency metrics should play a formal role in informing health policy. To achieve this, more efficiency metrics need to be collected, made readily available and updated on a regular basis. Enhancing comparability is essential. While there has been progress harmonizing data and definitions (for example, SHA) there remain gaps in practice, especially for health outcome data.

Additionally, while studies using aggregate data provide useful insight into health system performance, these metrics might mask important differences and issues. Many of these aggregate level studies produce inconsistent results whereby countries are deemed efficient in one model but inefficient in another. Researchers should focus less on trying to develop the correct models, and instead search for robustness across multiple analytical approaches. Our assessment also suggests the need to continue to focus on more micro level analyses. Technical developments, such as better data links within and across countries could help to facilitate data availability. Other developments include the expanded use of DRGs and case vignettes as instruments to compare the costs of similar types of care. Clarity is also needed to determine whether it is the production of health that is most valued, or the containment of costs. If it is the former, it is worth understanding how successfully other policies – not just those directly related to the health system – improve health.

The appeal of international comparisons of health care efficiency is clear, despite the many challenges. Overall, we do not find evidence that any countries consistently perform efficiently based on the studies reviewed in this chapter, suggesting a long way to go before definitive assessments of health system efficiency are achievable. To ensure that international health system efficiency metrics do not misinform policy decisions, it is essential for continued efforts to enhance data quality, availability and comparability.

References

Afonso A, St Aubyn M (2005). Non-parametric approaches to education and health efficiency in OECD countries. *Journal of Applied Economics*, 8(2):227–246.

Bellanger MM, Or Z (2008). What can we learn from a cross-country comparison of the costs of child delivery? *Health Economics*, 17(Suppl. S1):S47–S57.

Busse R (2012). Do diagnosis-related groups explain variations in hospital costs and length of stay? Analyses from the EuroDRG project for 10 episodes of care across 10 European countries. *Health Economics*, 21(Suppl. S2): 1–5.

Busse R, Schreyögg J, Smith PC (2008). Variability in healthcare treatment costs amongst nine EU countries: results from the HealthBASKET project. *Health Economics*, 17(Suppl. S1):S1–S8.

Cylus J, Papanicolas I, Smith PC (2015). Using data envelopment analysis to address the challenges of comparing health system efficiency. *Global Policy*.

Davis K et al. (2014). Mirror, mirror on the wall: how the performance of the U.S. health care system compares internationally. New York, The Commonwealth Fund (http://www.commonwealthfund.org/~/media/files/publications/fund-report/2014/jun/1755_davis_mirror_mirror_2014.pdf, accessed 22 July 2016).

Diez Roux AV (2011). Complex systems thinking and current impasses in health disparities research. *American Journal of Public Health*, 101(9):1627–1634.

Epstein D, Mason A, Manca A (2008). The hospital costs of care for stroke in nine European countries. *Health Economics*, 17(Suppl. S1):S21–S31.

European Commission (EC) (2015). Comparative efficiency of health systems, corrected for selected lifesyle factors: Final report. (http://ec.europa.eu/health/systems_performance_assessment/docs/2015_maceli_report_en.pdf, accessed 22 July 2016).

Evans DB et al. (2001). Comparative efficiency of national health systems: cross national econometric analysis. *BMJ*, 323(7308):307–310.

Fattore G, Torbica A (2008). Cost and reimbursement of cataract surgery in Europe: a cross-country comparison. *Health Economics*, 17(Suppl. S1):S71–S82.

Feachem RGA et al. (2002). Getting more for their dollar: a comparison of the NHS with California's Kaiser Permanente. *BMJ*, 324(7330):135–141.

Garber AM (2003). Comparing health care systems from the disease-specific perspective. In: *A disease-based comparison of health systems: what is best and at what cost?* Paris, OECD Publishing.

Gravelle H et al. (2003). Comparing the efficiency of national health systems: a sensitivity analysis of the WHO approach. *Applied Health Economics and Health Policy*, 2(3):141–147.

Hadad S, Hadad Y, Simon-Tuval T (2013). Determinants of healthcare system's efficiency in OECD countries. *European Journal of Health Economics*, 14(2):253–265.

Häkkinen U et al. (2013). Health care performance comparison using a disease-based approach: the EuroHOPE project. *Health Policy*, 112(1–2):100–109.

Häkkinen U et al. (2014). Quality, cost, and their trade-off in treating AMI and stroke patients in European hospitals. *Health Policy*, 117(1):15–27.

Hollingsworth B (2008). The measurement of efficiency and productivity of health care delivery. *Health Economics*, 17(10):1107–1128.

Hollingsworth B, Wildman J (2003). The efficiency of health production: re-estimating the WHO panel data using parametric and non-parametric approaches to provide additional information. *Health Economics*, 12(6):493–504.

International Monetary Fund (IMF) (2015). Republic of Slovenia. Technical assistance report: establishing a spending review process. IMF Country Report No. 15/265. (https://www.imf.org/external/pubs/ft/scr/2015/cr15265.pdf, accessed 22 July 2016).

Joumard I, André C, Nicq C (2010). Health care systems: efficiency and institutions. Economics Department Working Papers, No. 769. Paris, OECD Publishing (http://www.oecd.org/officialdocuments/publicdisplaydocumentpdf/?doclanguage=en&cote=eco/wkp(2010)25, accessed 22 July 2016).

Koechlin F, Lorenzoni L, Schreyer P (2010). Comparing price levels of hospital services across countries: results of pilot study. OECD Health Working Papers, No. 53. (http://www.oecd.org/officialdocuments/publicdisplaydocumentpdf/?cote=DELSA/HEA/WD/HWP(2010)4&docLanguage=En, accessed 22 July 2016).

Koechlin F et al. (2014). Comparing hospital and health prices and volumes internationally: results of a Eurostat/OECD project. OECD Health Working Papers, No. 75. Paris, OECD Publishing (http://ec.europa.eu/eurostat/documents/728703/728971/OECD-health-working-papers-75.pdf/a6e22472-95c4-4e77-bdb0-db3af4668e7f, accessed 22 July 2016).

Linna M, Häkkinen U, Magnussen J (2006). Comparing hospital cost efficiency between Norway and Finland. *Health Policy*, 77(3):268–278.

Medin E et al. (2011). Cost efficiency of university hospitals in the Nordic countries: a cross-country analysis. *European Journal of Health Economics*, 12(6):509–519.

Mobley LR, Magnussen J (1998). An international comparison of hospital efficiency: does institutional environment matter? *Applied Economics*, 30(8):1089–1100.

Moran V, Jacobs R (2013). An international comparison of efficiency of inpatient mental health care systems. *Health Policy*, 112(1–2):88–99.

National Audit Office (2012). Healthcare across the UK: a comparison of the NHS in England, Scotland, Wales and Northern Ireland. London, TSO (https://www.nao.org.uk/wp-content/uploads/2012/06/1213192.pdf, accessed 22 July 2016).

Organisation of Economic Co-operation and Development (OECD) (2000). A system of health accounts. Paris, OECD Publishing (https://www.oecd.org/els/health-systems/1841456.pdf, accessed 2 August 2016).

OECD (2004). The OECD Health Project. Towards high-performing health systems. Paris, OECD Publishing (https://www.oecd.org/els/health-systems/31785551.pdf, accessed 22 July 2016).

OECD (2013a). OECD Health Statistics Data. (http://www.oecd.org/els/health-systems/health-data.htm, accessed 2 August 2016).

OECD (2013b). *Cancer care: assuring quality to improve survival*. Paris, OECD Publishing (https://www.oecd.org/els/health-systems/Focus-on-Health_Cancer-Care-2013.pdf, accessed 22 July 2016).

OECD (2015). Cardiovascular disease and diabetes: policies for better health and quality of care. OECD Health Policy Studies. Paris, OECD Publishing (http://www.oecd.org/publications/cardiovascular-disease-and-diabetes-policies-for-better-health-and-quality-of-care-9789264233010-en.htm, accessed 22 July 2016).

OECD, EU (2014). Health at a glance: Europe 2014. Paris, OECD Publishing (http://www.oecd.org/health/health-at-a-glance-europe-23056088.htm, accessed 22 July 2016).

Pritchard C, Wallace MS (2011). Comparing the USA, UK and 17 Western countries' efficiency and effectiveness in reducing mortality. *JRSM Short Reports*, 2(7):60.

Puig-Junoy J (1998). Measuring health production performance in the OECD. *Applied Economics Letters*, 5(4):255–259.

Retzlaff-Roberts D, Chang CF, Rubin RM (2004). Technical efficiency in the use of health care resources: a comparison of OECD countries. *Health Policy*, 69(1):55–72.

Spinks J, Hollingsworth B (2009). Cross-country comparisons of technical efficiency of health production: a demonstration of pitfalls. *Applied Economics*, 41(4):417–427.

Steinmann L et al. (2004). Measuring and comparing the (in)efficiency of German and Swiss hospitals. *European Journal of Health Economics*, 5(3):216–226.

Street A et al. (2012). How well do diagnosis-related groups explain variations in costs or length of stay among patients and across hospitals? Methods for analysing routine patient data. *Health Economics*, 21(Suppl. S2):S6–S18.

Varabyova Y, Müller JM (2016). The efficiency of health care production in OECD countries: a systematic review and meta-analysis of cross-country comparisons. *Health Policy*, 120(3):252–263.

Varabyova Y, Schreyögg J (2013). International comparisons of the technical efficiency of the hospital sector: panel data analysis of OECD countries using parametric and non-parametric approaches. *Health Policy*, 112(1–2):70–79.

WHO (2000). The World Health Report 2000. Health systems: improving performance. Geneva, WHO (http://www.who.int/whr/2000/en/whr00_en.pdf?ua=1, accessed 22 July 2016).

Chapter 8

Efficiency measurement for policy formation and evaluation

Anita Charlesworth, Zeynep Or and Emma Spencelayh

8.1 Introduction

All health care systems are looking for ways to improve efficiency as they come under increasing pressure to control the growth in health care expenditure. To support sound decision-making, the use of efficiency metrics in assessing and evaluating system reform and policy interventions is critical. However, the use of robust evidence and, more specifically, the use of efficiency metrics in policy formation, vary across countries. In all countries policy decisions are based on a mixture of things, including societal values, fiscal priorities, public opinion and political ideology. Moreover, compared with other sectors, measuring efficiency in the health sector is complicated because of market characteristics specific to health. A proper efficiency evaluation in the health sector requires an analysis of health outcomes as well as service outputs, but this is not always straightforward.

This chapter looks at the role that efficiency metrics can play in shaping and evaluating policy choices in middle- and high-income countries using a conceptual policy development framework against which a number of country examples are appraised. Country examples compare the role of efficiency metrics across the stages of the policy cycle, following the ROAMEF (rationale, objectives, appraisal, monitoring, evaluation and feedback) model, which is a stylized framework for rationale policy development (Figure 8.1).

In practice, policy development diverges from this cycle, which is highly stylized and excludes key factors such as political context, values and events (Hallsworth, Parker & Rutter, 2011). The model is used here as a theoretical framework rather than a description of policymaking in practice. Following the six stages of the ROAMEF cycle, we examine the formation and implementation of a number of policies which feature commonly in strategies designed to improve health system performance in middle- and high-income countries.

Figure 8.1 *The ROAMEF cycle*

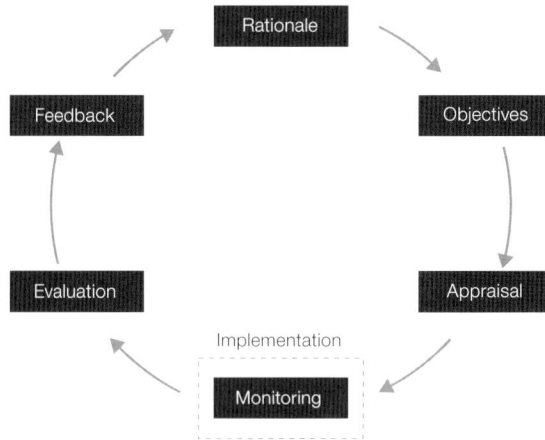

Source: HM Treasury (2011).

The OECD (2010) has distinguished three broad sequences of reform over the last few decades, separating macroeconomic policies aimed to restrain expenditure (prices and volume); microeconomic policies tackling demand (gatekeeping, care coordination, disease prevention); and supply (improving provider payment, purchasing systems, and so on). With regard to improving system performance, Roberts et al. (2004) identified five main policy levers: finance, payment, organization, regulation and provider behaviour.

In this chapter we examine the role of efficiency metrics in relation to five policy domains that are common issues in most health care systems and cover a broad range of the policy levers identified by the OECD and Roberts et al. (2004):

- the definition of the publicly funded health basket (regulation);
- cost sharing arrangements (finance);
- hospital reorganization (organization);
- provider payment reforms (payment); and
- public reporting of health care data (provider behaviour).

In each domain, we first outline recent or common policies introduced with the goal of improving technical and allocative efficiency (TE and AE), recognizing the rationale and objectives for each. We then examine the available evidence on the efficiency of these policies before their implementation and the process of evaluating the impact afterwards in selected countries. We have not conducted a systematic review of the evidence on efficiency but highlight key findings from recent literature and evidence scans. We focus on the efficiency metrics that are available in different countries, how/if these metrics are used at different stages of the policy development cycle, whether there are any common features of policies where efficiency metrics have a more or less prominent role in policymaking, and what implications this may have for the future development of efficiency measurement.

8.2 The definition of public health basket and regulation of reimbursement

8.2.1 Rationale for intervention

As resources are limited, it is important to ensure that the money being spent on health care is providing adequate quality and value. The definitions of the health services and products reimbursed from the public purse, and their prices, are crucial for assuring AE. Comparative effectiveness analysis is a way to better assess the value of health care treatment options (see Chapter 6). The assessment of costs and benefits of different health services and products can help identify the most cost-effective courses of treatment and thus increase the quality and value of health care with a given budget. However, reimbursement decisions take place in a social and political context and the consideration of efficiency is not always obvious. For example, in considering whether to introduce population health screening programmes (Box 8.1), policymakers have to weigh up the potential benefits against the potential harms, and consider the opportunity costs involved in introducing a resource-intensive intervention. There are a range of tools such as HTA which can help policymakers to determine the relative effectiveness and cost–effectiveness of different interventions.

8.2.2 The role of the HTA in supporting reimbursement decisions

This section focuses specifically on the role of the HTA and the different international approaches to dealing with cost–effectiveness and effectiveness in defining and regulating the health care included within the publicly funded benefit basket.

The WHO defines the HTA as the systematic evaluation of the impacts of health technology (including drugs, medicines, vaccines, procedures and systems). Its main purpose is to inform technology-related policymaking in health thereby improving the uptake of cost-effective technologies and prevent the uptake of those which are of less certain value (WHO, 2011).

The use of the HTA is common place in developed countries. In Europe, a HTA Network has been established to enhance cooperation between countries.[16] However, it can be argued that there is a constant tension between economic and scientific considerations given the need to control costs (Pugatch & Ficai, 2007).

---

16 See http://ec.europa.eu/health/technology_assessment/policy/network/index_en.htm (accessed 21 July 2016).

Box 8.1 *Population screening programmes*

Screening programmes in the general population are a strategy to support the early detection of cancer. Screening takes place across a healthy population and involves the mass application of tests to identify individuals who potentially have a symptomatic disease to support earlier diagnosis and treatment. The World Health Organization (WHO) suggests that screening programmes should only be undertaken where the prevalence of a disease is high enough to justify the effort of screening, the effectiveness of the testing process has been demonstrated and there are sufficient resources (both human and equipment) to cover a high proportion of a target group and to provide follow-up care (WHO, 2002). The screening criteria developed by Wilson and Jungner in the 1960s have become known as the 'classic criteria' and, in addition to the factors identified above by the WHO, include a criterion related to cost–effectiveness (i.e. that the cost of screening including diagnosis and treatment of those patients diagnosed should be economically balanced in relation to possible expenditure on medical care as a whole). (Wilson & Jungner, 1968)

While screening potentially offers benefits in the form of earlier diagnosis and treatment of cancer, it is a costly process at a system level and there are potential disadvantages to individual patients. There may be overtreatment of individual patients, unwarranted reassurance to those receiving a false-negative test and unwarranted anxiety and inappropriate treatment of those with false-positive tests (Holland, Stewart & Masseria, 2006). For example, in France, generalization of prostate cancer screening via the dosage of the prostate specific antigen has not been approved by the National Health Authority because of concerns about the diagnosis of cancer cases (false-positives) and surgical interventions on tumours, the majority of which would not have become symptomatic.

The role of screening as an appropriate, cost-effective intervention has been subject to increasing debate for some established programmes such as cervical or breast cancer screening. While breast and cervical cancer screening programmes are very common across the health systems of high- and middle-income countries, there are important differences; for example, the target population varies significantly across different countries and the evidence base on whether the potential benefits outweigh the harms is not universally accepted.

The Euroscreen Working Group conducted a systematic literature review of European trend studies ($n=17$), incidence-based mortality studies ($n=20$), and case-control studies ($n=8$), and estimated the reduction in breast cancer mortality for women invited for screening against those not invited and for women screened against those who were not screened. It was suggested that the best European estimate for breast cancer mortality reduction was 25–31% for women invited for screening and 38–48% for those actually screened (Broeders et al., 2012), that the chance of saving a woman's life by population-based mammography screening of appropriate quality was greater than that of overdiagnosis, and was contributing to the overall decline in the mortality rate across Europe for breast cancer (Paci, 2012).

However, another study, which reviewed seven trials involving 600 000 women who were randomly assigned to receive screening mammograms or not, suggested that breast cancer mortality was an unreliable outcome that was biased in favour of screening, that the trials with adequate randomization did not find an effect of screening on total cancer mortality, including breast cancer after 10 years or on all-cause mortality after 13 years, and further suggested that for every 2000 women invited for screening over a 10-year period, one would avoid dying of breast cancer, 10 healthy women would be treated unnecessarily and more than 200 women would experience psychological distress because of false-positive findings (Gøtzsche & Jørgensen, 2013). In response, to address the debate, the NHS National Cancer Director, Professor Sir Mike Richards, announced in October 2011 that he was commissioning a review of breast screening.

The review was conducted by an independent expert panel which was tasked with studying all the latest evidence on breast screening to estimate the likely benefits and risks associated with routine screening. The panel concluded that the United Kingdom's breast screening programmes confer significant benefit and should continue. The review did not look at costs (Cancer Research UK, 2012).

There is widespread public interest in the role of screening and there can be pressure from the media and other stakeholders to develop new programmes (Holland, Stewart & Masseria, 2006) or to increase the target population. In England, a campaign was launched to lower the age of the target population for cervical cancer screening from 25 following the death of Jade Goody, a television celebrity, at the age of 27. The government reviewed the policy in the wake of widespread press attention but did not lower the standard age for screening on the basis of the high rates of false-positive results in women under the age of 25 (BBC, 2009). European guidelines suggest that cervical screening should start between the ages of 20 and 30 but preferably not before the age of 25 or 30 depending on the burden of the disease in the population and the available resources (Arbyn et al., 2010).

8.2.3 The role of efficiency measurement in the HTA

The HTA plays a crucial role in providing evidence to inform policy decisions on the reimbursement of health technology. At a basic level, the HTA seeks to understand whether a new technology is effective. In some countries the analysis will go further, to consider whether the technology is cost-effective when compared to other interventions for a similar condition. In other countries, such as the United Kingdom, the analysis is further extended to consider whether a given technology is cost-effective when compared to interventions for any condition, through comparing QALYs and analysing the cost–effectiveness of different interventions by determining the cost per QALY. This section does not focus on the methodological limitations of QALY and other cost-utility measures, but instead focuses on the higher-level policy issues regarding the relative importance of HTA in policy decision-making (see Figure 8.2 for a range of considerations for HTA).

Figure 8.2 *Range of considerations for HTA*

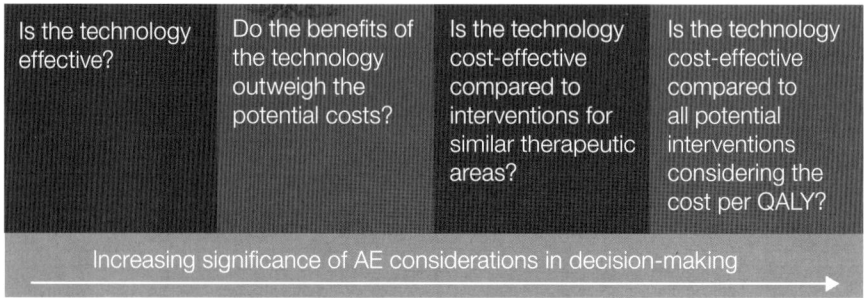

Is the technology effective?	Do the benefits of the technology outweigh the potential costs?	Is the technology cost-effective compared to interventions for similar therapeutic areas?	Is the technology cost-effective compared to all potential interventions considering the cost per QALY?

Increasing significance of AE considerations in decision-making →

Note: HTA = health technology assessment.

On the surface, the questions outlined in Figure 8.2 should lend themselves easily to using efficiency metrics as part of the decision-making process. The questions relate to a single issue, that is, the effectiveness or cost–effectiveness of an intervention. However, different approaches to the HTA have been adopted internationally.

One of the greatest areas of contention is the extent to which QALYs are used to determine the availability of different technologies and the extent to which it is fair to limit access based on a cost-per-QALY threshold. Table 8.1 shows some of the different approaches to determining reimbursement.

Table 8.1 *Use of cost–effectiveness thresholds in selected developed countries*

Country	Is a cost–effectiveness threshold used in access and reimbursement decisions?	
United Kingdom	Yes	Generally if a treatment costs >£20 000–30 000 per QALY, it would not be considered cost-effective (NICE, 2010).
France	No	The therapeutic value of a drug is assessed on its therapeutic benefit and on its added therapeutic value compared to other treatments. The added therapeutic value (ATV) represents the added health gain and plays a significant role in pricing decisions. Price negotiations follow the assessment of ATV. Drugs offering no ATV will only be added to the reimbursement list if they allow savings for the social security system (Sauvage, 2008). Since 2013, for drugs assessed as high ATV (therefore already accepted for reimbursement) manufacturers are asked to provide a cost-efficiency analysis (value per QALY). This information is only used in price negotiations, however, it is not clear how effectively, since the prices of these drugs are set by the pharmaceutical companies at the level of five comparative EU countries.
Germany	No	New drugs are assessed against appropriate comparators within the same therapeutic condition giving a reference price (IQWiG, 2009).
Australia	Not explicitly	The QALY is used in HTA but there are no fixed thresholds which represent an acceptable level of cost–effectiveness (Bulfone, Younie & Carter, 2009).
Ireland	Yes	Historically, the threshold has varied between €20 000 and €45 000 per QALY.*

Note: QALY = quality-adjusted life year;
* See National Centre for Pharmacoeconomics, http://www.ncpe.ie/about/ (accessed 21 July 2016).

Box 8.2 *Ireland: use of efficiency metrics in the HTA for ipilimumab*

The National Centre for Pharmacoeconomics (Ireland) (NCPE) conducts HTA of pharmaceutical products for the Health Service Executive (HSE) in Ireland. In September 2011, the NCPE concluded that Bristol-Myers Squibb Pharmaceuticals had failed to demonstrate the cost–effectiveness of ipilimumab for the treatment of advanced melanoma in adult patients who had received prior therapy and could not recommend the drug for reimbursement at the submitted price. The base case suggested that the drug would cost €85 000 per patient and the gross budget impact of ipilimumab therapy would range from €4.8 million to €7.4 million for 2012. In the base case, the increment cost per QALY gained with ipilimumab versus best supportive care was estimated at €147 899/QALY against a willingness to pay threshold of €45 000.

In May 2012, it was announced that the drug would be available as soon as an arrangement could be reached which would allow costs to be reimbursable following negotiations (O'Reilly, 2012). The drug was approved for reimbursement from 3 May 2012 (Dáil Éireann, 2012). It has been suggested that, following the negotiations, the cost be reduced to under €116 000 per QALY, which was still over the original threshold (Barry, 2013). In parallel, the HSE entered into negotiations with the Irish Pharmaceutical Healthcare Association (IPHA) to reach a new agreement on the cost of drugs, with potential savings in excess of €400 million over 3 years, and a separate agreement with the IPHA which would provide additional cost savings (An Roinn Sláinte, 2012).

Decisions on whether to fund new, innovative (but expensive) drugs can attract significant media attention and public pressure. For example, in Ireland in 2011, there was widespread controversy over the decision not to recommend ipilimumab for reimbursement. See the case in Box 8.2.

NICE is one of the best-known organizations assessing the cost per QALY gained when determining whether a new technology should be adopted by the NHS in England. NICE currently uses the QALY measurement to compare how much someone's life could be extended and/or improved before considering the cost per QALY gained. Generally, if a treatment costs more than £20 000–30 000 per QALY, it would not be considered cost-effective (NICE, 2010). However, NICE has not been immune to criticisms of rationing, and the concept of applying a value threshold in determining the availability of technologies is not universally accepted. On coming to power in 2010, the Conservative and Liberal Democrat coalition government proposed the creation of a Cancer Drugs Fund[17] to provide access to some cancer drugs for patients at the end of life. To date, £1 billion has been spent on drugs through the fund and four

---

17 The Cancer Drugs Fund was established in 2011 and is due to continue until 2016. It provides additional funding for cancer drugs in England which have not been approved by NICE.

drugs – bevacizumab, abiraterone, bendamustine and cetuximab – have accounted for around half of the spending. Most of the drugs have been examined by NICE and rejected on the grounds that they do not reach NICE's cost–effectiveness threshold level because of a combination of low effectiveness and high cost (HM Government, 2010).

Unlike the United Kingdom system, some countries have taken an active stance against the QALY threshold. For example, in the USA, the Patient Protection and Affordable Care Act (2010) prohibits the Patient-Centered Outcomes Research Institute from developing or employing dollars-per-QALY as a threshold to establish what type of health care is cost-effective or recommended, nor can a QALY threshold be used to determine coverage, reimbursement or incentive programmes under the Medicare Programme. It could also be argued that, aside from ideological issues, a cost–effectiveness threshold would be less likely to work in the USA given the diverse spread of payers and the complexity of health care delivery (Sullivan et al., 2009).

In Germany, the Institute for Quality and Efficiency in Health Care (IQWiG) examines the benefits and disbenefits of interventions.[18] IQWiG's functions are advisory in nature and its recommendations are not binding. Constitutionally, statutory health insurance (SHI) beneficiaries may not be deprived of access to beneficial health technologies on cost alone and, before 2007, IQWiG's remit was limited to the assessment of clinical benefit (IQWiG, 2009). The Act to promote competition among the SHI funds came into force on 1 April 2007 and gave IQWiG additional powers to assess the benefits and costs of drugs. However, the Federal Joint Committee – Gemeinsamer Bundesausschuss (G-BA)[19] – requested that the assessment of benefits and costs be carried out by comparing competing health technologies in a given therapeutic area. This meant that decisions about the relative importance of conditions and funding decisions would not lie with the Institute (IQWiG, 2009).

In practice, new drugs and medical interventions were covered by default and were only assessed by IQWiG if the G-BA requested an evaluation, which resulted in Germany having more new drugs available compared to other European countries but paying a high premium as a result (Nasser & Sawicki, 2009). From 1 January 2011, the G-BA and IQWiG were required to conduct benefit assessments of newly authorized drugs. Within three months of market authorization, the G-BA assesses the benefit of the new

---

18 See the IQWiG timeline (https://www.iqwig.de/en/about_us/iqwig_timeline.3252.html, accessed 8 August 2016).

19 The G-BA determines which services and technologies are to be reimbursed by the SHI funds and comprises physicians, dentists, hospitals and health insurance funds in Germany.

drug against appropriate comparators (in practice, this is delegated to IQWiG). After another three months, the G-BA makes a decision on the benefits case and pricing structure for the new medicine. Within six months, if additional benefit is proved, the reimbursement price is negotiated. If a medicine is not found to have additional benefit, it is allocated to a reference price group. Reference prices determine the maximum amount statutory health insurers will pay (G-BA, 2011).

While it is acknowledged that there are multiple approaches to HTA, there appears to be relatively little evidence relating to the effectiveness of HTA as a process (Wilsdon & Serota, 2011) and HTA reports do not typically define what they are hoping to achieve over and above the assessment of a given technology (Garrido, 2008). In March 2010, a new European project – the European Consortium in Healthcare Outcomes and Cost-benefit Research – was established to compare the health system organizations of the 27 Member States and to study the robustness of health outcomes used by HTA authorities in Europe. The final report suggested that HTAs expressed as the number of QALYs or cost per QALY were inconsistent and that European HTA agencies should use other methods. Instead of using the QALY, the report recommended that cost–effectiveness analyses should be expressed as a cost per relevant clinical outcome (Beresniak et al., 2013). However, the findings were not accepted by NICE, with its Chief Executive suggesting that there needed to be a measure which could be applied across all diseases and conditions to ensure that the costs to the NHS were justified by improvements in quality of length of life (NICE, 2013).

8.3 Cost sharing arrangements

All health care systems include some element of user charges and copayment for some services as part of the system of financing health care. Across the OECD in 2011, the proportion of health care expenditure funded by out of pocket (OOP) payments was around 20%. Among middle- and high-income countries, the reliance on OOP payments is lower than in low-income economies but it still varies considerably, with countries such as France, New Zealand and the United Kingdom below 10% yet Australia, Portugal, Spain and Switzerland at, or above, 20% (OECD, 2013). The Commonwealth Fund survey examined the performance of the health care system in 11 high-income countries. As Table 8.2 shows, in many high-income countries, significant minorities of patients still report cost issues as a barrier to accessing or completing medical care (Davis et al., 2014).

Table 8.2 *Cost-related access problems in 11 health care systems (percentage of surveyed patients/physicians reporting problems)*

	Australia	Canada	France	Germany	Netherlands	New Zealand	Norway	Sweden	Switzerland	United Kingdom	USA
Did not fill a prescription; skipped recommended medical test, treatment or follow-up; or had a medical problem but did not visit doctor or clinic in the past year because of cost	16	13	18	15	22	21	10	6	13	4	37
Patient's insurance denied payment for medical care or did not pay as much as expected	15	14	17	14	13	6	3	3	16	3	28
Patient had serious problems paying or was unable to pay medical bills	8	7	13	7	9	10	6	4	10	1	23
Physicians think their patients often have difficulty paying for medications or OOP costs	25	26	29	21	42	26	4	6	16	13	59
OOP expenses for medical bills >$1000 in the past year (USD equivalent)	25	14	7	11	7	9	17	2	24	3	41

Source: Davis et al. (2014).
Notes: OOP = out of pocket; USD = US dollar.

8.3.1 The rationale and objectives of user charges and copayments

The rationale for user charges in both insurance and tax-based health care systems is fundamentally the same: first, there is the financial objective of reducing insurance premiums and tax. The second rationale is to improve AE – tackling the incentive to overconsume. User charges are designed to reduce the problem of moral hazard[20] and the potential overconsumption of health care. Reducing consumption can improve efficiency if it reduces patients' use of clinically ineffective services but, if it reduces the use of cost-effective services, particularly prevention, it may be inefficient (Schokkaert & Van de Voorde, 2011). Some countries have been reforming their systems of copayment with the goal of improving AE. A prominent example is the series of innovations introduced in the USA under the banner of value-based insurance design (VBID) (Robinson, 2010).

8.3.2 The evidence of the efficiency impact of user charges and copayments

The empirical evidence suggests that user charges reduce the consumption of health care services in middle- and high-income countries, with primary care services having higher elasticity (more sensitive to price). Policymakers often rely

---

20 Moral hazard is a situation in which people or organizations may increase their risk-taking or consumption above allocatively efficient levels because all or part of the costs will be borne by others.

on user charges to slow the growth in health spending (Mladovsky et al., 2012). However, the potential for significant cost savings or enhanced efficiency from extending copayments and user charges is generally considered to be limited. User charges increase the financial burden on households (Wagstaff et al., 1992) and studies show that, in general, they do not differentiate effectively between cost-effective and low-value care. Moreover, they are particularly likely to reduce use among lower-income individuals, higher-need older people and chronically ill patients, even when the level of user charges is low (Gemmill, Thomson & Mossialos, 2008; Newhouse, 1993).

Increasing user charges in primary or ambulatory care may worsen health outcomes. Although frequently motivated by a desire to increase revenue or reduce cost, in some cases increasing user charges may have the opposite effect through increased spending in more expensive acute, emergency care. As a result, restricting user charges to low-value services and ensuring there are exemptions or caps for poorer households or regular users of care is more likely to enhance efficiency. However, it may not always be possible to identify low-value care and the transaction costs involved may be significant (Bach, 2008; Braithwaite & Rosen, 2007; Goldman, Joyce & Zheng, 2007; Thomson, Foubister & Mossialos, 2009; Trivedi, Rakowski & Ayanian, 2008).

8.3.3 The impact of efficiency measures on user charges and copayment decisions

Since the economic crisis in 2008, many countries faced with large fiscal deficits have increased user charges to reduce pressures on public funds, and private and social insurers have increased copayments to reduce the pressure on premiums. Across Europe, countries have increased or introduced user charges for a range of health services including ambulatory care, emergency department visits, pharmaceuticals and for specific services such as in vitro fertilization (IVF), physiotherapy, some mental health services and some vaccines (Mladovsky et al., 2012).

Measures of revenue raising

The 2008 economic crisis has seen countries prioritizing revenue raising as a response to burgeoning fiscal deficits. A recent review of international responses to austerity looked at the experience of five European countries following the recession of 2008 (Ellin et al., 2014). It found that in each country there had been a combination of changes to user charges, copayments and deductibles, and, in some countries, restrictions to the health basket. Table 8.3 shows the principal changes introduced in each country.

Table 8.3 *Changes to user charges, copayments, deductibles and the health basket in five European countries following the 2008 recession*

Country	Features of the response to austerity
Ireland	• Introduced new charges, including across a range of services for those without medical cards (two thirds of the population).
Spain	• Undocumented migrants and adults aged ≥26 who have not made social security contributions are excluded from receiving all but basic emergency care. • Introduced new charges and copayments, mainly for medicines. Older people on a higher income now pay 10% of the cost of medicines while others pay between €8 and €60 per month, depending on their pension.
Portugal	• Significant increases in user charges for medicines and services, although retaining financial incentive for people to access care in primary settings. • Exemption threshold raised, increasing the proportion of the population exempt from charges from 45–50% to 70%.
Netherlands	• Reductions in eligibility for long-term care and exclusion of specific services (for example, basic mobility aids, IVF) from mandatory coverage. • Mandatory deductibles increased from €170 to €350 between 2008 and 2013. • Copayments introduced for long-term care and physiotherapy.
Denmark	• Eligibility limited for certain procedures and surgeries (for example, gastric bypass). • Reimbursements restricted for dental care.

Source: Ellin et al. (2014).
Note: IVF = in vitro fertilization.

Beyond Europe, other countries have plans to increase copayments, principally for fiscal objectives. Faced with health care costs rising to 5.3% in 2012–2013, the Australian government proposed the introduction of a new copayment for visits to a GP, out-of-hospital pathology tests and imaging, from July 2015. The Federal Budget set out proposals to extend copayments from April 2015 under the Medicare program, with an A$7 fee for GP copayments which would be applicable to the poorest in society. However, there are plans to introduce a safety net with a cap introduced following the first 10 visits for key groups including pensioners, those on a low income and children under 16 (Johnson, 2014). Much of the political debate following the announcement has focused on the potential system impact of increased use of alternative services and the concern that there are other policies to support the financial sustainability of the health system which may be more effective (Consumers Health Forum of Australia, 2014). This highlights the need for policy to focus not just on the net efficiency impact of a specific policy but on its comparative efficiency and the potential opportunity cost of pursuing one option over another.

In Germany, the €10 fee per quarter for visits to a GP was abolished in 2012, 8 years after it was introduced, following a number of studies which suggested that that it was not effective in reducing demand for health care (Schreyögg & Grabka, 2010). Although the failure to achieve these objectives was cited as a reason for abolishing the copayment, there was no formal efficiency metric put in place when the payment was introduced to support a robust evaluation of the reform's impact.

Consideration of allocative efficiency

There is evidence to suggest that decisions on copayments and user charges are also influenced by concerns about AE. Switzerland is reforming its coinsurance rates to provide incentives for people to switch from traditional insurance plans to models of insurance with a managed care approach, which are considered to promote more efficient use of health resources. Under these reforms, coinsurance rates for those who opt for traditional insurance plans will rise from 10 to 15%, encouraging people to opt for managed care plans which will retain the lower coinsurance rate.

Perhaps the biggest development in the attempt to use copayment reform to support AE is the VBID concept, which was introduced in the USA over a decade ago. It describes a series of reforms to a number of health insurance plans in the USA that reduce copayments with the aim of encouraging patients to comply with recommended medication or treatment, to improve the proactive management of patients' conditions and minimize the costliest medical interventions. VBID focuses on conditions and treatments with well-established clinical evidence, particularly chronic conditions such as hypertension, asthma and diabetes. Over the past decade, the VBID concept has expanded to include incentives for other types of evidence-based services.

Following encouraging reports from early adopters of VBID, and the endorsement of the concept by a number of influential bodies in the USA, the 2010 Affordable Care Act adopted the VBID concept in its requirement that health insurance plans cover preventive services rated A or B by the 13 US Preventive Services Task Forces without a copayment option for the patient. The required preventive services include blood pressure screening, colorectal cancer screening and screening for sexually transmitted infections. The Act also allows the Secretary of the US Department of Health and Human Services to establish guidelines to permit a health insurance plan to use VBID (NCSL, 2016). Although the imperative to improve the AE of health spending was a key motivation behind the expansion of VBID in US health plans, there is no evidence of the development or use of systematic, consistent metrics of AE either by health plans or government bodies.

8.4 Hospital organization

Across health care systems over the last 20 years there has been a reduction in the number of curative hospital beds and a consolidation of hospitals, with an increasing number of hospitals merging into fewer, larger providers (Dash, Meredith & White, 2012; OECD, 2014). Over the last two decades, the average number of curative beds per 1000 population fell from 4.7 to 3.3.

8.4.1 The rationale and objectives of hospital mergers

The rationale for merger is often linked to concerns about the efficiency of the hospital sector. The hypothesized efficiency benefits are concentrated on different types of economies of scale and scope, either in terms of cost or quality. Table 8.4 outlines the common efficiency-related benefits claimed for hospital mergers.

Table 8.4 *Efficiency-based objectives frequently cited in support of hospital mergers*

Capturing the cost benefits of economies of scale and scope	Capturing the quality benefits of economies of scale and scope	Capturing the education and research benefits of economies of scale and scope
• Reduce duplication, lower administrative and management costs; • Strengthen the buying power of the hospital as a purchaser of goods and services; • Spread the cost of common resources (theatres, diagnostic equipment) across a larger volume and range of patient.	• Achieve the volume of patients needed for high-quality care; • Enable co-location of diagnostic, treatment and rehabilitation services (for example, for stroke and major trauma); • Support specialization of services to concentrate expertise; • Enable continuity of care with 24/7 services.	• Enable effective and efficient medical education and training; • Support research clusters to develop centres of excellence and multidisciplinary research.

Source: Authors' analysis.

However, mergers may also be motivated by the desire to increase the market power of the hospital. The benefit to the hospital of increased market power is traditionally defined in terms of higher profits arising from higher prices for health services. In many countries though, health care prices are fixed so that competition between hospitals is based on quality. In these health systems, mergers which increase market concentration pose a potential risk to quality incentives within the system (Gaynor, Laudecella & Propper, 2012).

In some cases, mergers arise from financial or clinical failure – a hospital is in deficit or struggling to deliver an acceptable quality of care and merger with another hospital is the failure regime in a sector where exit is very difficult. In 2009, faced with financial problems, the GasthuisZusters Antwerpen Hospital Group was formed from three hospitals (with 1100 beds) and four elderly care centres (with 300 residents) in the greater Antwerp region of Belgium. In Germany, an increasing number of public hospitals have been sold to private hospital chains, a trend driven mainly by budget deficits in regional and municipal governments (Schulten, 2006).

Systematic reviews of the relationship between outcomes and volumes suggest that for some services at least (for example, complex surgery), there is a relationship between the frequency with which the surgeon performs a procedure and quality (Halm, Lee & Chassin, 2002). There is a strong clinical consensus that higher volumes lead to better patient outcomes but, in some cases, there is limited evidence to support this consensus and there remains little evidence on specific volume thresholds (Glanville et al., 2010).

8.4.2 *The evidence of the efficiency benefits of mergers*

Although the objective of mergers is frequently to improve the efficiency of care (either in terms of quality or cost) the evidence of the impact of mergers on cost and quality is mixed, dated and limited. In terms of cost, a systematic review conducted in 1997 concluded that there was some evidence for economies of scale up to around 200 beds but also evidence of diseconomies of scale above 600 beds (Posnett, 1999). In some countries there are relatively few hospitals with fewer than 200 beds (Hong Kong, New Zealand and the United Kingdom). Other countries still have a significant number of small hospitals and merger activity does seem to be focused on consolidation among small providers (American Hospital Association, 2013).

Research on the impact of hospital volume on outcome shows that the volume/outcome relationship depends on the procedure/condition studied and often disappears above a small threshold. Gaynor (2004, 2006) provides a good summary of that literature. Overall, over time, the disparity in outcomes between low- and high-volume hospitals has narrowed, and outcomes have improved significantly for all hospitals. Given these improvements, lower minimum volume standards may be advisable in less populated areas (Ho, 2000).

Much of the empirical research is focused on the US health system. Studies of mergers in the USA suggest that hospital mergers generally increase prices and have no effect on quality (Vogt & Town, 2006; Weil, 2010). There is limited evidence on the impact of mergers in other countries and, critically, in systems with regulated prices. One exception is a recent study that looked at the effects of hospital mergers in the NHS in England. Using a number of measures including financial performance, productivity, waiting times and clinical quality, researchers found little evidence that mergers achieved the anticipated gains (Gaynor, Laudecella & Propper, 2012).

8.4.3 *The role of efficiency measurement in the decision-making process*

Hospital mergers can either be initiated by the organizations themselves or, in many cases, result from system-level planning exercises. A number of countries (including Germany, the Netherlands, the United Kingdom and the USA) approach hospital consolidation from the perspective of their general merger control regimes. In the Netherlands, the Competition Authority has responsibility for deciding merger cases but receives advice from the specific health regulator, the Health Authority, to identify whether there is an efficiency/public interest case for the merger based on the effects on patients in terms of affordability, quality and accessibility (Canoy & Sauter, 2009). For countries which take a market regulation approach to mergers, there is a significant evidence challenge in defining the relevant market for health services (both the geography and the relevant range of services) and then in assessing the potential loss of efficiency (in terms of cost or quality) from a merger proposal.

In some cases, governments have initiated major structural and institutional changes through national or local planning initiatives. The Ontario province of Canada established a programme of hospital reconfiguration motivated, in part, by financial and efficiency concerns. In 1994–1995, the government of Ontario had an operating deficit of CAD10.2 billion on revenues of CAD46 billion, or 22% of its budget. It set up a statutory body – the Health Services Restructuring Commission – with a legislative mandate to make binding decisions on the restructuring of hospitals across the province. It led to the amalgamation of 44 hospitals into 14 new organizations, the takeover of four hospitals by other hospital corporations, and the directed closure of 27 public hospitals (Rochon, 2010).

Denmark has undertaken an ambitious programme of hospital reconfiguration. In 2007, as part of a wider programme of structural reform of the Danish government, the Danish Health and Medicines Authority (DHMA) saw its role expanded from being a health sector regulator to a body with responsibilities for planning specialist functions across Denmark's hospitals. The DHMA issued guidance on standards for specialization to the five Danish regions and required them to submit plans to meet these standards, and to bid for capital resources from a 10-year DKK40 billion national investment fund for hospitals

(OECD, 2013). This programme of reform is expected to see the number of acute hospitals in Denmark fall from 40 in 2006 to between 20 and 25 in 2015 (Olejaz et al., 2012).

Decisions about hospital mergers and reconfigurations are often motivated by the desire to implement standards or guidelines developed by medical associations. A recent study in the United Kingdom reviewed a large number of guidance documents produced by Royal Colleges and other medical associations on the configuration of A&E and supporting services (Goudie & Goddard, 2011). They found that while there was a broad consensus about the need for a set of core services to be co-located with emergency services, there was less information on the minimum scale of provision. The authors comment that:

> *The evidence to support the guidance does not appear to draw upon economic evaluation. There is a high degree of circularity of argument as many documents cite other similar documents rather than primary sources. Expert opinion is a prevalent theme within the types of guidance cited and very often it is deemed to be 'self-evident' that a particular organisation of services is required. Whilst this evidence may well be valid, it is not usually based on economic analysis.*
> (Goudie & Goddard, 2011)

The Danish reforms to stimulate consolidation of specialist services referred to earlier also relied heavily on expert opinion. Clinical expert groups were used to determine which services should be considered specialist, and the appropriate volumes and co-location of services (OECD, 2013). The use of expert opinion is, in part, a response to limitations in the evidence base on economies of scale and scope in health care but it is also used to build support for change. Hospitals are arguably the most visible organizations within health care systems; they account for a significant proportion of health spending, their clinicians provide much of the professional leadership, and they have a significant impact on the overall provision of health care. As a result, decisions about hospital services are highly politically sensitive in most countries, regardless of the mix between public or private ownership and funding (McKee & Healy, 2002).

In many countries, clinical leadership and support for change is often seen as crucial to implementing otherwise highly contentious reforms. Many countries, including France and Germany, have introduced volume (compulsory) thresholds in the past decade, mainly with the goal of improving quality of care. In Germany, legislation in 2002 allowed the contracting parties in the German health system to determine minimum volume standards for planned care. In 2003 the compulsory health insurance funds proposed a list of 10 minimum volumes and, in 2004, these were introduced for five procedures by the G-BA (which includes the National Association of Doctors and Dentists, the German Hospital Federation and the health insurance funds). Annual minimum volume standards were implemented for five surgical procedures: kidney, liver and stem cell transplantation, and complex oesophageal and pancreatic interventions. In 2006, a minimum volume standard of 50 procedures per year was introduced for total knee replacement operations (de Cruppé et al., 2007).

To mitigate the potential negative effects of mergers, regulatory authorities have tried to impose behavioural remedies on hospitals seeking to merge; however, this is often difficult to enforce. Determining whether merged hospitals have, in practice, exercised market power is difficult in health systems where hospitals compete for patients on the basis of quality rather than price. In hospital systems with competition based on quality rather than price, post-merger attempts to enforce behavioural remedies may therefore not be an effective means of responding to a loss of efficiency. More fundamentally, unwinding a hospital merger is likely to be deeply problematic. Seeking to undo a merger may be an even less effective remedy as it introduces new risks of additional costs and quality failures.

8.5 Provider payment

Provider payment can be a powerful tool to promote efficient health care provision. Ideally, payment systems should encourage good quality of care while at the same time promoting the efficient use of resources at the health system level. In practice, different payment mechanisms (block, capitation, cost per case or fee for item of service) provide different incentives for providers, some of which may be conflicting with the goal of greater efficiency. Within each type of payment method there are variants that may create a different set of incentives, and several payment methods may be used in combination to mitigate unintended consequences that may be generated by each method individually. It is important to be aware of typical reactions triggered by each payment scheme and evaluate/measure the impact in terms of efficiency, quality and equity of access. This section looks at two popular payment mechanisms widely used in industrialized countries – DRG-based payment and P4P – to examine what evidence is used to justify or establish their efficiency and what metrics are used to monitor their impact on efficiency following implementation.

8.5.1 Rationale and objectives of activity-based payment

Activity-based payment, where hospital funding is linked to activity defined by DRGs, is widely considered a potential solution for improving efficiency in the hospital sector (O'Reilly et al., 2012). As a payment mechanism, it provides incentives to increase the number of patients that hospitals treat (compared to global budgets), and reduce inputs per case and/or improve the efficiency of the input mix. Like any other forms of payment, it can also generate perverse effects that have been largely described in the literature (Cots et al., 2011; Ellis & McGuire, 1996). Patient selection, specialization towards standardized care procedures, multiplication of high-intensity (better remunerated) procedures and upcoding are among the examples most often reported. Furthermore, the efficiency sought at the individual provider level may not always be compatible with the system-wide objective of assuring best allocation of resources in the health system, across different services, to achieve the best possible outcomes (AE). Hospitals can overprovide certain treatments/tests, modify the composition of services or abandon (when they can) certain activities considered unprofitable. This can also create problems in access to some services.

8.5.2 *The evidence of the efficiency benefits of DRG payment*

Empirical evidence on the impact of DRG payment on efficiency is surprisingly scarce. The majority of the earlier academic studies focused on technical efficiency (TE) (or productivity) looking at the relationship between hospital outputs and inputs, using empirical techniques called frontier modelling to identify the best output–input relationship to establish how much the efficiency levels of given hospitals deviate from the frontier values (Kautter, 2011). DEA is the most common metric used since it allows for flexible specification of hospital production (see Chapter 5). All these studies measure efficiency from the hospital perspective, and use either the number of discharges within each DRG or an aggregated discharge measure, adjusting for the hospital case mix, for defining outputs (Street, O'Reilly & Ward, 2011).

Despite the obvious trade-off between care quality and efficiency, quality is rarely and only partially taken into account in the analyses. In a few studies where outcomes (beyond outputs) are considered, they are always measured by inpatient mortality rates. Hospital inputs are often measured by partial indicators such as labour/physician FTEs or, less commonly, by running costs and medical expenses. Results from these earlier studies are rather mixed. The link between TE gains and DRG payment has not been demonstrated in many countries, including the Austria and the USA. However, in others, such as Norway, Portugal and Sweden, DRG payment was associated with greater TE in hospitals, although studies from Sweden showed that initial efficiency improvements were subsequently negated when activity ceilings were imposed on hospitals (Street, O'Reilly & Ward, 2011). Impact on cost efficiency, studied to a much lesser extent, appears to be mostly insignificant, except in Sweden (Gerdtham et al., 1999; Street, O'Reilly & Ward, 2011).

There is limited evidence on the impact of DRG payment on overall cost efficiency at the hospital sector level; however, DRGs are associated with higher hospital expenditure, including higher administration costs and hospital volumes (O'Reilly et al., 2012). Moreno-Serra & Wagstaff (2010) showed that the introduction of DRG payment (over global budgets) was associated with higher spending in central and eastern Europe and in Asia, with higher hospital volume but also lower amenable mortality, in particular for cerebrovascular diseases. It is difficult to attribute changes in outcomes to payment reform because of simultaneous changes in the health care contexts. In England, Farrar et al. (2009) showed that there was little measurable change in quality of care in terms of in-hospital mortality, 30-day post-surgical mortality and emergency readmissions after treatment for hip fracture, while average length of stay and unit costs decreased significantly in areas where DRG payment was introduced.

8.5.3 *The role of efficiency measurement in the decision-making*

Despite the weaknesses of the evidence base on efficiency and numerous studies pointing the perverse effects of DRG payment (Cots et al., 2011), countries that introduced DRG payment relatively recently often lack thorough monitoring and evaluation of its impact.

In most countries, payers and purchasers use partial efficiency metrics with average length of stay and hospital volume (number of cases) the most common indicators. For example, in France, the official monitoring and evaluation of the efficiency of the payment reform consisted of measuring the number of hospital cases in major categories and the average length of stay (for all stays). The rise in the number of hospital stays (not-weighted), given the overall hospital sector budget, is taken as a sign of higher efficiency; however, recent research suggested that DRG creep (substantial upcoding of activity) and induced demand may be a real problem for sector-wide efficiency (Or et al., 2013). Patient outcomes and quality metrics, such as 30-day readmission rates and complication/mortality after surgery, are not monitored regularly in France.

In all countries, average length of stay is used as a key indicator of efficiency. The significant reduction in average length of stay after the introduction of the DRG payment in many countries is seen as a sign of greater efficiency. However, providers can also discharge patients to be readmitted again or transfer patients prematurely to other institutions or home. Early analysis of the readmission rates in the USA suggested some evidence that hospitals modified their coding practices under DRG payment to readmit patients into higher-priced diagnoses

(Cutler, 2006). This, in turn, impacted Medicare's payment policy, which adjusted payments to discourage inappropriate discharges. Several European countries have been inspired by Medicare in monitoring readmission rates and not paying for readmissions within 30 days of discharge. But, the definition of avoidable readmission, how readmissions are counted and the non-payment policy vary widely across countries.

Activity-based payments encourage hospitals to optimize the use of their resources based on the theoretical model of so-called yardstick competition.[21] Economics literature has largely shown that yardstick competition is efficient only if prices are set correctly. This requires that managers and regulators know each hospital's cost function, that is, they can compare cost components of different hospitals (per case mix-adjusted stay) and determine benchmarks. However, in many European countries, such as France, Germany and Italy, unit cost data are not available for all hospitals and/or not used for benchmarking, partly because of the difficulties in measuring and standardizing hospital costs across providers (see Chapter 4). In the USA, the Medicare Payment Advisory Commission established efficiency rankings based on outcome measures (such as mortality, readmission, and so on) and inpatient costs, adjusting for factors beyond a hospital's control, which do not reflect efficiency (MedPAC, 2009). In contrast, in France, the policy of price convergence between public and private hospitals without using the same costing methodology, nor adjusting for factors beyond hospitals' control, has created distrust and distorted the discussion on efficiency differences between providers.

In most countries, DRG prices are set using average cost data from a sample of hospitals. Some argue that, for improving system-wide efficiency, a better option is to adjust prices for encouraging medical practice considered high quality and efficient, moving away from pricing based on observed costs per case. Evaluations of episodes of care incorporating pre- and post-hospital services (radiology examinations, physical therapy) can also be beneficial for establishing efficiency margins for given conditions/patient groups (see Chapter 3). In England, best practice tariffs have recently been introduced for selected areas (including cholecystectomy, hip fractures, cataracts and stroke) where significant unexplained variation in clinical practice is observed and clear evidence of what constitutes best practice is available (DoH, 2014). For example, best practice tariffs are set to incentivize day case activity for cholecystectomy while, for cataracts, the price covers the entire pathway, so that commissioners encourage best practice pathways where patients are treated in a joined-up and efficient manner.

---

21 Yardstick competition is the system of using comparative information about organizations with local or sector-based monopolies to set prices or performance standards.

8.5.4 The rationale and objectives of P4P

Traditionally, payment systems are based on the quantity and intensity of services provided. While this may be appropriate in most situations, it is problematic where low-intensity care can provide better outcomes than high-intensity care and when service content can vary widely between providers. P4P rewards providers for achieving specified valued outcomes. Most approaches adjust payments to physicians and hospitals on the basis of a number of different quality measures but some schemes also consider efficiency of service provision. Ultimately, P4P programmes aim to increase the provision of quality care by containing or reducing health care costs over the long-term.

Payments may be made at the individual, group or institutional level. Performance may be measured using benchmarks or relative comparisons (Kautter, 2011). The results of any P4P scheme, in terms of efficiency, depend on the performance measures used (the definition of quality and outcomes) and the reimbursement rules for providers, as well as the governance arrangements ensuring the system is functioning as intended without creating perverse effects.

8.5.5 The evidence of the efficiency benefits of P4P

There is some evidence that P4P programmes can improve quality and facilitate cost savings, although unintended or negative effects have also been reported. The variety of programmes and lack of proper evaluation makes it difficult to establish firm conclusions on the efficiency benefits from P4P programmes.

Several reviews concluded that the evidence is mixed with regard to P4P effectiveness, often finding a lack of impact on provider behaviour or inconsistent effects, albeit with a few exceptions (Houle et al., 2012; Van Herck et al., 2010). For example, Curtin et al. (2006) suggested a 2.5-fold return on investment for each US dollar spent on a P4P programme for diabetes in a US health maintenance organization. An evaluation from China's Ningxia Province (a predominantly rural area in the north-west of the country) suggested that capitation with P4P can improve drug prescribing practices by reducing overprescribing and inappropriate prescribing (Yip et al., 2014). The authors carried out a matched-pair, cluster-randomized experiment between 2009 and 2012 to evaluate the effects of P4P on antibiotic prescribing practices, health spending, outpatient visit volume and patient satisfaction. They found that the intervention led to a reduction of approximately 15% in antibiotic prescriptions and a small reduction in total spending per visit without any effect on other outcomes.

On P4P schemes for hospitals in the USA, a report on the Premier Project by Kahn et al. (2006) found that the cost (bonus expenses) of the programme was higher than financial penalties recovered from the hospitals. In England, the evaluation of the P4P for hospitals, which is broadly similar to the US scheme, showed that the P4P did not significantly reduce mortality in targeted conditions and that there is a statistically significant increase in mortality for non-incentivised conditions (Kreif et al. 2015).

8.5.6 *The role of efficiency measurement in the decision-making*

P4P has been increasingly seen as the solution to problems in health service delivery, not only in high-income settings but also in low- and middle-income countries. Most P4P schemes target GPs with the objective of improving health promotion and prevention rates, as well as the organization of medical practice. The evaluation of most of the schemes, however, has been limited. Often there is no control group and it is just presumed that one can compare before and after to capture the effects of P4P.

For example, New Zealand started its Performance Based Management (PBM) programme in 2006 within its Primary Health Organizations (PHOs), which are non-profit organizations that provide primary health care services (Buteow, 2008). In 2007 over 98% of New Zealanders enrolled in the PBM programme. The P4P scheme was one component of the health sector overall quality framework, and aligned with other initiatives to improve health outcomes and reduce inequalities. Financial incentives, relatively small, aimed to provide some additional resources to enhance primary care. While all performance indicators (mostly process indicators such as vaccination and screening rates) showed modest progress (Cashin, 2011), there has been no rigorous evaluation of the impact of the PBM and it is hard to demonstrate the link between the payments and the progress made (value for money).

In France, in an attempt to improve the quality and efficiency of primary care, the National Health Insurance Fund (HIF) introduced a P4P scheme in 2009 – contracts for improved individual practice (CAPI). These contracts for GPs were initially signed on a voluntary basis without altering the existing FFS scheme. The contract aimed to encourage prevention (vaccination for older patients, breast cancer screening), adherence to guidelines (diabetes management) and reduce inappropriate prescribing, in particular reducing the prescription of vasodilators (overprescribed despite being proven ineffective) and benzodiazepines (potentially dangerous and addictive) for older people. There was also a specific objective to improve efficiency by increasing generic prescribing rates. The first contracts could provide up to €7000 annually if 100% of the targets were achieved.

Analysis of the results by the HIF after one year of implementation showed modest improvement along performance indicators in all domains. However, data also showed that the results for prevention and diabetes have been improving for all GPs, and the difference between those who signed CAPI and others was not significant. No cost–effectiveness analysis was performed and the overall cost of the programme is not known. Nevertheless, the HIF decided to generalize the P4P scheme to all GPs in 2011 and broadened the objectives (related to organization of office practice, computer use in prescription and electronic data). Since 2012, with the payment for public health objectives, all physicians, including specialists, are covered by the P4P.

8.6 Public reporting of health care data

The role of information as a tool to influence both provider and patient behaviour has been increasingly recognized as having great potential to contribute to health system efficiency. While initiatives are bourgeoning, this is an area that is somewhat untested (Smith, 2012).

8.6.1 Rationale for intervention

A central pillar of the health information agenda has been the drive to improve the transparency of performance data at an organizational and service level. For example, the Tallinn Charter, signed by Member States of the WHO European Region, committed members to the promotion of transparency and to be accountable for health system performance to achieve measureable results (WHO, 2008). The growth in performance measurement and reporting can, in part, be attributed to pressure to contain costs and the parallel drive to empower patients, and the improvements in technology which allow more sophisticated approaches to data collection (Smith et al., 2008). However, this drive towards transparency is not universally popular. Health systems have had to balance the potential benefits of data transparency with the needs of those professionals working within the system.

Public reporting of such data might have a number of different purposes:

- to identify and prevent failure in care quality;
- act as a lever to drive up quality;
- facilitate patient choice;
- provide public reassurance; and
- provide accountability to system payers and customers (Nuffield Trust et al., 2013).

Efficiency measures will play an important role in all five objectives, although the methods for incorporating quality into efficiency measurement are still developing and different actors (such as providers, insurers and consumers) will each have different perspectives on what constitutes efficient service delivery (McGlynn et al., 2008).

The construction and presentation of performance information will depend on its purpose. Policymakers, in choosing to present new data, should be mindful of their audience and the potential trade-off between high-level summative measures and granular data (Pearse & Mazevska, 2010). For example, data aimed at improving service-level performance will need to be sufficiently granular to enable clinicians to make comparisons with their peers, but this might be inappropriately complex for members of the public who might benefit from high-level, easily digestible information.

8.6.2 *The evidence of the efficiency benefits of public reporting of health care data*

Many middle- and high-income countries have developed sophisticated registries or data sets which allow comparisons across providers with a degree of public transparency. For example, in Germany, all hospitals approved to provide care to SHI members must provide data on approximately 300 quality measures to the AQUA Institute for Applied Quality Improvement and Research in Health Care. (The G-BA has commissioned the AQUA Institute with nationwide cross-sectoral health care quality assurance.) These data returns are a key part of the Sektorübergreifende Qualitätssicherung im Gesundheitswesen (Cross-sectoral Quality in Health Care) programme which aims to provide formative feedback to health care providers to stimulate performance improvement; citizens are also the intended users (Szecsenyi et al., 2012). Performance results are then fed back to hospitals, allowing for peer comparison. From 2011, a structured quality dialogue has been initiated in circumstances where a hospital's performance suggests a quality deficiency (Institute for Applied Quality Improvement and Research in Health Care, 2012).

The use of public reporting as a means to encourage quality improvement is based on the principle that publicly reported performance metrics motivate providers to improve based on a range of factors including, among others, professional reputation and market forces. Krumholz et al. (2008) suggested that publicly reported efficiency measures should integrate quality and cost data but warned that an emphasis on restraining costs without thorough consideration of the consequences could undermine health outcomes, thereby leading to higher costs in the future. In addition, the drive to publish publicly available information on a specific topic area or intervention may not always be underpinned by robust evidence. For example, hospital trusts in England now have to publish their staffing ratios but NICE did not find evidence to suggest that there should be a single nursing staff-to-patient ratio (NICE, 2014) (see Box 8.3).

Box 8.3 *England: safer staffing ratios*

In November 2013, the Department of Health announced that, in England, it would be compulsory from June 2014 for NHS hospital trusts providing acute inpatient services to publish ward level information on staffing levels. Hospital trusts would be required to publish planned nursing and midwifery staffing levels each month and, every six months, trust boards would be required to undertake a detailed review of staffing levels. NICE was asked to produce independent, evidence-based guidance documents setting out the evidence on safe staffing levels and would review tools to set safe staffing levels (DoH, 2014).

NICE reviewed the evidence and did not recommend a mandatory minimum staffing level for adult inpatient wards, suggesting that there was no single nursing staff-to-patient ratio that could be applied across all such wards. However, NICE did recommend that if the available registered nurses for a particular ward were caring for more than eight patients during day shifts, additional monitoring should be implemented. As part of its recommendations, NICE identified considerable gaps in the evidence base regarding safer staffing levels including a lack of high-quality studies exploring and quantifying the relationship between staffing levels and outcomes relating to patient safety, quality and satisfaction. NICE also suggested that the lack of data collection in relation to the wide variety of outcome variables at ward level ruled out detailed economic analysis of patient outcomes in relation to the numbers of nursing staff on the ward (NICE, 2014).

There is evidence to suggest the public reporting of performance does have an impact on the performance of providers in health (Hibbard, Stockard & Tulser, 2003; Shekelle et al., 2008) although evidence is not fully conclusive (Ketelaar et al., 2011). Box 8.4 demonstrates how policymakers can use performance metrics in practice to inform decision-making. However, distinguishing the impact of public reporting of efficiency measures from other dimensions of performance is challenging and the use of efficiency measurement lags far behind quality measurement in health care (Hussey et al., 2009).

There is also evidence to suggest that consumers have been slow to use the increasingly comprehensive information that is available to them (Hibbard, 2008), which may diminish the effectiveness of public reporting. Presenting information on efficiency to the public can be challenging. For example, some consumers might equate high cost with high quality and low cost with low quality (Hibbard et al., 2012). This is echoed by learning from Aligning Forces for Quality, a quality improvement programme in the USA funded by the Robert Wood Johnson Foundation, which highlights the practical challenges of presenting cost and efficiency measures to the public (Aligning Forces for Quality, 2011). Focus groups were conducted as part of the programme ($N=8 \times 2$) and found that consumers find it difficult to access and understand information on the cost of

Box 8.4 *Finland: the PERFECT (PERFormance, Effectiveness, and Costs of Treatment) project*

The PERFECT project monitors the content, quality and cost–effectiveness of treatment episodes in specialized medical care* in Finland, assessing factors that influence variation between regions and service providers. For selected disease groups and procedures, comparative data on procedures and patients are created through combining the data sets from different registries (National Institute for Health and Welfare, 2013).

The project has developed protocols for eight diseases or procedures which are either very common, have a high economic burden or are resource-intensive: AMI; revascular procedures – percutaneous transluminal coronary angioplasty, CABG; hip fracture; breast cancer; hip and knee joint replacements; very-low-birth-weight (VLBW) infants; schizophrenia; and stroke (Häkkinen, 2011).

Use of metrics to inform policymaking

As part of the PERFECT Project, researchers studied the effects of hospital birth levels and time of birth on mortality, morbidity and cost–effectiveness, for very-low-gestational-age (VLGA) or VLBW infants.

Five university hospitals had a neonatal intensive care unit (NICU) of level IIIB or higher. Sixteen additional hospitals with a level IIB (or higher) rating routinely delivered VLGA/VLBW infants. It was discovered that the one-year mortality of liveborn VLBW/VLGA infants was higher if born in level II versus level III hospitals.** The findings contributed to a change in legislation that required these babies to be treated in university hospitals (OECD, 2013).

The researchers also investigated the cost–effectiveness of caring for VLGA/VLBW infants. Despite high initial costs, the researchers found that the care of VLGA/VLBW infants was already cost-effective by four years of age and cost–effectiveness could be further improved by reducing long-term morbidities. This project quantified the effect of prematurity-related morbidities on the cost per QALY. Long-term morbidities were strongly associated with prolonged initial hospitalization and increased the need for hospital care after initial discharge (Lehtonen et al., 2011).

* In 2013 there were 320 municipalities in Finland (http://www.localfinland.fi/en/Pages/default.aspx). Each municipality must be a member of one of the 20 hospital districts (excluding the Åland Islands) which organize and provide specialist medical services for their member municipalities. Each hospital district has a central hospital. In total, there are five university-level teaching hospitals (Vuorenskoski, 2008).

** The American Academy of Pediatrics Committee on Fetus and Newborn defined levels of neonatal care in 2004. Level II care (special nursery care) would provide care for infants ≥32 weeks' gestation and weighing ≥1500 g who are stable or who are moderately ill. Level III care NICU units would provide comprehensive care for infants born <32 weeks' gestation and weighing <1500 g and infants born at all gestational ages and birth weights with surgical or medical conditions (American Academy of Pediatrics, 2004).

care and that consumer interest in applying cost information to decision-making depends on a range of factors including exposure to OOP costs, the severity and urgency of their condition and preconditions about provider quality (Aligning Forces for Quality, 2012).

8.7 Conclusion

Across the range of major health policies reviewed for this chapter, we find that questions of efficiency are very often a major part of the rationale for intervention. Sometimes this is implicit, but more often it is explicit. Despite the focus on efficiency in the rationale and objectives for policies across all areas, we find:

- little evidence that formal efficiency metrics are used in a systematic way in the development of policy; and
- little evidence that appropriate efficiency metrics are monitored in the evaluation of policy.

Although policies were often motivated by efficiency objectives, we find little evidence of systematic monitoring or evaluation of policies after implementation to establish whether the policy has delivered its objectives. As a result, where evidence suggests policies may not be improving efficiency, there is often policy stasis with continued reliance on policy tools that have been shown to have a limited or no effect.

A focus on efficiency and more formalized methods of considering these questions seems to be greatest in areas of policy where there is either a legal framework to policy implementation (merger control in some countries) or bodies independent of political processes, with a clear remit and framework to make decisions (HTA in some countries with formal HTA organizations).

Evidence on AE is much weaker than on TE although, for many middle- and high-income countries, questions of AE are a high priority given the pressures on health care systems from changing and increasing demands in the face of constrained resources.

In part this reflects a somewhat piecemeal approach to policy. We find relatively few examples of a systematic examination of the policy options to improve system efficiency and, as a result, much of the focus on efficiency is narrow and does not take account of the comparative effectiveness of different policies to improve efficiency.

Cross-national bodies have often led work on tools to improve policymaking in this area (see Chapter 7). For example, the OECD has a range of programmes of comparative analysis and cross-country learning on health system efficiency and fiscal sustainability. Its work on system efficiency attempted to compare countries using output-oriented DEA, which examined one output – life expectancy at birth – with two measures of input, health care spending and a composite measure of socioeconomic and lifestyle characteristics (Jourmand, André & Nicq, 2010). However, as the OECD work shows, developing overall metrics for system-level efficiency is difficult given the multiple objectives of health care systems and domains of quality, and also given that the validity of quantitative measures of relative efficiency may be challenged.

At the international level, in some specific policy areas, there have been targeted efforts to improve policymaking. There has been a growing focus on building capacity in policymakers to produce better regulation. For example, in 2012, the OECD Regulatory Policy Committee made a number of recommendations aimed at strengthening its members' capability for regulatory reform. The OECD's recommendations were consistent with the ROAMEF cycle and emphasized the importance of integrating regulatory impact assessment into the early stages of policy design, carrying out programme review (which would include further cost–benefit analysis) and publishing reports on the performance/effectiveness of interventions (OECD, 2012). However, as the case studies in Boxes 8.2–8.4 show, there is somewhat limited monitoring and use of efficiency metrics across the ROAMEF cycle.

Policy questions relating to single, discrete issues or issues where effective distribution of a finite budget is an overt aim, appear to lend themselves more easily to the use of efficiency metrics in decision-making. However, it is clear that policymakers do not make decisions based on efficiency metrics alone. For example, the case study in Box 8.2, which focused on the introduction of ipilimumab in Ireland, demonstrates that public opinion is a significant factor in decision-making. The role of cost-utility metrics, such as the QALY in HTA and reimbursement policy, polarizes opinion. While economists can demonstrate the relative value of an intervention on a cost-per-QALY basis, it is ultimately for policymakers to decide whether treatment for certain conditions has a higher social value and whether it is socially acceptable to impose a threshold on treatment costs. For a process so closely tied to evidence-based decision-making, the variation in approach is significant, as are the moral and ethical considerations of limiting the availability of medicine or technologies on the grounds of cost. As rising demand continues to place pressure on health care resources, it may be increasingly difficult for policymakers (particularly those representing public payers) to avoid valued-based comparisons across therapeutic areas.

Decisions on complex and controversial policy proposals will be based on a wide range of factors including societal and sector considerations (see Figure 8.3).

Figure 8.3 *Factors that can influence decision-making among policymakers*

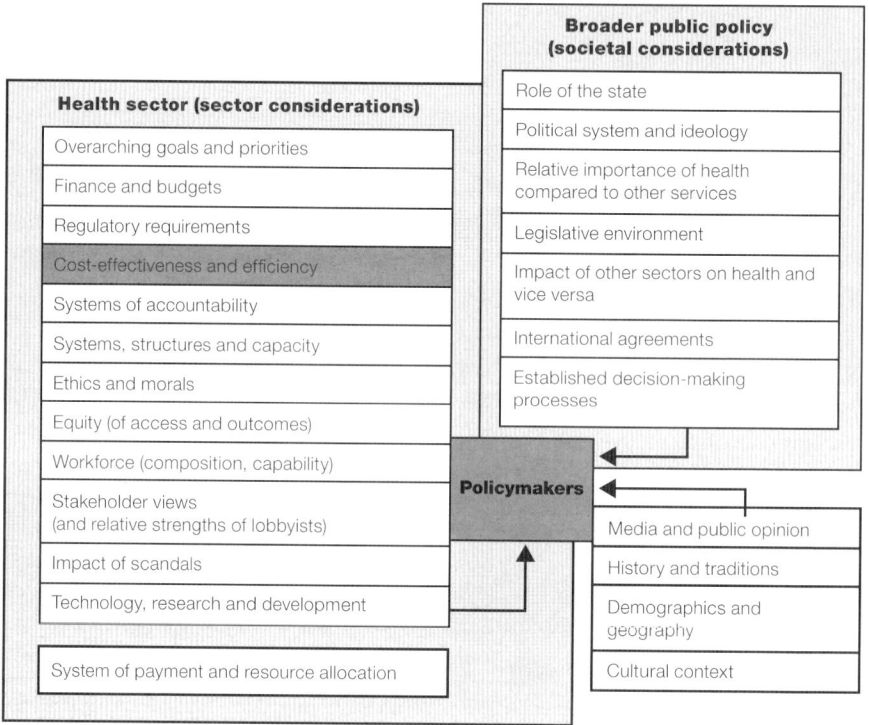

This decision-making process is equally challenging when considering wide-scale structural reform, particularly where a decision might be highly controversial or political in nature. It is in these cases in particular where the discontent between policy and research interests can be at its starkest. Policymakers need timely, concise and context-specific input, whereas research approaches often require time to produce evidence that is relevant and robust (Garrido, 2008). In such cases, decisions can sometimes be taken with limited reference to efficiency metrics. As an example, one assessment focusing on the introduction of a provider ratings regime made no attempt to quantify the expected benefits despite introducing a policy that would potentially impact over 21 500 providers of health and long-term care (DoH, 2014).

A key issue is the availability and accessibility of underlying data to construct meaningful efficiency metrics. Often policymakers use what is available as metrics rather than investing in new, specific data and monitoring. For example, both DRG-based payment systems and P4P have a conceptual appeal. It seems logical that payment should be related to demonstrated performance on the objectives established by payers. However, these general schemes for payment need to be carefully adapted to pursue specific policy objectives and ensure their efficiency, and only a small number of partial efficiency measures are used for evaluating such payment schemes. In many European countries where activity-based payment has been introduced, hospital costs and care quality are not tracked sufficiently. Obtaining access to itemized hospital cost data is a lengthy process for researchers in many countries. The evaluation of most of the P4P schemes concentrate on monitoring the process variables that are part of the payment scheme without properly assessing the associated costs. Potential perverse effects (unintended consequences) of these schemes (for example, patient selection, induced demand) are rarely studied since this often requires data beyond those collected routinely within these schemes.

A second issue is the mutualization of the knowledge and information on well-established efficiency metrics to evaluate policy. Without robust measures it is not possible to provide sound analysis or to find the right policy direction to take. For example, despite the bulk of evidence on their costs, France does not regularly monitor hospital adverse events as a quality measure. This means that hospitals having adverse events are better remunerated, since these are coded as CCs which receive a significantly higher tariff.

The other key issue is that the evidence on efficiency is often not clear-cut and the policy implications are open to different interpretations. For example, in relation to payment reform, all payments models have pros and cons that should be identified, monitored and compensated for. The payment reforms aiming to reinforce efficiency of specific providers often ignore results at the system level for AE, and efficiency is not the sole objective of the payment system. Many countries have objectives that relate to transparency, accountability and equitable funding (O'Reilly et al., 2012).

There will always be circumstances where decision-makers want to try something new – perhaps an intervention with a limited evidence base – or need to respond quickly to a scandal or pressing policy issue. However, it is critical that sufficient attention is placed on the monitoring, evaluation and feedback stage of the ROAMEF cycle and that proper consideration is given to the use of efficiency metrics to support these stages.

References

Aligning Forces for Quality (2011). Lessons learned in public reporting: crossing the cost and efficiency frontier. Princeton, NJ, Robert Wood Johnson Foundation (http://forces4quality.org/af4q/download-document/3021/Resource-RegTable_CostEfficiency.pdf, accessed 22 July 2016).

Aligning Forces for Quality (2012). Consumer beliefs and use of information about health care cost, resource use, and value. Findings from consumer focus groups. Princeton, NJ, Robert Wood Johnson Foundation (http://forces4quality.org/af4q/download-document/6224/Resource-rwjf402126.pdf, accessed 22 July 2016).

American Academy of Pediatrics (2004). Levels of neonatal care. *Pediatrics*, 114(5):1341–1347. (http://pediatrics.aappublications.org/content/pediatrics/114/5/1341.full.pdf, accessed 7 August 2016).

American Hospital Association (2013). How hospital mergers and acquisitions benefit communities. (http://www.aha.org/content/13/13mergebenefitcommty.pdf, accessed 22 July 2016.)

An Roinn Sláinte (Department of Health) (2012). New drug deal worth €400 million over three years says Minister Reilly. (http://health.gov.ie/blog/press-release/new-drug-deal-worth-e400-million-over-three-years-says-minister-reilly/, accessed 7 August 2016).

Arbyn M et al. (2010). European guidelines for quality assurance in cervical cancer screening. Second edition: summary document. *Annals of Oncology*, 21(3):448–458.

Bach PB (2008). Cost sharing for health care. Whose skin? Which game? *New England Journal of Medicine*, 358(4):411–413.

Barry M (2013). The patient and health technology assessment: challenges and opportunities. ISPOR 16th Annual European Congress, 2–6 November 2013, Dublin. (http://www.ispor.org/congresses/Dublin1113/presentations/FirstPlenary-Michael-Barry.pdf, accessed 22 July 2016).

BBC (2009). Smear test age limit to remain. *BBC News*. (http://news.bbc.co.uk/1/hi/health/8116962.stm, 22 July 2016).

Beresniak A et al. (2013). Final report summary: ECHOUTCOME (European Consortium in Healthcare Outcomes and Cost–Benefit Research). (http://cordis.europa.eu/result/rcn/57938_en.html, accessed 22 July 2016).

Braithwaite RS, Rosen AB (2007). Linking cost sharing to value: an unrivalled yet unrealized public health opportunity. *Annals of Internal Medicine*, 146(8):602–605.

Broeders M et al. (2012). The impact of mammographic screening on breast cancer mortality in Europe: a review of observational studies. *Journal of Medical Screening*, 19(Suppl. 1):S14–S25.

Bulfone L, Younie S, Carter R (2009). Health technology assessment: reflections from the Antipodes. *Value in Health*, 12(Suppl. 2):S28–S38.

Buteow S (2008). Pay-for-performance in New Zealand primary health care. *Journal of Health Organization and Management*, 22(1):36–47.

Cancer Research UK (2012). The 2012 breast screening review. (http://www.cancerresearchuk.org/about-cancer/type/breast-cancer/about/screening/breast-screening-review-2012, accessed 7 August 2016).

Canoy M, Sauter W (2009). Hospital mergers and the public interest: recent developments in the Netherlands. (https://www.nza.nl/1048076/1048181/Research_paper_Hospital_Mergers_and_the_Public_Interest.pdf, accessed 23 July 2016).

Cashin C (2011). New Zealand: Primary Health Organization (PHO) Performance Program: Major developments in results-based financing in OECD countries, country summaries. The World Bank.

Consumers Health Forum of Australia (2014). Better bang for your buck. (https://www.chf.org.au/pdfs/chf/HealthVoices_APRIL14_WEB.pdf, accessed 23 July 2016).

Cots F et al. (2011). DRG-based hospital payment: intended and unintended consequences. In: Busse R et al., eds. *Diagnosis-related groups in Europe: moving towards transparency, efficiency and quality in hospitals*. Maidenhead, Open University Press (http://www.euro.who.int/__data/assets/pdf_file/0004/162265/e96538.pdf, accessed 7 August 2016).

Curtin K et al. (2006). Return on investment in pay for performance: a diabetes case study. *Journal of Healthcare Management*, 51(6):365–374.

Cutler DM (2006). *The economics of health system payment. De Economist*, 154(1):1–18.

Dáil Éireann (House of Representatives) (2012). Written answers: anti-cancer drugs. (http://oireachtasdebates.oireachtas.ie/debates%20authoring/DebatesWebPack.nsf/takes/dail2012051000150#, accessed 2 August 2016).

Dash P, Meredith D, White P (2012). *Marry in haste, repent at leisure: when do hospital mergers make strategic sense*. Health Systems and Service Practice. London, McKinsey & Company.

Davis K et al. (2014). Mirror, mirror on the wall. How the performance of the US health care system compares internationally. New York, The Commonwealth Fund (http://www.commonwealthfund.org/~/media/files/publications/fund-report/2014/jun/1755_davis_mirror_mirror_2014.pdf, accessed 22 July 2016).

de Cruppé W et al. (2007). Evaluating compulsory minimum volume standards in Germany: how many hospitals were compliant in 2004? *BMC Health Services Research*, 7:165.

Department of Health (DoH) (2014). Hard truths: the journey to putting patients first. Volume one of the Government response to the Mid Staffordshire NHS Foundation Trust Public Inquiry. (https://www.gov.uk/government/uploads/system/uploads/attachment_data/file/270368/34658_Cm_8777_Vol_1_accessible.pdf, accessed 23 July 2016).

Ellin J et al. (2014). *International responses to austerity: an evidence scan*. London, The Health Foundation.

Ellis RP, McGuire TG (1996). Hospital response to prospective payment: moral hazard, selection, and practice-style effects. *Journal of Health Economics*, 15(3):257–277.

Farrar S et al. (2009). Has payment by results affected the way that English hospitals provide care? Difference-in-differences analysis. *BMJ*, 339:b3047.

Federal Joint Committee (G-BA) (2011). The benefit assessment of pharmaceuticals in accordance with the German Social Code, book five (SGB V), section 35a. (http://www.english.g-ba.de/benefitassessment/information/, accessed 23 July 2016).

Garrido MV (2008). *Health technology assessment and health policy-making in Europe: current status, challenges and potential*. Observatory Studies Series No 14. Copenhagen, WHO Regional Office for Europe on behalf of the European Observatory on Health Systems and Policies (http://www.euro.who.int/__data/assets/pdf_file/0003/90426/E91922.pdf, accessed 23 July 2016).

Gaynor M (2004). Quality and competition in health care markets: what do we know? What don't we know? *Économie Publique*, 15(2):87–124.

Gaynor M (2006). What do we know about competition and quality in health care markets? (http://www.bristol.ac.uk/media-library/sites/cmpo/migrated/documents/wp151.pdf, accessed 7 August 2016).

Gaynor M, Laudecella M, Propper C (2012). Can governments do it better? Merger mania and hospital outcomes in the English NHS. *Journal of Health Economics*, 31(3):528–543.

Gemmill MC, Thomson S, Mossialos E (2008). What impact do prescription drug charges have on efficiency and equity? Evidence from high-income countries. *International Journal for Equity in Health*, 7:12.

Gerdtham UG et al. (1999). Internal markets and health care efficiency: a multiple-output stochastic frontier analysis. *Health Economics*, 8(2): 151–164.

Glanville J et al. (2010). *The impact of hospital treatment volumes on patient outcomes*. York, York Health Economics Consortium (http://webarchive.nationalarchives.gov.uk/20130513202829/http://www.ccpanel.org.uk/content/CCP01_The_impact_of_hospital_treatment_volumes_on_patient_outcomes.pdf, accessed 23 July 2016).

Goldman DP, Joyce GF, Zheng Y (2007). Prescription drug cost sharing: associations with medication and medical utilization and spending and health. *JAMA*, 298(1):61–69.

Gøtzsche P, Jørgensen KJ (2013). *Screening for breast cancer with mammography (review)*. The Cochrane Collaboration. London, John Wiley & Sons (http://nordic.cochrane.org/sites/nordic.cochrane.org/files/uploads/ResearchHighlights/Screening%20for%20breast%20cancer%202013%20CD001877.pdf, accessed 23 July 2016).

Goudie R, Goddard M (2011). *Review of the evidence on what drives economies of scope and scale in the provision of NHS services, focusing on A&E and associated hospital services*. London, Office of Health Economics (https://www.ohe.org/sites/default/files/Review%20of%20evidence%20on%20what%20drives%20economies%20of%20scale%202011.pdf, accessed 23 July 2016).

Häkkinen U (2011). The PERFECT project: measuring performance of health care episodes. *Annals of Medicine*, 43(Suppl 1):S1–S3.

Hallsworth M, Parker S, Rutter J (2011). *Policy making in the real world: evidence and analysis*. London, Institute for Government (http://www.instituteforgovernment.org.uk/sites/default/files/publications/Policy%20making%20in%20the%20real%20world.pdf, accessed 23 July 2016).

Halm EA, Lee C, Chassin MR (2002). Is volume related to outcome in health care? A systematic review and methodological critique of the literature. *Annals of Internal Medicine*, 137(6):511–552.

Hibbard JH, Stockard J, Tusler M (2003). Does publicizing hospital performance stimulate quality improvement efforts? *Health Affairs*, 22(2):84–94.

Hibbard JH (2008). Using systematic measurement to target consumer activation strategies. *Medical Care Research and Review*, 66(Suppl. 1):9S–27S.

Hibbard J et al. (2012). An experiment shows that a well-designed report on costs and quality can help consumers choose high-value health care. *Health Affairs*, 31(3):560–568.

HM Government (2010). *The Coalition: our programme for government*. London, The Cabinet Office (https://www.gov.uk/government/uploads/system/uploads/attachment_data/file/78977/coalition_programme_for_government.pdf, accessed 23 July 2016).

HM Treasury (2011). *The Greenbook: appraisal and evaluation in central government*. London, The Stationery Office.

Ho V (2000). Evolution of the volume-outcome relation for hospitals performing coronary angioplasty. *Circulation*, 101(15):1806–1811.

Holland W, Stewart S, Masseria C (2006). *Policy brief: screening in Europe*. Copenhagen, World Health Organization on behalf of the European Observatory on Health Systems and Policies.

Houle SK et al. (2012). Does performance-based remuneration for individual health care practitioners affect patient care? A systematic review. *Annals of Internal Medicine*, 157(12):889–899.

Hussey P et al. (2009). A systematic review of health care efficiency measures. *Health Services Research*, 44(3):784–805.

Institute for Applied Quality Improvement and Research in Health Care (2012). *German hospital quality report 2011*. Göttingen, AQUA Institute GmbH.

Institute for Quality and Efficiency in Health Care (IQWiG) (2009). General methods for the assessment of the relation of benefits to costs. Cologne, IQWiG (http://www.ispor.org/peguidelines/source/Germany_AssessmentoftheRelationofBenefitstoCosts_En.pdf, accessed 23 July 201).

Johnson C (2014). Concern sickest to be hurt most by GP co-payment. ABC Health and Wellbeing. The Pulse. (http://www.abc.net.au/health/thepulse/stories/2014/05/15/4005271.htm, accessed 23 July 2016).

Joumard I, André C, Nicq C (2010). *Healthcare systems: efficiency and policy settings*. Paris, OECD Publishing.

Kahn CN 3rd et al. (2006). Snapshot of hospital quality reporting and pay-for-performance under Medicare. *Health Affairs*, 25(1):148–162.

Kautter J (2011). Incorporating Efficiency Measures into Pay for Performance. In: Cromwell J et al., eds. *Pay for performance in health care: methods and approaches*. Research Triangle Park, NC, RTI Press.

Ketelaar NA et al. (2011). Public release of performance data in changing the behaviour of healthcare consumers, professionals or organisations. *Cochrane Database of Systematic Reviews*, 11:CD004538.

Kreif et al.(2015) *Examination of the synthetic control method for evaluating health policies with multiple treated units*. Health Economics. ISSN 1057-9230 DOI: 10.1002/hec.3258

Krumholz HM et al. (2008). Standards for measures used for public reporting of efficiency in health care: a scientific statement from the American Heart Association Interdisciplinary Council on Quality of Care and Outcomes research and the American College of Cardiology Foundation. *Journal of the American College of Cardiology*, 52(18):1518–1526.

Lehtonen L et al. (2011). PERFECT preterm infant study. *Annals of Medicine*, 43(Suppl 1):S47–S53.

McGlynn EA (2008). *Identifying, categorizing, and evaluating health care efficiency measures: final report*. AHRQ publication No. 08-0030. Rockville, MD, Agency for Healthcare Research and Quality.

McKee M, Healy J (2002). *Hospitals in a changing Europe*. Maidenhead, Open University Press.

Medicare Payment Advisory Commission (MedPAC) (2009). Report to the Congress: Medicare Payment Policy. Washington, DC, MedPAC (http://medpac.gov/documents/reports/march-2009-report-to-congress-medicare-payment-policy.pdf, accessed 7 August 2016).

Mladovsky P et al. (2012). Health policy responses to the financial crisis in Europe. Policy Summary 5. Copenhagen, WHO Regional Office for Europe on behalf of the European Observatory on Health Systems and Policies (http://www.euro.who.int/__data/assets/pdf_file/0009/170865/e96643.pdf, accessed 24 July 2016).

Moreno-Serra R, Wagstaff A (2010). System-wide impacts of hospital payment reforms: evidence from Central and Eastern Europe and Central Asia. *Journal of Health Economics*, 29(4):585–602.

Nasser M, Sawicki P (2009). Institute for Quality and Efficiency in Health Care: Germany. *Issue Brief (Commonwealth Fund)*, 57:1–12.

National Conference of State Legislature (NCSL) (2016). Value-based insurance design. (http://www.ncsl.org/research/health/value-based-insurance-design.aspx, 24 July 2016).

National Institute for Health and Welfare (2013). PERFECT: PERFormance, Effectiveness and Cost of Treatment episodes. (https://www.thl.fi/en/web/thlfi-en/research- and-xpertwork/projects-and-programmes/projects/21963, 2 August 2016).

Newhouse JP (1993). Free for all? Lessons from the RAND Health Insurance Experiment. Cambridge, MA, Harvard University Press.

National Institute for Health and Care Excellence (NICE) (2010). Measuring effectiveness and cost effectiveness: the QALY. London, NICE.

NICE (2013). National Institute for Health and Care Excellence. Centre for Health Technology Evaluation. Consultation Paper: Value Based Assessment for Health Technologies. London, NICE (https://www.nice.org.uk/Media/Default/About/what-we-do/NICE-guidance/NICE-technology-appraisals/VBA-TA-Methods-Guide-for-Consultation.pdf, accessed 24 July 2016).

NICE (2014). Safe staffing for nursing in adult inpatient wards in acute hospitals. Safe staffing guideline 1. London, NICE (https://www.nice.org.uk/guidance/sg1/resources/guidance-safe-staffing-for-nursing-in-adult-inpatient-wards-in-acute-hospitals-pdf, accessed 24 July 2016).

Nuffield Trust (2013). *Rating providers for quality: a policy worth pursuing? A report for the Secretary of State for Health*. London, Nuffield Trust.

Organisation for Economic Co-operation and Development (OECD) (2010). *Value for money in health spending*. OECD Health Policy Studies. Paris, OECD Publishing.

OECD (2012) Recommendation of the Council on regulatory policy and governance. (http://www.oecd.org/governance/regulatory-policy/49990817.pdf, accessed 7 August 2016).

OECD (2013) *Strengthening Health Information Infrastructure for Health Care Quality Governance Good Practices, New Opportunities and Data Privacy Protection Challenges*. OECD Health Policy Studies. Paris, OECD Publishing.

OECD, EU (2014). Health at a glance: Europe 2014. Paris, OECD Publishing (http://www.oecd.org/health/health-at-a-glance-europe-23056088.htm, accessed 7 August 2016).

Olejaz M et al. (2012). Denmark Health System Review Health Systems in Transition. *Vol.* 14 No. 2. Copenhagen, WHO Regional office for Europe on behalf of the European Observatory on Health Systems and Policies (http://www.euro.who.int/__data/assets/pdf_file/0004/160519/e96442.pdf, accessed 24 July 2016).

Or Z et al. (2013). Activité, productivité et qualité des soins des hôpitaux avant et après la T2A, Document de travail IRDES, No 56. (http://www.irdes.fr/EspaceRecherche/DocumentsDeTravail/DT56SoinsHospitaliersT2A.pdf, accessed 24 July 2016).

O'Reilly et al. (2012). Paying for hospital care: the experience with implementing activity-based funding in five European countries. *Health Economics, Policy, and Law*, 7(1):73–101.

Paci E (2012). Summary of the evidence of breast cancer service screening outcomes in Europe and first estimate of the benefit and harm balance sheet. *Journal of Medical Screening*, 19(Suppl. 1):5–13.

Patient Protection and Affordable Care Act (2010). (http://www.gpo.gov/fdsys/pkg/BILLS-111hr3590enr/pdf/BILLS-111hr3590enr.pdf#page=623, accessed 24 July 2016).

Pearse J, Mazevska D (2010). *The impact of public disclosure of health performance data: a rapid review*. Haymarket, NSW, The Sax Institute (https://www.saxinstitute.org.au/wp-content/uploads/12_The-impact-of-public-disclosure-of-health-performance-dat.pdf, accessed 8 August 2016).

Posnett J (1999). Is bigger better? Concentration in the provision of secondary care. *BMJ*, 319(7216):1063–1065.

Pugatch MP, Ficai F (2007). *A healthy market? An introduction to health technology assessment*. London, Stockholm Network.

Roberts MJ et al. (2004). *Getting health reform right: a guide to improving performance and equity*. New York, Oxford University Press.

Robinson JC (2010). Applying value-based insurance design to high-cost health services. *Health Affairs*, 29(11):2009–2016.

Rochon M (2010). Restructuring health and hospital services: the Ontario experience. (http://www.nuffieldtrust.org.uk/sites/files/nuffield/mark_rochon_restructuring_health_and_hospital_services.pdf, accessed 24 July 2016).

Sauvage P (2008). Pharmaceutical pricing in France: a critique. *Eurohealth*, 14(2):6–8. (http://apps.who.int/medicinedocs/documents/s20974en/s20974en.pdf, accessed 24 July 2016).

Schokkaert E, Van de Voorde C (2011). User charges. In: Glied S, Smith PC, eds. *The Oxford Handbook of Health Economics*. Oxford, OUP.

Schreyögg J, Grabka MM (2010). Copayments for ambulatory care in Germany: a natural experiment using a difference-in-difference approach. *European Journal of Health Economics* 11(3):331–341

Schulten T (2006). Liberalisation, privatisation and regulation in the German healthcare sector/hospitals. Düsseldorf, Hans-Böckler-Stiftung (http://www.boeckler.de/pdf/wsi_pj_piq_sekkrankh.pdf, accessed 24 July 2016).

Shekelle P et al. (2008). *Does Public Release of Performance Results Improve Quality of Care?* London, The Health Foundation.

Smith P (2012). What is the scope for health system efficiency gains and how can they be achieved? *Eurohealth incorporating Euro Observer*, 18(3). (http://www.euro.who.int/__data/assets/pdf_file/0017/174410/EuroHealth-v18-n3.pdf, accessed 24 July 2016).

Street A, O'Reilly J, Ward M (2011). DRG-based hospital payment and efficiency: theory, evidence and challenges. In: Busse R et al., eds. *Diagnosis-related groups in Europe moving towards transparency, efficiency and quality in hospitals*. European Observatory on Health Systems and Policies series. Maidenhead, Open University Press (http://www.euro.who.int/__data/assets/pdf_file/0004/162265/e96538.pdf, accessed 24 July 2016).

Sullivan S et al. (2009). Health technology assessment in health-care decisions in the United States. *Value in Health*, 12(Suppl. 2):S39–S44.

Szecsenyi J et al. (2012). Tearing down walls: opening the border between hospital and ambulatory care for quality improvement in Germany. *International Journal for Quality in Health Care*, 24(2):101–104.

Thomson S, Foubister T, Mossialos E (2009). *Financing health care in the European Union. Challenges and policy responses.* Copenhagen, WHO Regional Office for Europe on behalf of the European Observatory on Health Systems and Policies (http://www.euro.who.int/__data/assets/pdf_file/0009/98307/E92469.pdf, accessed 24 July 2016).

Trivedi AN, Rakowski W, Ayanian JZ (2008). Effect of cost sharing on screening mammography in Medicare health plans. *New England Journal of Medicine*, 358(4):375–383.

Van Herck P et al. (2010). Systematic review: effects, design choices, and context of pay-for-performance in health care. *BMC Health Service Research*, 10:247.

Vogt WB, Town R (2006). How has hospital consolidation affected the price and quality of hospital care? Policy brief No. 9. Princeton, NJ (http://www.rwjf.org/content/dam/farm/reports/issue_briefs/2006/rwjf12056, accessed 24 July 2016).

Vuorenskoski L (2008). Health systems in transition. Finland: health system review. European Observatory on Health Systems and Policies. Copenhagen, WHO Regional Office for Europe on behalf of the European Observatory on Health Systems and Policies (http://www.euro.who.int/__data/assets/pdf_file/0007/80692/E91937.pdf, accessed 24 July 2016).

Wagstaff A et al. (1992). Equity in the finance of health care: some international comparisons. *Journal of Health Economics*, 11(4):361–387.

Weil T (2010). Hospital mergers: a panacea? *Journal of Health Services Research & Policy*, 15(4):251–253.

WHO (2002). National cancer control programmes: policies and managerial guidelines. 2nd edn. Geneva, WHO (http://www.who.int/cancer/media/en/408.pdf, accessed 24 July 2016).

WHO (2008). The Tallinn Charter: health systems for health and wealth. Copenhagen, WHO Regional Office for Europe (http://www.euro.who.int/__data/assets/pdf_file/0008/88613/E91438.pdf, accessed 24 July 2016).

WHO (2011). *Health technology assessment of medical devices*. WHO Medical device technical series. Geneva, WHO.

Wilsdon T, Serota A (2011). *A comparative role and impact of health technology assessment*. London, Charles River Associates.

Wilson JMG, Jungner G (1968). *Principles and practice of screening for disease*. Geneva, WHO.

Yip W et al. (2014). Capitation with pay-for-performance improves antibiotic prescribing practices in rural China. *Health Affairs*, 33(3):502–510.

Chapter 9

Efficiency measurement for management

Alec Morton and Laura Schang

9.1 Introduction

The previous chapter discussed the use of efficiency analysis tools to guide policy formulation and development. While few readers will doubt that clear, consistent policy direction is necessary for the delivery of productivity improvements, it is not sufficient. To lead to action on the ground, policy interventions have to influence the behaviour of the staff who see and treat patients, and deliver public health and social care programmes. In this chapter, we discuss the challenges facing management as it seeks to use the analytical tools discussed elsewhere in this volume to secure efficiency improvements.

It should be emphasized that the environment of the working manager is very different from the environment of the policymaker, and even more so that of the academic researcher (Mintzberg, 1973). Unlike academic researchers (at least those unburdened with management responsibilities), managers in general and in the health service in particular, typically describe a significant part of their time as being occupied with responding to sporadic, unanticipated and urgent problems, and filtering information, either through attending mostly irrelevant meetings or scrolling through a seemingly endless flow of emails to head off incipient crises. Unlike policymakers, managers have relatively limited and weak levers for driving and securing change; for example, they have to operate within the existing financial settlement, with institutions and staff facing incentives designed into their existing mandates and terms of employment. Moreover, the elevated social status of medical professionals means that health care managers have more circumscribed authority than managers in most other industries.

In short, with very limited time and capacity, managers have to make decisions about what evidence (if any) they look at and believe, what expertise they draw on, and how they search for solutions and present them in a persuasive way. Efficiency analysis tools can have a role in this process if they can provide a plausible framework for interpretation, and can form an element in articulating the case for change. For example, several authors have noted that frontier-based methods (DEA and SFA), despite their popularity in academic circles, have received much less attention in the practitioner world, where the most popular efficiency analysis tools are episode and population costing systems (Hollingsworth & Street, 2006; Hussey et al., 2009). It is plausible that what academics see as a strength of DEA, that it aggregates multiple inputs and outputs in a single efficiency measure, is, from a managerial point of view, a weakness, as it distracts attention from the question of where the problems actually lie and where one should search for ideas for improvement.

In the first part of the chapter we present two frameworks which can help us understand how managers might think about evidence and solutions to efficiency problems in different settings. The first framework, Cynefin, is borrowed from knowledge management and provides a perspective on the role of evidence in efficiency analysis; the second, grid-group cultural theory, is drawn from the sociology of risk and provides a perspective on the role of culture and ideology in the search for solutions. In the second part of the chapter we discuss how efficiency analysis can support three key tasks for managing the system. We structure our discussion roughly using the classical Simonian tripartite classification of the stages of decision (Simon, 1977): intelligence, the stage in which one establishes that one has a problem; design, the stage in which one develops alternative solutions; and choice, the stage at which on decides which solution to implement. We review managerial tools that are available to support each of these activities and reflect on what the Cynefin and grid-group cultural theory frameworks can tell us about how they are to be used.

9.2 Who are managers?

In the general management literature, there have been several attempts to define management, from Henri Fayol's description of management as involving planning, organizing, commanding, coordinating and controlling, through to Mintzberg's analysis of the interpersonal, information and decisional components of the manager's job, to Stewart's framework which involves looking at the managerial role in terms of its demands, constraints and choices which it affords (Wren, 2005). From a health care point of view, these definitions highlight that managers are typically not involved in primary production, that is, treating and caring for the sick. For this reason, managers can be controversial figures in health care systems. In the United Kingdom, governments regularly launch rhetorical attacks on bureaucrats, while lauding front-line professionals, even as they create new regulatory responsibilities and structures.

Even though health care managers do not enjoy the same generally positive public image as others in the medical workforce, they are present in all systems and recent evidence suggests that the quality of management is an important driver of system performance (Dorgan, 2010). Managers operate in different contexts and institutions, including purchasing organizations (for example, regional health care authorities, sickness funds) or provider organizations (for example, hospitals, physician networks). While the specific tasks differ between contexts, we take the view that management is essentially about making decisions within the scope and remit the manager enjoys through his position in the system hierarchy (Simon, 1977). Decision-making is, clearly, a process that is not exclusive to management. However, it is fundamental to any managerial role and independent of the context in which managers operate and so provides a useful framework that is independent of the specifics of any given managerial role (for example, whether the manager is working in a hospital or in a purchasing organization). In this chapter, we follow Herbert Simon's (1977) famous model that distinguishes between three roles in the managerial decision-making process: intelligence, design and choice.

An important defining feature of the manager's job in health care (and indeed in other professional services) is that there are parts of the production process which necessarily remain somewhat opaque to the manager. Thus, while one would hope and expect that a modern manager in health care would typically have access to reasonably reliable and timely information about costs, throughput and quality, interpreting that information and determining what actions are implied can be less than straightforward, compared to the case of simpler production facilities (Morton & Cornwell, 2009). This observation is a theme of this chapter. (Of course, we do not mean to suggest that it is not worthwhile improving the quality and availability of data, merely to observe that no database will ever be sufficiently comprehensive to settle all possible management-related questions decisively.)

It is important to realize that managers have a different, and specifically a narrower, view of efficiency than policymakers. For both managers and policymakers, efficiency involves balancing inputs and outputs, but managers operate in a much more constrained environment. The manager of a hospital or insurer has virtually no ability to control demand (typically the service is free at the point delivery, or user fees are heavily regulated), certainly in the short-term; the technologies and services to be offered may be mandated by a centralized HTA agency; staffing levels may be determined by an external professional body; pay rates may be determined nationally through collective bargaining; a unionized and professional production staff may be extremely effective in resisting efforts to change work practices. In a system where there is an institutional separation between purchasers and providers, managers on the purchasing side may seek to extract efficiencies by shopping around, but this is only possible where there is real variety in the provider market. Considering all these constraints, it is remarkable that managers can find sufficient space for action to positively influence the delivery of services.

9.3 Frameworks for analysis

In this section, we present two frameworks that we use in our subsequent discussion: the Cynefin framework from the area of knowledge management, and grid-group cultural theory from the sociology of risk.

9.3.1 Cynefin

The Cynefin framework of Kurtz & Snowden (2003) – Cynefin is a Welsh word roughly meaning habitat – is framework for sensemaking rooted in the field of knowledge management and can help to illustrate the challenges managers face in translating information into action. The Cynefin framework seeks to classify particular domains of action in terms of the possibilities for knowledge that domain affords. As such, it is particularly useful for clarifying what kind of guidance evidence can and cannot be provided, and hence, how and when one might want to engage with experts. Central to the Cynefin framework are four domains:

- the known domain in which cause and effect is understood, solid and unquestioned evidence exists and predictive modelling is possible;
- the knowable domain in which cause-and-effect relationships exist but are not known, or not known widely; knowledge could in principle be acquired in this domain but it would be costly and difficult to do so;
- the complex domain in which events are one-offs and cause and effect can be discerned retrospectively;
- the chaotic domain in which causal mechanisms are unclear, even after the event.

Securing efficiency in the known domain is relatively straightforward: this is the domain where managers feel most comfortable. For example, one can manage by ensuring that best practice is being followed and reviewing delayed discharges to make sure that internal discharge processes and communication with providers who provide follow-up care are optimized. As one moves out of the known region, professional judgement becomes more important. In the knowable domain what constitutes good practice is more contested, and so more room has to be made for local knowledge: identifying the causes of elevated readmission rates may require investigating practices in the community outside the formal health care system. In the complex domain, attempts to manage by compliance with standards are often seen by those on the ground not only as constraining professional practice, but as part of a pre-emptive blame shifting exercise in anticipation of things going wrong, which, inevitably, happens. Last, in the chaotic domain, even the experts do not know what is going on. Prescribing generic antibiotics on a precautionary basis in an environment where access to testing facilities is limited and costly may seem to make sense on cost–effectiveness grounds, but it is precisely such actions that create drug resistant pathogens which in turn generate large-scale new illness and cost (Laxminarayan et al., 2013). Where there is the possibility of chaotic behaviour, managers have to recognize that the problem is beyond their responsibility and outside help (fundamental scientific expertise, policy intervention) needs to be called on. Ultimately, such problems have to be tackled at a higher system level, but where the higher levels of this system fail to take appropriate action, it will be left to managers on the ground to pick up the pieces.

9.3.2 Grid-group cultural theory

Grid-group cultural theory, a model of culture popular in the sociology of risk (Thompson, Ellis & Wildavski, 1990), can be applied to health services to gain further insights into managers' individual views of how the health system works and their place within it. It is useful because it provides a framework for explaining the kind of ideology people use when conceptualizing solutions to efficiency problems. Grid-group cultural theory is based on a 2 × 2 classification system: the two dimensions are the extent to which an individual identifies with a larger social unit (group) and the extent to which individual choice is experienced as being constrained by external forces (grid).

Individuals inhabiting each of the four cells of the matrix are referred to as:

- Individualists (low-grid, low-group): people in this cell do not identify strongly with larger groups and reject external constraints. They see relationships as expedient and subject to negotiation. Their natural form of social organization is the market.
- Egalitarians (low-grid, high-group): people in this cell identify strongly with others but reject external constraints. They view relationships as intrinsically important but reject status distinctions. Their natural form of social organization is the commune.
- Hierarchists (high-grid, high-group): people in this cell identify strongly with others and accept external constraints. They view both relationships and social roles as important. Their natural form of social organization is the bureaucracy.

- Fatalists (high-grid, low-group): people in this cell experience social constraints but do not identify with larger groups. For them, the world is arbitrary and relationships are problematic and frustrating. Their natural form of social organization is the prison.

To see how this might be relevant in an organization seeking to make efficiency improvements, consider the case of the surgical department of a hospital that has been experiencing cost overruns. What kind of solutions might first come to mind to the responsible manager? The individualist's preferred solution is to actively use performance incentive payments to increase surgical throughput: if that does not work, they will outsource diagnostics. Such solutions require the ability to benchmark externally, that is, to know whether incentive payments will increase output or whether outsourcing will improve results. It would be helpful to know what the performance of other comparable institutions is. The egalitarian wonders why so many patients show up in such poor shape and have such weak support networks that they often have to be readmitted shortly after discharge. They advocate an asset-based approach to build individual and community capacity, and thus to manage demand. This line of reasoning leads one to require broader information about the patient journey between different care providers, and thus demands the ability to link data across multiple care encounters. The hierarchist just wants to make sure that everyone is doing their job and following best practice. They carefully study the guidelines and launch a new round of clinical audit. This presupposes that good-quality clinical guidance has been produced at the centre (and costed to ensure that it is actually deliverable). The fatalist responds by fiddling the figures, reasoning that this is what everyone else does anyway.

9.4 Managerial roles for efficiency analysis in intelligence, design and choice

The following section considers the different roles managers need to adopt to ensure efficiency improvements, while also considering the tools available to assist them in these roles and the challenges they may face in implementing them. In the view of this chapter, management consists, essentially, of making decisions. Depending on the context, these may be decisions about the structure of service delivery or about the allocation of health care staff. Following Herbert Simon (1977), managerial decision-making in a context of health system efficiency involves three fundamental roles:

1. the diagnosis of an efficiency problem;
2. the design of a solution; and
3. the choice of the appropriate response.

9.4.1 Intelligence: diagnosing the efficiency problem

Before thinking about solutions to efficiency problems, the logical first step is to diagnose where the problems lie – this is the intelligence phase. An efficiency problem in managing health services could take two forms: perceived excessive costs for the observed level of output (or, conversely, perceived underproduction for a given level of spending); and a wrong mix of outputs being produced (reflecting problems of technical efficiency (TE) and allocative efficiency (AE), respectively; see Chapter 1). From a managerial perspective, the promise of efficiency measurement lies in its potential to point towards areas of concern and thus enable further targeted analysis and action.

Managers may discover that they have an efficiency problem through either what one might think of as external or internal avenues: they may be told by some powerful stakeholder that they have to improve efficiency (while being given the same or less money) or there may be an exogenous shock (like an epidemic) that results in a spike in demand or resource consumption, requiring efficiency improvements if the system is to be kept in financial balance. Alternatively, they may discover efficiency problems through internal monitoring of their own performance. As the second avenue relates to actions that are within management control, we focus in this chapter on the internal monitoring route to problem discovery. One would expect that the better an organization is at internal monitoring, the abler it will be to predict and respond to efficiency problems forced on it by external parties or events.

In this section, we discuss which efficiency measures, such as variations in clinical practice and outcomes, can support managers in identifying that they have a problem. In a systematic review of efficiency measures, Hussey et al. (2009) found that most measures that are actually used by health service managers consist of ratios, based on single metrics for inputs and outputs. An example of a ratio-based measure is severity-adjusted average length of stay (the ratio of total days of hospital care to discharges, adjusted for patient severity). A popular approach to use such measures is to assemble them in dashboards. These business tools colour-code trends, for instance, in red (reflecting poor or worsening efficiency requiring priority attention), amber (reflecting poor or worsening efficiency requiring close monitoring) and green (reflecting adequate levels of efficiency). However, key challenges lie in the subjective choice about the level of efficiency that is interpreted as requiring immediate attention, as opposed to continued monitoring only.

Econometrical or mathematical programming methodologies, such as SFA and DEA, respectively, which have generated much academic research (see Chapter 5) are hardly used by practising managers (Hussey et al., 2009). While these approaches allow for the analysis of multiple metrics of inputs, outputs and explanatory variables, which are aggregated into a single number of system or organizational efficiency, they tend to require controversial methodological choices, in particular about the sets of weights used to combine multiple metrics into a single composite measure (Goddard & Jacobs, 2009). As such, composite metrics treat the health system as a black box and do not pinpoint the precise areas where targeted intervention is needed. They tend to have limited relevance for managers who must design and choose between specific actions to be taken. An emerging alternative to this, however, is the use of ratio-based efficiency analysis (REA; Salo & Punkka, 2011). REA is similar to DEA, but instead of forcedly assigning a single efficiency rank to each entity studied, the method enables the generation of ranking intervals and dominance relations. REA thus provides managers with a transparent indication of uncertainty about their organization's relative position and about the degree to which action is warranted (Schang et al., 2016).

In some health systems, applying external pressure for action to improve efficiency has been pursued in the form of public reporting of measures of efficiency. A pertinent example at the system level is the analysis of geographical variations in health system performance, promoted especially by John Wennberg and colleagues in the USA and increasingly also by governments and academic institutions in several European countries including Germany, Italy, the Netherlands, Spain and the United Kingdom, and other OECD countries such as Australia, Canada and New Zealand.[22] This research has shown persistent variations in health outcomes, activity and expenditure across geographical regions and health care providers (for a systematic review, see Corallo, 2014). Many of the indicators used can be interpreted as partial measures of efficiency, because they focus, for instance, on rates of avoidable hospital admissions. The underlying rationale, from a health system efficiency perspective, is that resources are misallocated as patients consume expensive hospital care, although high-quality primary care might have prevented their admission in the first place. When multiple measures of variation in cost and outcomes are put together, the analysis of variations can be understood as a form of benchmarking (for an extended discussion of benchmarking in health care, see Neely, 2013): if comparable regions seem to have better outcomes (lower costs) for a given level of spending (output), then there may be scope in the other regions to release resources to be invested in areas of higher-value care.

To provide useful information for local managers working in a time-pressured environment, evidence of variations needs to be translated into tools that can

---

22 For more information, see the website of the Wennberg International Collaborative (http://wennbergcollaborative.org/index.php, accessed 21 July 2016).

relatively quickly and easily be applied by users without advanced levels of statistical knowledge, such as in the form of visual aids. An example from England are the spend and outcome tools (SPOTs) that adapt the familiar idea of cost–effectiveness analysis planes, often used in HTA, for system-level analyses. SPOTs plot a local health economy's outcomes against costs in specific areas (for example, cancer, circulatory diseases, mental health) relative to other local health systems. Positions in the South/East quadrant (bottom right; higher cost/worse outcome) can provide a strong case for further enquiry and action to move closer to the better-performing systems. Positions in the North/East (top right; higher cost/better outcome) and South/West (bottom left; lower cost/worse outcome) quadrants may reflect, but also provoke, a reconsideration of current priorities for investment, for instance, through a more detailed priority-setting exercise (see section 9.3) focused on the relative value gained from different interventions in these areas. An indicative SPOT display for a fictional public health programme is shown in Figure 9.1.

Figure 9.1 *SPOT display for a fictional public health programme*

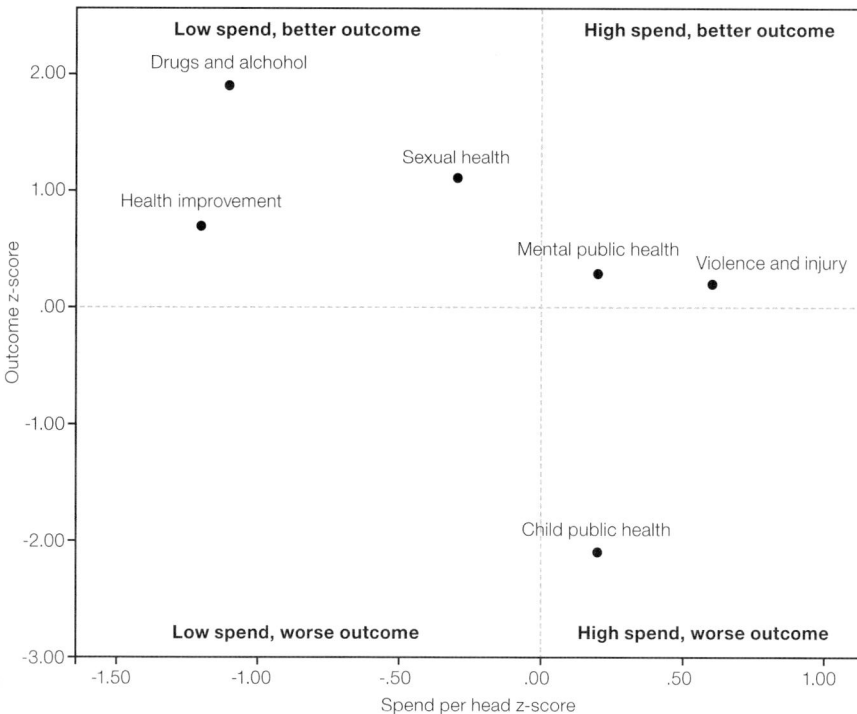

Notes: The z-score measures the distance from the mean value (either positive or negative); the units are standard deviations. SPOT = spend and outcome tool.

In practice, however, many hurdles need to be overcome before such tools can be used by health service managers. Our evaluation of the NHS Atlas of Variation in Healthcare England (Schang et al., 2014) highlighted the following practical challenges: many managers were simply not aware of this information, despite it being distributed as a paper copy to all Chief Executives and Directors of Public Health; information was sometimes not accepted as valid because of known measurement and coding issues; there were doubts over the perceived applicability of the data in providing a rounded picture of performance; and some organizations could not use the information because of capacity constraints or because the next year's priorities had already been agreed and contracts had already been signed when the data were published.

In terms of Cynefin, when thinking about the efficiency metrics available to managers, some information will fall into the known domain, such as cost–effectiveness evidence, where good and bad performance can be identified. However, most efficiency metrics fall within the knowable or complex domains. In these domains, performance indicators are likely to represent what Carter, Klein & Day (1995) termed tin openers – in themselves inaccurate pictures of performance, but useful triggers for further investigation to clarify causes and consequences – rather than dials – good measures that can be judged against normative standards. For instance, when comparing rates of hip replacement across regions, much more detailed analysis at provider and patient levels of analysis is required to examine to what extent higher rates of surgery reflect comparative inefficiency rather than valued activities justifiable by, say, higher levels of medical need or patient preferences. Diagnosing problems simply in terms of the empirical distribution of performance thus can be problematic. It ignores that best performance is not always known or knowable, and that even organizations leading the top end of the distribution may have substantial scope for improvement.

The grid-group cultural framework can also provide a perspective on how different health care systems assign a different locus of ownership to managerial tools for problem diagnosis. For example, the NHS Atlas of Variation in Healthcare is clearly targeted at managers and clinicians within established organizations in charge of allocating resources for health care across sectors, thus reflecting a more hierarchist view of diagnosing problems and searching for solutions. In contrast, in Germany, in the absence of an institution with cross-sectoral responsibility for health system planning (Ettelt et al., 2012), attempts to disseminate information on variations have taken a more individualist perspective by targeting patients and consumers of health services (Nolting, 2011) with a view to empowering them to question advice given to them by medical professionals. However, for moving beyond problem diagnosis towards leading change, a stronger group element that involves coordinated action between different stakeholders may be helpful (see Box 9.1) (Nuti & Seghieri, 2014).

Box 9.1 *Managing system efficiency in Italian regions*

Years of experience in performance management at a regional level in Italy have suggested that the strong focus on regular discussion between managers from different regions and academic researchers, combined with tangible incentives, such as linking parts of chief executives' remuneration to performance outcomes, were key elements in sustaining commitment to change. Starting in 2004, the Tuscany regional health authority entrusted the Laboratorio Management e Sanità of Scuola Superiore Sant'Anna (MeS Lab) to design a multidimensional performance evaluation system that includes indicators of elements of efficiency (outputs and financial sustainability). Indicators are selected through an interaction process between the MeS Lab research team and the regional representatives. To provide decision support for each health care provider, results are discussed in systematic and consensus-based meetings between the top management and regional administrators every three months. Starting in 2006, performance results are also linked to the remuneration of chief executives. Combined with a striking visual reporting system (the target diagram), which highlights multidimensional aspects of performance and the public disclosure of the performance results, the Tuscan system has been shown to successfully improve overall regional performance and has been adapted to other Italian regions.

Source: Nuti & Seghieri (2014).

9.4.2 Design: Process improvement methodologies

Having diagnosed an efficiency problem, the next stage is to design solutions, typically involving some form of service reconfiguration of the services under the manager's area of responsibility. Operations management concepts drawn from philosophies such as lean thinking, Six Sigma, total quality management and the like are often promoted as providing guidance on how to reconfigure services to improve patient flow, and thus simultaneously reduce cost and drive up quality (Hopp & Lovejoy, 2013; Ronen & Pliskin, 2006; Vissers & Beech, 2005). A critical idea behind these improvement philosophies is to concentrate on optimizing processes and flow of patients along these processes rather than optimizing single, isolated steps. For example, one operations management principle is to focus on the bottleneck activities in the process, as it is these that constrain throughput and driving waiting times. This is change number 8 of the NHS Modernisation Agency's (2004) 10 high-impact changes.

Several stories of the transformative power of these concepts exist, for example, Bolton NHS Foundation Trust's lean transformation of its trauma service (Fillingham, 2007) or the Glasgow Royal Infirmary's re-engineered fracture clinic (Vardy et al., 2013). See Box 9.2 for a description of the latter. The message that comes across clearly from these accounts, and the broader academic literature (Radnor, Holweg & Waring, 2012; Waring & Bishop, 2010), is that these concepts, while potentially powerful, are not plug and play. To realize benefits requires deep engagement with the concepts, significant expertise about the idiosyncrasies of the local process and the strategic vision and communication skills to build a case for change and sell it to an often sceptical audience.

A different approach to improve efficiency in health service operations is shared decision-making. This approach has emerged in response to evidence of wide variations in the provision of so-called preference-sensitive care where the best choice depends on patients' preferences over the benefits, harms and scientific uncertainties associated with each option (O'Connor, Llewellyn-Thomas & Flood, 2004). Since doctors or scientific committees do not know these preferences (Folland & Stano, 1990), shared decision-making seeks to involve patients in the decision-making process. For example, in the treatment for osteoarthritis, hip replacement surgery is but one of many other medical, pharmaceutical and physiotherapeutic options and shared decision-making would seek to communicate the range of options and help patients clarify their personal

---

Box 9.2 *Fracture clinic redesign at Glasgow Royal Infirmary*

In 2010, Glasgow Royal Infirmary introduced a new set of procedures for the management of undisplaced fractures, referred to as a Virtual Fracture Clinic. The overall concept was to reduce unwarranted variation by simplifying and standardizing non-operative, orthopaedic trauma outpatient care (>75% of all limb fractures). The modern literature supports this redesign, as many stable, minor injuries can be managed safely with early mobilization and self-care. It was agreed that the experienced A&E team should provide treatment and information for simple injuries without routine orthopaedic review in about one third of cases. All other injuries are fully treated in A&E, and where appropriate allowed home to be reviewed virtually (without patients in attendance). The X-rays and clinical records are reviewed electronically by an Orthopaedic Consultant and nurse the following day, including weekends. All patients are then telephoned by the specially trained, experienced nurse and treatment is discussed. This may consist of purely advice, but if required an appointment at the most appropriate time and subspecialty clinic is arranged. Only about one third of people who were previously routinely reviewed are required to attend for a face-to-face appointment. Patient satisfaction with the clinical outcomes and new process is excellent, and it saves valuable time for both clinical teams and patients. Direct staffing costs for the first attendance are 50% less than in a traditional system, that is, the quality of patient care has been significantly improved while greatly reducing the cost.

Source: Jenkins et al. (2016); Vardy et al. (2013).

preferences so that the best strategy can be agreed on. Among the benefits that are claimed to flow from the implementation of shared decision-making are improvements in AE, that is to say, before producing outputs one verifies that these outputs are actually valued by the intended beneficiary. In the case of BPH, for example, experiences show that many patients who are fully informed of the likely consequences, good and bad, of different treatment modes, elect not to have surgery (Wennberg, 2010).

Implementation of shared decision-making has tended to follow two routes: reforming education and training systems for health professionals; and empowering patients to become more reflective of their personal preferences. To streamline the process, patient decision aids (PDAs) have been developed for use before or during clinical consultations to guide patients through a structured package of information about options, questions about personal values and trade-offs.[23] According to a recent Cochrane review, PDAs consistently improve patient knowledge of options and outcomes and enable more accurate perceptions of outcome probabilities when compared to usual care (Stacey, 2011). In practice, however, perceived time constraints remain the most commonly reported barrier, among health professionals, to their widespread implementation (Légaré et al., 2008). This is particularly challenging since PDAs appear to have a variable effect on the time required for consultations; when patients prepare using a decision aid, this can shorten but also lengthen subsequent consultations (Stacey, 2011). Although strides have been made towards shared decision-making in cultural and organizational contexts as diverse as Canada, China, Germany, Norway, the United Kingdom and the USA (Légaré et al., 2008), available studies show that professionals frequently question the applicability of PDAs to meet the needs of their populations and that progress hinges on the willingness of both patients and professionals to engage in the process (Stacey, 2011).

9.4.3 Choice: priority-setting and resource allocation

The term priority-setting and resource allocation (PSRA) is often used in health care to describe the activity of deciding what to do, that is, which treatments should be funded, what service reconfigurations should be undertaken and so on. (The somewhat more dramatic term rationing is sometimes also used.) PSRA represents a natural follow-up activity to performance measurement and the design of service reconfigurations: if performance measurement represents the intelligence phase of the decision-making process, and lean and shared decision-making have an important role in generating ideas about how services might be reconfigured, then PSRA represents the choice phases, where decisions about which service improvements to implement are actually made. For example, in

---

23 A range of PDAs for chronic and non-urgent conditions can be accessed, for example, via the website of the Ottawa Hospital Research Institute: https://decisionaid.ohri.ca/AZlist.html (accessed 21 July 2016).

the intelligence phase, you might realize that you have efficiency problems in your diabetes and childhood mental health services; in the design phase, you might work out and cost strategies for addressing these problems through service reconfiguration; and in the choice phase, you might decide which of these two clinical areas to target.

PSRA has become increasingly well-established in many jurisdictions at the policy level in many European countries, through HTA agencies like NICE in England, the Scottish Medicines Consortium in Scotland, the HAS in France and the IQWiG in Germany (see Chapter 6). Such agencies typically draw more or less explicitly on the ideas of economic evaluation presented in Drummond (2005) and Gold et al. (1996), based around trading off health gain, captured in QALYs, against cost. A variant of the economic evaluation approach, generalized cost effectiveness analysis, has been promoted by the WHO and has received some attention in developing countries (Tan-Torres Edejer et al., 2003).

Even in jurisdictions like England, where there is a strong central HTA agency, there is still considerable scope for decision-making at the local management level. This may be because there is as yet no published policy on guidance on some particular technologies which the local provider wishes to use or because some of the options being considered are not the kind of things that are susceptible to HTA (for example, closure of a small, inefficient and unsafe, but popular, A&E). Alternatively, it could be because local circumstances mean that because the assumptions about cost or population health underpinning published, policy-level technology assessments do not apply locally (for example, the ethnic mix means that the local population has a high prevalence of sickle cell anaemia, making it cost-effective to invest in specialized services; providing a small island-based population with timely access to CT scans may not be cost-effective, making it problematic to offer thrombolysis as a treatment for ischaemic stroke).

The closest thing to a process template for PSRA at the local level is PBMA (Mitton & Donaldson, 2004; Peacock, 2010). Accounts of PBMA emphasize that PSRA involves providing both a modelling framework for eliciting and organizing judgements about the reasons for doing different treatments, and process ground rules. For example, multicriteria decision analysis, in which stakeholders are invited to score the performance of packages of activity against various objectives, is often presented as a practical and accessible modelling framework, which is simpler and more flexible than full-scale health economic modelling (see Peacock, Carter & Edward, 2007 or Wilson, Rees & Fordham, 2006 for examples). In a similar way, the accountability for reasonableness framework (a collection of principles relating to transparency, relevance of argumentation and openness to appeals) is often presented as a process model (Daniels & Sabin, 2008).

Recently, work sponsored by the Health Foundation and involving the authors has taken a somewhat different approach from the standard PBMA paradigm (Airoldi, 2013; Airoldi & Morton, 2011; Airoldi et al., 2014). Proponents of the socio-technical allocation of resources (STAR) approach share the view of the advocates of PBMA that providing decision support has a substantive and process component. The philosophy behind the STAR approach is that the analysis framework of health economics with its focus on monetary cost and individual health benefits provides the soundest and most compelling framework for resource allocation for population health. Recognizing how this modelling framework is used at the policy level for national HTA decisions is far too complex, costly and demanding of specialized skill to implement at the local level, STAR provides a parsimonious health economics model that can serve as a framework for organizing locally available evidence, expert assessments and value judgements (see Box 9.3).

Box 9.3 *STAR for health care purchasers and clinical experts*

STAR refers to an approach to health care prioritization based on a concept of decision-making as having both a social and technical dimension in the spirit of Phillips, Bana & Costa (2007). At the core of the STAR approach are decision conferences, facilitated participative modelling workshops, where participants representing diverse viewpoints and interests in the system – managers, hospital doctors, GPs, nurses and allied health professionals, finance and public health specialists, and patient representatives – are guided through a set of structured assessments of population-level costs and benefits associated with particular courses of action. The philosophy of STAR is that while clinical evidence is critical to making decisions, decisions never drop out of analysis; decisions must ultimately be taken on the basis of expert judgements of facts and values. Thus, while STAR workshops rely on preparatory data gathering, which is tabled at the workshop, the process stresses visual interactive tools to help all workshop participants understand both the scale of costs and benefits associated with particular options on the table, and the efficiency or so-called bang for the buck of these options. STAR has been deployed in several primary care trusts in England (as the commissioning organizations were called at the time), with documented stories of impact on the Isle of Wight and in Sheffield. STAR has also worked with IMPRESS, a clinical expert group, to arrive at commissioning guidelines for chronic obstructive pulmonary disease (COPD). These guidelines were glowingly reviewed in the BMJ by Gray & El Turabi (2012) who stated that "the tool used by IMPRESS … should be adopted and adapted by all clinical communities of practice to estimate and visualise the marginal benefits of all aspects of care for the benefit of patients".

Sources: Airoldi (2013); Airoldi et al. (2014); IMPRESS (2012).

As we have noted earlier, different health care activities are located in different domains of the Cynefin spectrum. One might then expect that the differing nature of the evidence base between, for example, public health interventions (more knowable) than surgical interventions (more known) would present a challenge to would-be priority setters. In our experience, this is indeed a salient feature of the management of PSRA. A common concern heard from Directors of Public Health is that they believe that rebalancing their portfolio towards the preventive and away from the acute side is the right thing to do for their local population. However, the evidence is all for the acute interventions. Indeed, one of the strengths of the STAR approach, which recognizes the validity of expert judgement as an input, is that it enables a discussion of the relative merits of acute versus preventive interventions within a common framework.

Grid-group cultural theory also offers an interesting perspective on priority-setting. Most PSRA methods, as noted earlier, have a strong group element: they are intended as participatory frameworks. How far that participation extends, however, varies from application to application. For example, the main workshop event in the application reported by Airoldi et al. (2014) involved 25 stakeholders: the eight executive directors of the health authority, nine commissioning managers, three patient and public representatives, four clinical experts and one representative of social services. In another application, the group members were all members of a clinical expert group (IMPRESS) who wished to issue commissioning guidance on COPD (IMPRESS, 2012). Grid-group cultural theory highlights how intense participation is; which constituencies are included will be culturally driven and culturally dependent.

9.5 Recommendations for practice

In this section, we give some examples of tasks that might face managers tasked with achieving efficiency improvements, and reflect on how the frameworks we have presented might give insight into how to go about tackling these tasks.

9.5.1 Task 1: designing a set of efficiency indicators

Efficiency indicators should be designed with a view in mind of the extent to which the aspects of efficiency being measured are under the control of the organization being assessed. As the Cynefin framework suggests, if a performance measurement framework contains a small number of efficiency measures where the causal links between action and performance are clear, this may stimulate the evaluated organization to identify efficiency improvements through redesigning processes; however, if many indicators are not of this type, then the risk is that managers in the organization will be overwhelmed by the resulting ambiguity. This may result in unintended and unproductive effects, such as cynicism and gaming.

Following from this, a key insight offered by grid-group cultural theory is that if efficiency indicators are to be used to drive performance improvements, this should be done in a way that is appropriate with the prevailing culture. To enable low-grid managers, that is, managers who feel constrained by external factors – for example, because they feel that a poor efficiency metric is capturing a factor outside their control (such as poor hospital outcomes reflecting patient lifestyles) – then processes should be put in place for managers to communicate these concerns to other stakeholders and to policymakers. This in turn should feed back to an improvement in the measurement and monitoring frameworks in place at both organizational and system levels.

Grid-group cultural theory can also provide us with some insights regarding the best types of incentives likely to work in organizations, or to incentivize the management of organizations. In low-group settings, that is, when managers do not identify as part of the larger health system, performance management systems that rely heavily on extrinsic motivators, such as targets or financial rewards, may be appropriate. On the other hand, in high-group settings, where managers view themselves as part of a wider system, the danger is that such motivators may undermine intrinsic motivation and engender cynicism and game playing; in this instance, a more developmental approach may be appropriate. Of course, the use of extrinsic versus intrinsic motivators may be implemented in a deliberate attempt to change culture, but managers who do so should be mindful that both high- and low-group cultures are viable and can support high performance in the right circumstances.

9.5.2 Task 2: using analytical methods to identify process improvements

In some cases, the process improvements that can support greater efficiency may be obvious: reducing unnecessary diagnostic tests and substituting generic for branded pharmaceuticals are simple and easy to implement. However, often in health care, quite detailed investigations (clinical trials, detailed costing or simulation studies) are needed to establish whether one intervention is more cost-effective than another. Moreover, it may be difficult to pinpoint sources of inefficacy in systems that are quite complex and fragmented. For example, it may be that a very efficient hospital exists within a very inefficient health system. While the hospital itself may be providing the best treatment with the resources it has, outcomes may not appear good because of inefficiencies elsewhere in the system (such as poor prevention, for example).

The Cynefin framework recognizes this complexity. Some causal connections between action and outcome are obvious and it requires only minimal action to decide what to do, whereas in other settings the link is less clear and significant investigative work may be required. Moreover, Cynefin reminds us that there are limits to what can be achieved by analysis. For example, in an environment without good diagnostic coding or data linking, it may be simply impossible to know whether introducing a management programme in primary care for adults with respiratory problems, such as COPD or asthma, does actually reduce emergency admissions. The existence of these limits of analysis highlights that management operates in an environment that is significantly constrained by policy choices, and sometimes the most appropriate action – indeed the only possible response with any chance of effectively addressing the problem – may be to escalate the problem to a higher system level.

Equally, grid-group cultural theory highlights the importance of cultural fit when analytical methods are used as a tool of communication and persuasion. Analytical methods by their nature are somewhat opaque: accepting conclusions that flow from such methods requires taking on trust that the method has been implemented competently and in good faith. High-grid cultures, where managers feel they are constrained by external factors, will deal with this by having standards and checklists for analysis (such as the checklists for economic evaluation that currently seem popular). In high-group cultures, on the other hand, the focus will be on the personal standing of the analyst. In cultures that are neither high-grid nor high-group, if analytical methods can be used as a tool of persuasion, the modelling methods chosen will have to be very accessible (for example, painstaking documentation, visual interactive displays to communicate the model structure and workings) and people whose behaviour is to be changed will have to be given the time and opportunity to study and convince themselves, if change efforts are to have any chance of being successful. Therefore, the appropriate choice of analytical method depends on careful attention to what is considered as persuasive by the stakeholders who bear the responsibility for implementing any resultant action.

9.5.3 Task 3: engaging stakeholders in decision-making

Cynefin highlights the importance of thinking through why one wants to involve stakeholders in decision-making. In some environments, where causes are known and straightforward, involvement of stakeholders might be essentially a communication campaign: in this case, involvement could be relatively light touch. In other environments, where causes are unknown or knowable, involving stakeholders could be a good way to get a better understanding of causal relationships, particularly where relationships are not captured in data. In the rare case where the environment is genuinely chaotic, all that one can reasonably hope for from the involvement of stakeholders may be that this kick-starts the process of sensemaking, as problems involving chaotic systems cannot, in the memorable quote of Einstein, "be solved at the same level of thinking as created them".

Grid-group cultural theory also offers potentially useful insights into the question of how intensively to involve stakeholders in decision-making. Fatalistic stakeholders will not participate usefully in engagement, unless they can be transformed into stakeholders of some other type. Individualistic stakeholders may participate in engagement but must be managed. The danger is that such stakeholders will never be able to step out of their role as lobbyists for special interests. In hierarchist and egalitarian cultures, there will be different expectations about who should be included and involved: hierarchists will be happy with a decision in which those with relevant expertise and formal leadership roles have been consulted, whereas egalitarians will want to see evidence that the process includes those who are most likely to be affected by the decision on the ground, including grass roots staff and patients.

9.5.4 Task 4: communicating recommendations through guidelines and protocols

An important idea in Cynefin is that not all knowledge claims are equal: it is now a commonly accepted principle in guideline development that guidelines should include some indication of the strength of the evidence underpinning a particular recommendation, so that those charged with implementing guidance can make a properly sensitive and contextualized judgement about whether to follow a particular piece of recommendation. Initiatives like GRADE (Guyatt et al., 2008) are important precisely because the development of a standard system for communicating the strength of evidence behind a guideline is vital if busy clinicians (and managers) are to be able to quickly form an impression of how unconditional and binding (or how tentative and provisional) they should take a particular recommendation to be.

Similarly, grid-group cultural theory highlights that, in cultural terms, guidelines rely on implicit culture which is, at least to some extent, hierarchist: for guidelines to be accepted, readers must accept that guideline writers are offering legitimate and well-founded advice. To some extent, this hierarchism is inculcated into the medical profession through the process of professional education. However, there is also a significant individualist strand within medicine, and in different places and different specialities the balance will be struck differently. Grid-group cultural theory thus highlights the importance of being sensitive to such cultural differences, and not to assume that guidelines will be accepted enthusiastically everywhere.

9.6 Conclusion

A theme of this chapter has been that the use of efficiency analysis in the management setting has to be understood, as the Cynefin framework suggests, in terms of the affordances of the underpinning evidence; in some domains of health care, cause-and-effect relationships are clear, but in others this is less the case. Often, there is good compelling evidence for efficiency improvement which speaks for itself, but it is in the (common) situations where this is not the case that management judgement has to be brought to bear. While science can wait until the evidence is in before coming to a conclusion, and while policymakers can commission evidence reviews and hire experts, neither of these options are available to a manager who will face their board on Friday and is expected to present recommendations for action.

Another theme has been that that the cultural context of management determines how efficiency analysis tools are used, as highlighted by grid-group theory. This prevailing culture may be influenced by national institutional structures: for example, one might speculate that NHS-like systems with centralized lines of control and salaried health professionals may lead managers to think and act in more hierarchist and bureaucratic ways, while managers working in systems with independent and self-employed professionals may be more naturally inclined to adopt market-based or individualist solutions. At the policy level, decision-makers may have access to enough levers of power to believe that they can transform organizational culture: managers on the other hand must, to a much greater extent, work within the straitjacket which culture imposes.

In so far as neither the evidence base not the prevailing culture can be changed, our argument leads to the conclusion that to be usable and used, efficiency analysis tools have to fit with both that evidence base and cultural context: that is, they have to suggest or evoke arguments which are plausible in the light of the evidence, for solutions which are culturally acceptable. Although some tools explicitly and sometimes successfully seek to transform existing culture – for example, by building on ideas from other industries – it is likely that managers will need some prior common ground to anchor these ideas. Moreover, our argument suggests that it is not enough to have a technical modelling tool (SFA, MCDA), but one also has to have a process account of how such a tool can be used – how should supporting evidence be generated and whom should be involved in the interpretation of results and search for solutions.

The need to improve efficiency in health care – that is, to get more benefit for patients and populations with fewer resources – is going to sorely test health services in coming years. The tools and concepts of efficiency analysis have a part to play but managers have to engage with them in a way where they are realistic and sensitive to what these tools can and cannot offer, and whether they are able to do this will have a huge influence on the shape which our health services take over the next few years and decades. In our view this calls for a significant amount of dissemination activity by the research community via multiple channels (for example, discussions at key practitioner events and conferences, easily accessible web-based tools in addition to hard copies, and a continued stream of publications on efficiency and performance in health care) and co-production of knowledge through work with local stakeholders to help inform the case for change. We hope that volumes such as the present one can play a useful role in facilitating such discussions.

Acknowledgements

The authors would like to acknowledge the contribution of Dr Lech Rymaszewski, Consultant Orthopaedic Surgeon at the Glasgow Royal Infirmary and Gillian Anderson in drafting the text of Box 9.3.

References

Airoldi M (2013). Disinvestments in practice: overcoming resistance to change through a sociotechnical approach with local stakeholders. *Journal of Health Politics, Policy and Law*, 38(6):1149–1171.

Airoldi M, Morton, A (2011). Portfolio decision analysis for population health. In*: Salo A, Keisler J, Morton A, eds. *Portfolio decision analysis: methods for improved resource allocation*. New York, Springer.

Airoldi M et al. (2014). STAR—People-powered prioritization: a 21st-century solution to allocation headaches. *Medical Decision Making,* 34(8): 965–975.

Carter N, Klein R, Day P (1995). *How organisations measure success: the use of performance indicators in government*. London, Routledge.

Corallo AN et al. (2014). A systematic review of medical practice variation in OECD countries. *Health Policy*, 114(1):5–14.

Daniels N, Sabin JE (2008). *Setting limits fairly: learning to share resources for health*. Oxford, OUP.

Dorgan S et al. (2010). *Management in healthcare: why good practice really matters*. London, McKinsey and Company (http://cep.lse.ac.uk/textonly/_new/research/productivity/management/PDF/management_in_healthcare_Report.pdf, accessed 31 August 2016).

Drummond M (2005). *Methods for the economic evaluation of health care programmes*. Oxford, OUP.

Ettelt S et al. (2012). Assessing health care planning: a framework-led comparison of Germany and New Zealand. *Health Policy*, 106(1):50–59.

Fillingham D (2007). Can lean save lives? *Leadership in Health Services*, 20(4):231–241.

Folland S, Stano M (1990). Small area variations: a critical review of propositions, methods, and evidence. *Medical Care Review*, 47(4):419–465.

Goddard M, Jacobs R (2009). Using composite indicators to measure performance in health care. In: Smith P et al., eds. *Performance measurement for health system improvement: experiences, challenges, and prospects*. Cambridge, CUP.

Gold MR et al., eds. (1996). *Cost–effectiveness in health and medicine*. Oxford, OUP.

Gray M, El Turabi A (2012). Optimising the value of interventions for populations. *BMJ*, 345: e6192.

Guyatt GH et al. (2008). GRADE: an emerging consensus on rating quality of evidence and strength of recommendations. *BMJ*, 336(7650):924–926.

Hollingsworth B, Street A (2006). The market for efficiency analysis of health care organisations. *Health Economics,* 15(10):1055–1059.

Hopp WJ, Lovejoy WS (2013). *Hospital operations: principles of high efficiency health care*. Upper Saddle River, NJ, Pearson FT Press.

Hussey PS et al. (2009). A systematic review of health care efficiency measures. *Health Services Research*, 44(3):784–805.

IMPRESS (2012). IMPRESS guide to the relative value of COPD interventions. (http://www.impressresp.com/index.php?option=com_docman&Itemid=82#sthash.yjsqf2mF.dpuf, accessed 2 August 2016).

Jenkins PJ et al. (2016). Fracture clinic redesign reduces the cost of outpatient orthopaedic trauma care. *Bone and Joint Research*, 5(2):33–36.

Kurtz CF, Snowden DJ (2003). The new dynamics of strategy: sense-making in a complex and complicated world. *IBM Systems Journal*, 42(3):462–483.

Laxminarayan R et al. (2013). Antibiotic resistance: the need for global solutions. *The Lancet. Infectious Diseases*, 13(12):1057–1098.

Légaré F et al. (2008). Barriers and facilitators to implementing shared decision-making in clinical practice: update of a systematic review of health professionals' perceptions. *Patient Education and Counseling*, 73(3):526–535.

Mintzberg H (1973). *The nature of managerial work.* New York, Harper Collins Publishers.

Mitton C, Donaldson C (2004). Health care priority setting: principles, practice and challenges. *Cost Effectiveness and Resource Allocation*, 2(1):3.

Morton A, Cornwell J (2009). What's the difference between a hospital and a bottling factory? *BMJ*, 339:b2727.

Neely A (2013). Benchmarking: lessons and implications for health systems. In: Papanicolas I, Smith P, eds. *Health system performance comparison: an agenda for policy, information and research.* Maidenhead, Open University Press.

Nolting H (2011). Faktencheck Gesundheit. Regionale Unterschiede in der Gesundheitsversorgung, Gütersloh, Bertelsmann Stiftung.

Nuti S, Seghieri C (2014). Is variation management included in regional healthcare governance systems? Some proposals from Italy. *Health Policy*, 114(1):71–78.

O'Connor AM, Llewellyn-Thomas HA, Flood AB (2004). Modifying unwarranted variations in health care: shared decision making using patient decision aids. *Health Affairs*, (Suppl. Variation):VAR63–VAR72.

Peacock SJ et al. (2007). Priority setting in health care using multi-attribute utility theory and programme budgeting and marginal analysis (PBMA). *Social Science & Medicine*, 64(4):897–910.

Peacock SJ et al. (2010). Priority setting in healthcare: towards guidelines for the program budgeting and marginal analysis framework. *Expert Review of Pharmacoeconomics & Outcomes Research*, 10(5):539–552.

Phillips LD, Bana e Costa CA (2007). Transparent prioritisation, budgeting and resource allocation with multi-criteria decision analysis and decision conferencing. *Annals of Operations Research*, 154(1):51–68.

Radnor ZJ, Holweg M, Waring J (2012). Lean in healthcare: the unfilled promise? *Social Science & Medicine*, 74(3):364–371.

Ronen B, Pliskin JS (2006). *Focused operations management for health services organizations: linking efficiency and productivity.* San Francisco, CA, Jossey-Bass.

Salo A, Punkka A (2011). Ranking intervals and dominance relations for ratio-based efficiency analysis. *Management Science*, 57(1):200–214.

Schang L et al. (2014). From data to decisions? Exploring how healthcare payers respond to the NHS Atlas of Variation in Healthcare in England. *Health Policy*, 114(1):79–87.

Schang L et al. (2016). Developing robust composite measures of healthcare quality. Ranking intervals and dominance relations for Scottish Health Boards. *Social Science & Medicine*, 162:59–67.

Simon HA (1960). *The new science of management decision.* New York, Harper and Row.

Stacey D et al. (2011). Decision aids for people facing health treatment or screening decisions. *Cochrane Database of Systematic Reviews*, 10: CD001431.

Tan-Torres Edejer T et al., eds. (2003). *WHO guide to cost–effectiveness analysis.* Geneva, WHO (http://www.who.int/choice/publications/p_2003_generalised_cea.pdf, accessed 2 August 2016).

Thompson M, Ellis R, Wildavsky AB (1990). *Cultural theory.* Boulder, CO, Westview Press.

Vardy J et al. (2013). Fracture pathway redesign improves emergency department efficiency. *Emergency Medicine Journal*, 30:876.

Vissers J, Beech R, eds. (2005). *Health operations management.* London, Routledge.

Waring JJ, Bishop S (2010). Lean healthcare: rhetoric, ritual and resistance. *Social Science & Medicine*, 71(7):1332–1340.

Wennberg JE (2010). *Tracking medicine: a researcher's quest to understand health care.* Oxford, OUP.

Wilson EC, Rees J, Fordham RJ (2006). Developing a prioritisation framework in an English Primary Care Trust. *Cost effectiveness and Resource Allocation*, 4:3.

Wren DA (2005). *The evolution of management thought.* Hoboken, NJ, John Wiley & Sons.

Chapter 10

Conclusions

Jonathan Cylus, Irene Papanicolas, Peter C. Smith

10.1 Introduction

Measuring health system efficiency is not straightforward. While the basic notion of efficiency seems simple – maximizing output relative to input – it often becomes difficult to apply this concept to the health system. Among the many challenges faced in practice, there are challenges in ensuring that the systems, providers and patients evaluated are sufficiently comparable, and that resources are properly attributed to outputs and outcomes. Furthermore, the production processes underlying health systems are intrinsically complex and poorly understood, making it difficult to develop measures that reliably capture efficiency. International comparison is especially challenging, given the variations in institutional arrangements and the definition of what is considered to fall within the boundaries of the health system across countries.

Despite the complexities associated with developing robust measures, the demand for comparative efficiency metrics remains strong. Stakeholders, including ministries of finance, but also tax-paying citizens, want to know that their contributions to the health care system are not being wasted. Likewise, health service managers require tools that enable them to do more with their available resources. Therefore, it is important to continue seeking improvements to metrics, while recognizing their limitations and the potential for misinterpretations.

This concluding chapter considers some of the key themes that emerge from the different chapters in this volume, relating to the challenges in the measurement and use of efficiency indicators. Section 10.2 outlines the main challenges currently encountered when measuring efficiency, and considers how these challenges relate to our framework for thinking about health systems efficiency (see Chapter 1). Section 10.3 considers how one might appropriately interpret a selection of common efficiency metrics. Finally, Section 10.4 considers the lessons that emerge from this volume regarding the use of efficiency metrics and the potential for progress in using the information we have to make judgements about efficiency throughout the health system, and thereby improve policy and managerial decisions.

10.2 Revisiting the analytical framework: key challenges of efficiency measurement

Chapter 1 highlighted some of the complexities associated with developing and interpreting efficiency measures. To think about efficiency metrics, we introduced an analytical framework that considers five aspects of any indicator:

- what entity is being assessed?
- what are the outputs (or outcomes) under consideration?
- what are the inputs under consideration?
- what are the external influences on attainment?
- what are the links with the rest of the health system?

This volume has reviewed a series of topics that are important for measuring efficiency and has highlighted a number of challenges across these five areas. Certain challenges emerge as common themes across many of the chapters. Below we review these in turn, considering some of the insights offered from the contributions to this volume.

10.2.1 What entity is being assessed?

Efficiency analysis first requires one to choose the accountable entity to be scrutinized, whether it is an individual practitioner, team, provider organization or entire health system. As discussed in Chapter 1, this requires that the boundaries of any analysis are clearly drawn for all units being compared. When drawing these boundaries, it is important that two key issues are taken into account: 1) the boundaries are set in a way that ensures the entities being compared are similar; and 2) the boundaries drawn reflect entities that can be held accountable for any of the (in)efficiencies identified.

The issue of comparability is raised in many chapters. Chapter 2 considered the use of patient classification systems, such as DRGs, to create standardized units of health care output that can be compared to one another, particularly in terms of the costs of providing comparable output. Chapter 3 discussed the potential for even more refined patient classification using detailed registry data, which can allow analysts to categorize full episodes of an individual's care across multiple providers. While expanding the boundaries of analysis beyond a single provider, such as a hospital, is exciting, it may still be more useful in practice to restrict analysis to specific entities that can be held accountable for any observed variations. Chapter 7 explored the challenges associated with conducting efficiency comparisons across health systems, where these challenges are further compounded by differences in populations (and burdens of illness) as well as in the provision of health care so that data on inputs and outputs are often not comparable.

Many chapters note that existing metrics are by-products of institutional arrangements in the system, such as existing payment structures. For example, Chapter 2 again noted that many outputs reflect units of reimbursement (such as DRGs), while Chapter 4 noted that much of the existing cost data also reflects billing systems. As a result, the units compared are often those for which there are data available, but not necessarily across the specific units that can be held accountable for existing (in)efficiencies. For example, in many systems administrative, hospital-level data are used to conduct efficiency analyses across hospitals. However, the detection of inefficiency at a local hospital does not necessarily mean that the local entity should be held responsible for that inefficiency. It is often the case that the inefficiency arises from constraints imposed on the local organization or practitioner by higher levels of authority, such as the use of clinical guidelines, legal requirements, performance targets and financing mechanisms. It is important that, as well as identifying the nature and magnitude of inefficiency, the analysis also correctly identifies the source ultimately responsible for the causes of inefficiency.

10.2.2 *What are the outputs (or outcomes) under consideration?*

As noted in the framework in Chapter 1, two fundamental issues regarding outputs need to be considered in the context of efficiency analysis: 1) how should the outputs of the health care sector be defined; and 2) what value should be attached to these outputs. We have touched on the first issue earlier, which relates in part to establishing clear boundaries to define the entity whose outputs (or outcomes) are being measured.

As discussed in Chapter 2, as more health systems have adopted DRGs as a patient classification tool, there has been a growing interest in using these instruments for efficiency measurement. DRGs are useful for comparing similar types of patients and for aggregating hospital output to account for differences in case mix across providers. However, a challenge in using DRG systems to compare efficiency is that they are not designed to capture information on health outcomes, making it difficult to account for variations in quality of care.

Nevertheless, the chapter highlighted that it is conceivable that the basic idea of patient classification systems could be attached to measures of health improvement, at least for certain high-volume cases that have predictable health outcomes. For example, it should be feasible to develop systems that define groups of patients with similar characteristics (for example, based on diagnosis, severity and functional status) who would be likely to benefit in a similar way from particular types of treatment (medical or surgical procedures). Such an approach could advance measurement of effectiveness and move health systems towards more cost-effective delivery of care. The increased use of electronic health records, linked data sets and registries, capturing entire patient treatments, offers some scope for developing more complete efficiency metrics, capable of assessing the relative merits of alternative approaches to care.

To this end, Chapter 3 considered the potential of using registry data to develop efficiency metrics. Registry data contains detailed patient information, which can be used to more accurately group similar types of patients based on characteristics like diagnosis and treatment. However, even with registry data, there are important limitations that make it challenging to measure efficiency. One such challenge is that, as with DRGs, there are limited outcome indicators available in registry data. These indicators are usually confined to mortality or the occurrence of adverse events, such as a complication or reoperation. Thus, the actual effectiveness of a treatment (that is, change in health status) must often be inferred indirectly (for example, if a patient is not readmitted over a given time period, it might be assumed that their treatment was successful). In the future, the use of PROMs might offer greater scope for improved quality measurement if these are included in registries (Smith & Street, 2013).

A particular challenge, rarely mentioned in the chapters, is the production of joint outputs with other organizational entities, such as the entity's contribution to integrated care for a patient across a range of providers. In some ways, this challenge is a prime reason for pursuing the linked data systems discussed in Chapter 3, but it may be the case that meaningful efficiency measurement can only be secured once a purchaser is made accountable for the entire package of care that a patient receives. At present, little work has been done on purchaser efficiency.

10.2.3 What are the inputs under consideration?

Another challenge in measuring efficiency and constructing adequate efficiency measurement is in the measurement of inputs. A number of challenges exist in developing suitable cost data. Often, the costs data available in a country are heavily influenced by the existing regulatory structures in place. For example, the payment of hospitals using DRG groups influences both the unit being costed and the costing calculations themselves.

As noted in Chapter 3, one of the challenges in using registry data approaches to measure efficiency is the lack of suitable cost information available. Cost structures in health care are intrinsically complex, and in most cases it is difficult to attribute costs directly to individual patients. Instead, costs are typically drawn from the existing payment structures in place, which can be summed to provide estimates of the cost of treatment overall. Using these normative cost estimates complicates efficiency comparison, since the input costs are based on the outputs produced rather than the inputs used to provide treatment, frustrating the objective of much efficiency analysis.

Chapter 4 highlighted issues in relation to the measurement of health care costs, and outlined the basic steps that must be taken to create a costing system that can appropriately attach costs to objects of interest, such as patients. The authors argued that systems need to shift away from volume-based costing methods to better capture service use. New costing system designs need to focus on developing greater levels of detail in the measurement of resources, cost pools and cost objects.

10.2.4 What are the external influences on attainment?

Indicators of the entity's efficiency are usually represented by a ratio of some input (or inputs) to some output (or outputs). To secure comparability across entities, it is usually necessary to adjust either inputs or outputs for variations in the uncontrollable external factors that affect the performance of providers and practitioners.

Chapters 2, 3 and 4, which considered different tools for the measurement of inputs and outputs, also emphasized the importance of identifying and controlling for external influences. Methods such as case mix adjustment can be used to adjust for different factors, depending on the specific purpose of the evaluation. For example, when attempting to compare unit costs across providers, case mix adjustment can be used to adjust for differences in the risk of the populations that different providers are serving, which may require them to provide treatment that is more or less expensive than average. Another use of case mix adjustment may be in the comparison of outcomes across different providers, where differences in the characteristics of the population may influence mortality observed across these providers.

Chapters 5 and 6 discussed the methods that combine health care inputs and outputs into efficiency metrics. Chapter 5 discussed the potential for using frontier methods, such as DEA and SFA, to assess how effectively a unit of production, such as a hospital, uses its inputs, such as staff and drugs, to produce outputs, such as the quantity of patients treated. Chapter 6 explored the use of CEA to consider allocative efficiency (AE), that is, to examine the extent to which available resources are allocated across and between inputs so as to maximize health outcomes. Both chapters noted that while these methods have the potential to provide meaningful insights, they will be sensitive to the assumptions made by analysts, and the quality of the data used to measure inputs and outputs. In particular, one issue to consider is to what extent the observed inputs and outputs are influenced by external factors that need to be adjusted for before drawing conclusions about relative efficiency.

For example, Chapter 5 discussed some of the limitations of using an approach like DEA. Care must be taken in interpreting DEA results, because the efficiency frontier can be unduly influenced by stochastic variation, measurement error or unobserved heterogeneity in the data. As noted in the chapter, small variations among inefficient hospitals only affect the magnitude of the estimate for that hospital, but larger variations can move the frontier itself, affecting efficiency estimates for a range of hospitals. DEA is also sensitive to the number of input and output variables used; importantly, there is no agreed method to select the correct model specification. Chapter 5 concluded by outlining sets of guidelines for different users of these methods, which help to ensure these issues are considered.

Similarly, in Chapter 6, where the authors review cost–effectiveness analysis techniques and their potential for evaluating AE, they noted the importance of being able to consider external influences of attainment. Cost–effectiveness analysis is most commonly performed at the micro level, to evaluate individual treatment options; however, these methods can be applied at the macro level to compare different programmes of care or the optimal mix of health services. At all levels of analysis, adjustments must be made to control for any external influences that may influence observed outcomes and inputs, such as the case mix of patients. At the macro level, differences in policy constraints, environmental factors and determinants of demand for services must also be taken into account when interpreting results and making comparisons.

Chapter 7 also discussed how external factors may influence international comparisons of efficiency. In addition to controlling for the factors mentioned earlier, such as differences in populations, this chapter emphasized that different systems also have different organizational features that are likely to influence efficiency comparisons.

10.2.5 What are the links with the rest of the health system?

Finally, the last part of the framework presented in Chapter 1 considered the links across different components of the health system. Often efficiency analysis is performed at the practitioner or organizational level; yet, when these analyses are interpreted, they should not be considered in isolation from other parts of the health system. Chapters 8 and 9 considered the use of efficiency measures and analysis in policy formulation and health service management. Both these chapters highlighted the challenge of using efficiency information, which is often not straightforward and may be open to different interpretations.

Chapter 8 explored the role that efficiency metrics play in shaping and evaluating policy using different country examples. The authors considered a number of policies, ranging from payment reform to the definition of the health basket. One key conclusion that emerged when looking across these policies is the importance of considering how policies aimed at one sector, or efficiency metrics from one sector, may be influenced by links across the health system. For example, payment reforms aiming to reinforce efficiency of specific providers, such as DRGs or P4P, may be evaluated only within the sector they are introduced in, but how they influence AE across the system is not considered.

Similarly, Chapter 9 considered how managers may use efficiency information. In this chapter, the authors noted that some methods favoured by academics or policymakers, such as DEA or SFA, which aggregate multiple inputs and outputs in a single measure, may be unhelpful for managers who are looking for particular inefficiencies to target within their institution. However, they also noted the importance for policymakers to carefully consider the links across the system when evaluating organizational efficiency metrics, so that managers are not held to account for inefficiencies that arise from other areas. For example, a hospital may have a high length of stay for a number of reasons, one being inefficiency of the hospital, but another may be because of a lack of suitable discharge facilities for patients needing long-term care.

10.3 The role of simple metrics

While there is great value in using advanced metrics, such as frontier-based analyses, simple metrics that reflect discrete production processes can also be extremely useful. However, as with all efficiency metrics, they can only provide glimpses of inefficient processes; they should not be taken at face value without investigation. The challenge with most efficiency is to seek to explain unexplained variation. If we do not know why an indicator varies, then we cannot say what the root cause is, whether the variation is meaningful and how to respond. The seemingly simple measure of average length of stay as an indicator of efficiency can be useful, but is difficult to interpret without considering a range of other metrics. For example, having adjusted for variations in case mix, it may be necessary to explore further to see whether declines in length of stay have been accompanied by an increase in readmissions if patients are discharged too early. In summary, it is almost always essential to undertake contextual analysis and look at more than one indicator to understand any efficiency metric.

Therefore, efficiency metrics need to be accompanied by other relevant contextual metrics that can assist with further analysis. There is a currently a lack of agreed analytical frameworks to help analysts explore further when an entity performs poorly on a specific indicator. In the same vein, frameworks are needed to suggest potential policy levers when inefficiencies have been uncovered. In their absence, the evidence on efficiency is often not clear-cut and the managerial and policy implications are open to different interpretations.

To illustrate how analysts may want to approach interpretation of efficiency metrics, Boxes 10.1–10.6 review some common indicators of efficiency that are also often used as dashboard indicators or to benchmark different providers and/or countries. We consider the following questions for each:

1. What is the indicator?
2. What does it tell you and what does it not tell you?
3. What should you do next if you find variation?

Box 10.1 *Per-case expenditure*

What is it?

Per-case expenditure provides information on how much money is spent to deliver various health care services. Different health care services use very different types and amounts of inputs; as a result, we would not gain very much information by directly comparing the costs of a hip replacement with the costs of a hernia operation. To appropriately compare expenditure, two general approaches can be taken so that we are comparing like-with-like. If there is an interest in comparing aggregate expenditure, say, across hospitals, expenditure can be summed after using weights to account for differences in patient case mix; DRGs are a useful tool to account for differences in the intensity of services. Alternatively, while less common, to compare expenditure for specific types of care, vignettes that describe particular diagnoses, procedures and patient characteristics can be used to cost hypothetical episodes of care.

What does it tell you, and what does it not tell you?

Comparing expenditure gives a sense of whether too much is being spent to provide similar health care services. However, countries that spend the same amount of money delivering services do not necessarily provide equivalent services. It is very difficult to account for differences in quality of care by only comparing expenditure by case, so the assumption is that quality of care is uniform.

What should you do next if you find variation?

There are a number of reasons why per-case expenditure could appear too high. It is possible that input costs, such as provider salaries, or the prices of drugs and diagnostic tests are too high, or that too many inputs are being used to treat a condition. For example, providers may order unnecessary diagnostic tests that increase costs without additional health gains. Likewise, the indicator relies on the assumption that expenditure has been adjusted to render services fully comparable across systems, but this may not have been done sufficiently. It may be that health systems treat the same conditions using very different approaches or that costs have not been properly adjusted to account for regional differences in overall prices. Most importantly, there could be large differences in the quality of care provided; if a system is found to produce the same health services for a much lower expenditure, it is important to make sure that patients are having satisfactory health outcomes.

Box 10.2 *Duplicate tests*

What are they?

Duplicate testing indicators provide information on whether a particular test has been administered repeatedly to the same patient within a short period of time. The data are often collected through patient surveys, though they can also be collected using patient records.

What do they tell you and what do they not tell you?

Duplicate tests can be indicative of inefficient use of resources. Tests can be expensive and if the results of a test are already known, there might not be a good reason to conduct the test again. Alternatively, some tests may have high rates of false-positives or false-negatives, or be inconclusive; therefore, on some occasions, a provider might need to administer a second test to make an accurate diagnosis. Additionally, patients may require a test to be redone if enough time has passed since the last test and there is a possibility that the results have changed.

What should you do next if you find variation?

If patients are receiving the same tests more than once, it is important to find out where this is happening and what types of tests are being repeatedly administered. For example, it could be that patients are receiving the same tests in a hospital because patient records are not being shared across wards. Or, it could be that patients visit different primary care providers who are unaware that a patient has already been given a particular test in another setting, again because information is not being shared. Alternatively, it could be that tests are being repeated because of the possibility that the results have changed; this should be investigated before taking action that limits access to repeat testing.

Box 10.3 *Generic prescribing*

What is it?

Generic prescribing gives information on whether providers and pharmacists are prescribing and dispensing generic medicines more often than brand name medicines. Since generic medicines are typically less expensive than brand name drugs, if generic medicines comprise a large share of total medicines, it is indicative of greater efficiency.

What does it tell you and what does it not tell you?

The share of generic prescribing gives an indication of whether a system is obtaining medicines at low cost. However, although it is not really a problem in European countries, it is important to be sure that generic drugs are biologically equivalent to brand name drugs; otherwise, there may be differences in the quality of drugs. Also, patients may have health needs for which the most effective medicines are not yet available in generic form.

What should you do next if you find variation?

Generic prescribing is almost without fail a useful metric. However, if generic prescribing is low, there are various questions that must be asked to identify the causes. First, are providers rewarded for prescribing brand name drugs? If pharmacists receive higher margins for dispensing brand name drugs, or if pharmaceutical companies compensate providers for prescribing brand name drugs, they may be incentivized to offer them. Second, do patients believe that generic drugs are of lower quality? If patients have expectations that generics are not equivalent to brand name drugs, it is important to either improve patient information, or to reduce (or eliminate) copayments for generic drugs while raising (or instituting) copayments for brand name drugs.

Box 10.4 *Emergency readmissions*

What are they?

Emergency readmission measures, sometimes called unplanned readmissions, provide information on whether a patient has been readmitted for any cause to any hospital within a short period of time. Often, this period of time is around 30 days; however, in practice this can vary. These data are often reported in administrative data or patient records, and sometimes are adjusted for patient characteristics that make readmission more likely (such as patient's age or known comorbidities).

What do they tell you and what do they not tell you?

Emergency readmissions can be indicative of poor-quality care and an inefficient use of resources, which go towards treating the patient again. Emergency readmissions may be indicative of patients being discharged too early and/or receiving substandard care in hospital.

However, factors outside the hospital's control, such as other complicating illnesses, patient lifestyle choices and behaviours, and the care provided to patients after discharge, may also have an impact on emergency readmissions.

Finally, emergency readmissions may also be indicative of good care; if, for example, hospitals are better able to successfully treat very ill patients, and indeed save their lives, they are likely to have higher readmission rates than hospitals that have higher mortality rates.

What should you next if you find variation?

If providers, or indeed countries, have different readmission rates or if readmission rates change over time, it is important to find out which of these explanations may apply.

Before coming to the conclusion that providers with high emergency readmission rates are inefficient, it is important to rule out some of the other explanations outlined earlier. As a first step, it may be useful to explore the cause of readmissions for particular hospitals. Are they driven by particular clinical conditions or events? Do they change for particular subgroups of patients? Exploring the patient characteristics of different hospitals may also provide further information and help to ensure that a needier population does not account for the higher readmission rates. This should be done even if readmission rates are adjusted for patient characteristics; for example, it is likely that a hospital in a deprived area will have different readmission rates compared to a hospital in an affluent area, even when controlling for age and comorbidity. This may also capture other factors, such as the presence of a social network after discharge or the capacity of patients to manage their own care. Exploring whether the proportion of patients readmitted through the A&E department versus being transferred from other facilities may also help to better understand the nature of readmissions.

It may also be useful to explore the relationship between readmission rates and other measures of hospital quality, such as mortality rates or even process and throughput measures such as patient discharge consultations, medical errors, waiting times or length of stay.

To explore variation in readmission rates across countries, it may be useful to explore additional avenues. For example, it may be useful to ensure that readmissions are measured the same way, to ensure the time period; providers and conditions included in the national definitions are also consistent.

Box 10.5 *Average length of stay for particular conditions*

What is it?

As the name suggests, this measure provides information on the number of days per inpatient stay, on average. Average length of stay (LOS) in hospitals can be used both as a general measure (to cover all conditions), and by particular condition/treatment (for example, average LOS for hip replacement). Average LOS in hospitals as an indicator of efficiency relies on the assumption that with all other things being equal, a shorter hospital stay will imply reduced costs as the patient moves out of the expensive inpatient care setting.

What does it tell you and what does it not tell you?

Average LOS for particular conditions can help to highlight variations in resource use across providers. However, in most cases, it is not clear what an ideal length of time for the average LOS should be. It is commonly assumed that shorter LOS is more efficient, as a shorter stay implies reduced costs; however, this may not always hold true for a number of reasons, such as:

- Even within the same condition, cases are different in terms of their severity and the intensity of treatment. For example, it is likely that an older, frailer patient will need to stay in the hospital longer than a younger, healthier patient who underwent the same treatment.
- Shorter LOS may be inefficient in the long run. While discharging patients earlier may appear efficient in the short-term by cutting costs, it may result in increased probability of complications, or slower recovery, which can cost more in the long term either through expensive readmissions or accumulated outpatient services.
- Hospital costs are not the same across all days of an inpatient stay. It is likely that costs in the initial days of the stay are more expensive, as these are the days where diagnostic tests and/ or interventions are likely to occur. Later days may entail necessary bed rest and continuing medications, which will be cheaper.

What should you next if you find variation?

If providers, or indeed countries, have different average LOS, for particular conditions or overall, it is important to find out which of these explanations may apply.

Differences in LOS across providers may reflect differences in patient characteristics, such as age, severity of treatment or other factors. It is thus important to look at these characteristics before concluding that higher LOS is inefficient. However, longer LOS can also reflect inefficiencies; for example, it may be linked to administrative delays (such as delays in scheduling tests, coordinating care across providers, performing a treatment).

To explore variation in average LOS across countries, it may be useful to explore differences in health system structure and definitions. For example, care may be structured differently across countries such that rehabilitation is performed in hospitals in some countries, while in other countries it occurs in rehabilitation facilities. Indeed, it may also be that different countries employ different definitions for what they consider to be hospitals and thus do not record the same information for this indicator.

Other structural factors that may be important to consider are payment systems or targets. Different payment systems put in place to reimburse hospital stays, such as budgets, per diem payments or DRGs, produce different incentives for early or late discharge. For example, hospitals that are paid on a per diem basis can generate more income by discharging patients later than hospitals that are paid through budgets.

Box 10.6 *Operations per specialist*

What are they?

Operations per specialist provide information on the number of operations any one provider is performing. Particularly for conditions where there is high demand, it is assumed that if specialists are performing more operations they are more efficient.

What do they tell you and what do they not tell you?

This indicator makes some fundamental assumptions that may not always hold; it assumes that more operations is an efficient measure, that all operations require the same intensity of care and that specialists not performing operations are spending their time inefficiently.

While performing more operations may be indicative of high demand, it may also be indicative of supplier-induced demand where operations are not always entirely necessary. In this case more operations would be costly and without gain, thus inefficient.

Not all operations require the same intensity of care and/or preparation time. Some operations may take longer to be performed because of different patient characteristics, resulting in fewer operations overall.

Many specialists spend some of their time not conducting operations, but in other efficient pursuits. For example, if they are involved in teaching, they may be supervising operations. They may be preparing for operations by reviewing case files or recommending necessary tests and/or consulting with patients. Finally, they may spend time conducting research which can improve the efficiency of operations in the future.

What should you next if you find variation?

If there is large variation across providers in the number of operations they are undertaking, it is important to understand why this is happening. It may be that the prevalence of the illness for which the operation is conducted differs across the regions where the variation occurs. It may be because some of the specialists only conduct the operation on a particular subset of patients, or because they are engaged in other activities. However, it is also important to explore potential sources of inefficiency. For example, are fewer operations happening because of a lack of operating theatre space, or other clinical staff (such as anaesthetists or nurses)?

10.4 Promising opportunities for efficiency measurement

While there are a multitude of challenges associated with measuring efficiency in health systems, the chapters presented in this volume highlighted many methodological achievements and promising opportunities for the future. Here we discuss some of the ways in which efficiency measurement can continue to develop and become increasingly useful for policymakers and managers.

10.4.1 Greater attention to cost accounting data

Identifying the costs of health care is intrinsically complex, especially in the hospital sector. As discussed in Chapter 4, many hospital costs are fixed and shared across many patients. A central concern of cost and management accounting is determining how these fixed costs, which are often described as overheads, can be attributed to individual patient care. This is important, as the level of granularity of cost data can have a large effect on the costs that are attributed to patient care. Costs calculated at an aggregate level will reveal no differences in input resources used to treat patients with the same cost classification, even though patients may actually use very different types and levels of resources.

Depending on the system and local accounting capacity, there is a whole spectrum of potential costing mechanisms that could determine the cost data available. These range from 1) detailed patient level through 2) applying local unit costs to individual use through 3) local episode averages and then 4) national averages. The usefulness for efficiency analysis decreases as you move along this spectrum. If it is not possible to effectively capture variation between providers or patients in terms of costs (because these data are not captured) then the usefulness of any efficiency analysis is severely constrained.

More work is needed to fully understand how different costing mechanisms affect efficiency comparisons. To maximize the potential of the data, cost accounting should allow for calculation of costs at the level of individual patients. This is likely to be directly beneficial for patient care, but is also extremely important for evaluating the efficiency of care delivery. Moreover, more attention could be paid to assessing the level of overhead costs irrespective of how they link to patient care. For example, more comparisons of the drivers of administrative costs could be helpful to determine whether some overhead expenditure is unnecessarily high (or indeed inefficiently low).

10.4.2 Further exploiting patient registries by utilizing actual patient costs

While registry data are used most frequently to develop quality indicators, they are generally underused for efficiency comparisons. In part, this is because (as discussed earlier) available cost data are often simply the average prices paid for services, rather than the actual costs of care inputs. It is important that patient-level registry data are linkable to actual costs, rather than some type of normative or average costs.

One reason that registry data are often linked with output prices is that registries are generally maintained by payers. From the perspective of the payer, the cost of inpatient treatment is the price of payment. So, in fact, one could argue that when comparing the efficiency of, for example, health insurers (or health maintenance organizations), it can make sense to use the prices they pay as a proxy for costs. In principle, it should be possible to link data on actual costs to registers if hospitals have data on input costs and if they agree to share these data with the institution responsible for maintaining the register.

This may not be feasible for all types of care, however. Hospitals are the most common provider to have patient cost data available (and efficiency comparisons, in general). Outside of hospitals, this could be more problematic. There is in general very little reliable patient-level cost data available on the ambulatory care sector. So, cost data covering all sectors are likely to be unavailable. Yet, there exists enormous potential for better cost data from other care settings in the future, particularly as information systems improve and patient classification systems extend into providers beyond the hospital. For example, Australia, Canada and the USA have patient groupers for ambulatory settings, including home care and long-term skilled nursing care. As use of these types of patient classification systems becomes more widespread, they should be designed to be comparable across health systems.

10.4.3 Focus on improving outcome measurement

While there is significant potential for improving input data through better cost accounting data, and realized developments in output measures in the form of case mix adjustment of intermediate outputs, such as hospital inpatient stays, it remains difficult to capture comparable outcome measures. QALYs are in principle a widely accepted outcome measure. However, for many interventions they require modelling of future health trajectories, and their direct use for monitoring comparative efficiency is infeasible. Furthermore, there are no agreed ways to adjust them to account for equity or other variations in societal preferences, as explained in Chapter 6.

There has been recent progress in the use of PROMs to make comparisons across providers delivering a specific treatment (Smith & Street, 2013), and expanded use of PROMs in administrative databases would be a useful practical step for efficiency measurement. For chronic diseases, it would also be useful if health status were monitored over time in patient registries. As well as facilitating efficiency measurement, this may also contribute to better disease management.

10.4.4 Putting advanced methodological approaches to greater use, while recognizing the benefits of simple tools

Frontier-based methods, like DEA, are more often used by academics than by policy analysts, and are used even more rarely by managers. However, if used properly, DEA can be a valuable diagnostic tool. A number of guidelines to ensure that these types of methods are beneficial are included in Chapter 5. Among them is the importance of engaging with stakeholders at an early stage so that they fully understand the data and methods.

Many previous applications of DEA fail to provide good models for how DEA should be used. DEA has often been used in situations where the units (for example, countries) are not sufficiently comparable, for example, to compare efficiency across all EU countries (see Medeiros & Schwierz, 2015). This is an important issue, as it leads to an implausible production–possibility frontier and may render some producers inefficient that, in fact, are producing as well as could be expected given the circumstances in which they must operate. DEA is also not necessarily as useful when a large part of variation in outputs is the result of unobserved factors, since all unexplained variation will be ascribed to inefficiency, leading to implausible results and discrediting the technique. Most DEA studies have assessed inputs relative to outputs, which makes more conceptual sense than looking at inputs relative to outcomes, a large part of which may be beyond the control of health care institutions.

While advanced methodological approaches can certainly be put to better use, there is also much to be said for more use of simple metrics. For example, measures such as unit costs (despite the complexities associated with cost accounting discussed earlier) are transparent and can be extremely helpful to identify providers and countries that have unexplained variations. Such variations can then be analysed in more depth to identify their root cause (Reschovsky et al., 2014). The recently published Carter (2016) review in England also makes use of a number of simple metrics to compare acute care NHS hospitals. One such measure, referred to as care hours per patient day, reflects the ratio of total hours of nurses and support staff in a day to the number of inpatient admissions. The metric, which is simple enough to be calculated at ward, hospital, regional and national levels, assesses the efficiency of staff deployment levels. The report also proposes using purchasing price indexes to compare the prices paid for inputs across providers.

10.4.5 More attention should be paid to AE

Cost–effectiveness analysis has largely been used to make *ex ante* resource allocation decisions, for example, by setting a cost-per-QALY threshold. However, the principle of monitoring AE retrospectively has received relatively little attention, even though many policy decisions (for example, using HTA to make coverage decisions) and managerial decisions (for example, to reconfigure services) are primarily about AE. Increased use of retrospective AE analysis should therefore be encouraged. For example, it could inform metrics that reflect the extent of inappropriate care (which is not cost-effective or lies outside the chosen health benefits package). Such measures could reflect treatments that are inappropriate in their entirety, or treatments that are inappropriate for particular subgroups of patients. At the system level, AE indicators might seek to determine whether there is an optimal balance between broad sectors, such as prevention, disease management, and curative and ambulatory care.

10.4.6 Metrics should be designed (and presented) to meet the needs of different stakeholders

Metrics must not only be chosen based on whether they provide a clear indication of inefficient processes; they must also be geared towards the stakeholders that are best positioned to inform decisions and affect change. At the policy level, decision-makers may have access to a variety of levers that could transform health care production. Managers, on the other hand, are those on the ground, but may have relatively limited levers for driving and securing change. Usability of evidence depends on how much influence the audience of the evidence actually has over the processes that are evaluated. If managers have no control over prices, staffing, and so on, they are unlikely to pay much attention to a diagnosis that these are the prime causes of their organization's inefficiency.

Too little consideration has been given to the presentation of findings. This is an important area requiring attention, as presentation devices are the crucial link between data and decision-makers. Policymakers and managers can only respond to efficiency analyses if the materials are presented in a way that is insightful, actionable and designed to meet their specific needs. For example, managers working in a time-pressured environment need information to be translated into tools that can relatively quickly and easily be applied by users without advanced levels of statistical knowledge, such as in the form of visual aids. SPOTs are an example from England. As spelt out in Chapter 9, managers may not use efficiency metrics because they are not aware of the information, because they do not accept the data as valid, because they believe they cannot apply the findings to their work or because there are real constraints limiting change.

10.5 Concluding remarks

Increasing the use and understanding of efficiency evidence is important for sound policymaking and management. Currently, especially in countries with public funding challenges, many reforms are motivated by the nominal objective of improving efficiency. Yet, in many cases the data or analytical resources are not fit for purpose; in the absence of sound efficiency metrics, decision-makers may be tempted to implement crude expenditure reductions that indiscriminately affect both inefficient and efficient institutions and practitioners. On the other hand, slavish reliance on incomplete efficiency metrics – such as length of stay – may also lead to unintended consequences, for example, by shifting costs onto community services.

Better efficiency measurement and greater understanding of how to interpret efficiency indicators are essential for developing more focused and effective policies towards enhancing efficiency. To this end, the authors of Chapter 1 put forward a framework for scrutinizing efficiency metrics that comprised the following elements:

- the entity to be assessed;
- the outputs (or outcomes) under consideration;
- the inputs under consideration;
- the external influences on attainment; and
- the links with the rest of the health system.

We suggest that anyone considering the use of any efficiency metric for policy purposes undertakes a critical examination of the proposed metric along these dimensions. Doing so should then make it possible to examine questions such as:

- Is the correct actor being targeted for the efficiency metric under consideration?
- To what extent are the outputs of the entity fully captured in the metric?
- To what extent are the inputs of the entity fully captured in the metric?
- Are the external (uncontrollable) influences on attainment fully taken into account?
- Are there potential influences on the rest of the health system that the metric does not take into account?

Applying such a framework to evaluate an efficiency indicator invariably reveals that it is necessary to dig deeper to gain a full understanding of the reasons for the observed variations. In part, this reflects the fact that most efficiency metrics offer only partial glimpses into discrete production processes within the broader health system, rather than the efficiency of the health system in its entirety. One upside, however, of partial measures over more comprehensive metrics, is that the reasons for the observed variations may be relatively easier to identify and address. For example, simple metrics showing high rates of unnecessary diagnostic tests or low levels of substituting generic for branded pharmaceuticals are fairly straightforward to understand and react to. Nevertheless, often in health care, quite detailed investigations (clinical trials, detailed costing or simulation studies) are still needed to establish whether one intervention is more cost-effective than another.

Recognizing that there is no perfect system-wide efficiency indicator, there is great interest in identifying the right set of partial indicators that give the most complete snapshot of health system efficiency. The indicators included in Boxes 10.1–10.6 of this chapter provide a good starting-point. These are the type of indicator found in many systems. However, they are usually fashioned opportunistically from administrative data sources and not embedded within a systematic framework, or designed to improve decision-making at all levels. More generally, there cannot be a one-size-fits-all dashboard of efficiency metrics suitable for all health systems. To determine the appropriate metrics, it is necessary to have a clear understanding of the institutional arrangements, information resources and other design aspects of the health system and design a framework accordingly for analysis.

Efficiency metrics are of great importance for governing, managing and reforming any health system, and improving the management of its institutions. As a result, there is a massive agenda to improve their scope, comparability, timeliness, quality and usefulness. To prevent stakeholders from dismissing efficiency metrics as being irrelevant, based on poor data or analysis, or impossible to act on, engagement between analysts and decision-makers is necessary. Knowing the audience, their levels of autonomy and the levers they can pull, is therefore a key consideration for how efficiency metrics are chosen, and how the analyses are presented. There is a clear need for policymakers to set out clearly what they mean by efficiency, to give local decision-makers the leadership capacity and autonomy needed to pursue improved efficiency, and to put in place information systems that measure progress accurately and in a timely fashion. Only then will efficiency metrics play a more prominent role in policymaking and managerial decisions.

References

Carter (2016). Operational productivity and performance in English NHS acute hospitals: unwarranted variations. An independent report for the Department of Health by Lord Carter of Coles. (https://www.gov.uk/government/uploads/system/uploads/attachment_data/file/499229/Operational_productivity_A.pdf, accessed 22 July 2016)

Medeiros J, Schwierz C (2015). European economy. Efficiency estimates of health care systems. Economic Papers 549. Brussels, European Commission (http://ec.europa.eu/economy_finance/publications/economic_paper/2015/pdf/ecp549_en.pdf, accessed 22 July 2016).

Reschovsky JD et al. (2014). Geographic variations in the cost of treating condition-specific episodes of care among Medicare patients. *Health Services Research*, 49(1):32–51.

Smith PC, Street AD (2013). On the uses of routine patient reported health outcome data. *Health Economics*, 22(2):119–131.